NUCLEAR CARDIOLOGY

PRACTICAL APPLICATIONS

Notice

Medicine is an ever-changing science. As new research and clinical experience broaden our knowledge, changes in treatment and drug therapy are required. The authors and the publisher of this work have checked with sources believed to be reliable in their efforts to provide information that is complete and generally in accord with the standards accepted at the time of publication. However, in view of the possibility of human error or changes in medical sciences, neither the authors nor the publisher nor any other party who has been involved in the preparation or publication of this work warrants that the information contained herein is in every respect accurate or complete, and they disclaim all responsibility for any errors or omissions or for the results obtained from use of the information contained in this work. Readers are encouraged to confirm the information contained herein with other sources. For example and in particular, readers are advised to check the product information sheet included in the package of each drug they plan to administer to be certain that the information contained in this work is accurate and that changes have not been made in the recommended dose or in the contraindications for administration. This recommendation is of particular importance in connection with new or infrequently used drugs.

NUCLEAR CARDIOLOGY
PRACTICAL APPLICATIONS

Gary V. Heller, MD, PhD

Associate Director, Cardiology
Director, Nuclear Cardiology
Director, Cardiovascular Fellowship Program
Hartford Hospital
Hartford, Connecticut
Professor of Medicine and Nuclear Medicine
University of Connecticut School of Medicine
Farmington, Connecticut

Robert C. Hendel, MD

Professor of Medicine
Director, Nuclear Cardiology
Director, Coronary Care Unit
Section of Cardiology
Rush University Medical Center
Chicago, Illinois

McGraw-Hill
Medical Publishing Division

New York   Chicago   San Francisco   Lisbon   London
Madrid   Mexico City   Milan   New Delhi   San Juan
Seoul   Singapore   Sydney   Toronto

Nuclear Cardiology: Practical Applications

3 4 5 6 7 8 9 0   KGP/KGP   0 9 8 7 6 5

ISBN 0-07-138635-1

This book was set in Galliard by Rainbow Graphics.
The editors were Darlene Cooke and Michelle Watt.
The production supervisor was Richard Ruzycka.
Project management was provided by Rainbow Graphics.
The index was prepared by Oneida Indexing, Inc.
Quebecor World/Kingsport was printer and binder.
This book was printed on acid-free paper.

Library of Congress Cataloging-in-Publication Data

Nuclear cardiology : practical applications / edited by Gary V. Heller, Robert C. Hendel.
    p. ; cm.
  Includes bibliographical references and index.
  ISBN 0-07-138635-1
  1. Heart–Radionuclide imaging. I. Heller, Gary V. II. Hendel, Robert.
  [DNLM: 1. Cardiovascular Diseases—radionuclide imaging. 2. Heart–radionuclide imaging. WG 141.5.R3 N9637 2004]
RC683.5.R33N793 2004
616.1′207575–dc21
                                                      2003046418

DEDICATION

For Susan, Judy, Adam, and Jason with love and appreciation for their continuous support, and for our mentors who inspired us to write this book.

G.V.H. and R.C.H.

Contents

Color plates appear between pages 178 and 179.

Contributors

Mohammed Awaad, MD
Assistant Clinical Professor
Ohio State University
Cardiology Associates of SE Ohio
Zanesville, Ohio

Timothy M. Bateman, MD
Professor of Medicine
University of Missouri
Cardiovascular Consultants
Kansas City, Missouri

Anita Bhandiwad, MD
Beth Israel Deaconess Medical Center
Boston, Massachusetts

William E. Boden, MD
Chief, Division of Cardiology
Hartford Hospital
Professor of Medicine
University of Connecticut School of
Medicine
Hartford, Connecticut

James A. Case, PhD
Cardiovascular Imaging Technologies
Kansas City, Missouri

S. James Cullom, PhD
Cardiovascular Imaging Technologies
Kansas City, Missouri

Peter Danias, MD
Boston, Massachusetts

Andrea Fossati, MD
Champlain Valley Cardiovascular Associates
South Burlington, Vermont

Laura L. Ford-Mukkamala, DO
Associated Cardiovascular Consultants, PA
Cherry Hill, New Jersey

Michael S. Fowler, MD
Former Cardiovascular Fellow
Associates in Cardiovascular Medicine
Torrington, Connecticut

Vanessa Go, MD
Cardiovascular Associates
Denver, Colorado

Rory Hachamovitch, MD, MSc
Associate Professor of Medicine
Keck School of Medicine
University of Southern California
Division of Cardiovascular Medicine
Los Angeles, California

Thomas H. Hauser, MD
Beth Israel Deaconess Medical Center
Boston, Massachusetts

Gary V. Heller, MD, PhD

Associate Director, Cardiology
Director, Nuclear Cardiology
Director, Cardiovascular Fellowship
Program
Hartford Hospital
Hartford, Connecticut
Professor of Medicine and Nuclear Medicine
University of Connecticut School of
Medicine
Farmington, Connecticut

Robert C. Hendel, MD

Professor of Medicine
Director, Nuclear Cardiology
Director, Coronary Care Unit
Section of Cardiology
Rush University Medical Center
Chicago, Illinois

Susie Kim, MD

Aurora Denver Cardiology
Lone Tree, Colorado

Philip R. Liebson, MD

Professor of Medicine
Department of Medicine, Section of
Cardiology
Rush University Medical Center
Chicago, Illinois

April Mann, CNMT

Hartford Hospital
Hartford, Connecticut

Kourosh Mastali, MD

Fellow in Cardiology
John H. Stroger, Jr. Hospital of Cook County
Chicago, Illinois

Sachin Navare, MD

Cardiovascular Fellow
Division of Cardiology
Hartford Hospital
Hartford, Connecticut

Georgias Papaioannou, MD

Cardiovascular Fellow
Hartford Hospital
Hartford, Connecticut

Asad Rizvi, MD

Cardiology, PC
Hartford, Connecticut

Ahmad Salloum, MD

Coastal Cardiovascular Consultants, PA
Brick, New Jersey

Aaron Satran, MD

Cardiology Fellow
University of Louisville
Department of Medicine, Section of
Cardiology
Louisville, Kentucky

R. Jeffrey Snell, MD, FACC

Department of Medicine, Section of
Cardiology
Rush University Medical Center
Chicago, Illinois

Raymond Taillefer, MD

Professor of Nuclear Medicine
Université de Montréal
Montreal, Canada

Louise E.J. Thomson

Nuclear Medicine/Cardiac Imaging
S. Mark Taper Foundation Imaging Center
Cedars-Sinai Medical Center
Los Angeles, California

Muthu Velusamy, MD

Cardiology Consultants
Pensacola, Florida

Kim A. Williams, MD

Associate Professor, Section of Cardiology
University of Chicago
Chicago, Illinois

Preface

The field of nuclear cardiology, and specifically myocardial perfusion imaging, has demonstrated sustained growth for the last five years at a rate of approximately 10 to 15% per year. This owes to the increasingly recognized value of nuclear cardiology, particularly for clinical applications and patient management. As more physicians are ordering and using the test results, the need for practical information regarding nuclear cardiology has also increased. Although several textbooks in nuclear cardiology are available, none are targeted toward those who order the procedures. Our textbook has been designed for the consumers of nuclear cardiology, particularly primary care physicians, family care practitioners, general cardiologists, and others who require a practical understanding of this specialty. It has also been developed as an introduction to nuclear cardiology for house staff, radiology and nuclear medicine residents, and cardiology fellows.

Our book has been divided into three sections. The first section deals with the indications for myocardial perfusion imaging such as the evaluation of known or suspected coronary artery disease, preoperative risk assessment, and acute chest pain imaging in the emergency department. The second section is designed to provide the referring physician with more information on how the procedures are performed and their implications. Additionally, several chapters provide information about other imaging modalities. Finally, the technical aspects of many nuclear cardiology procedures are described in the third section, which is especially focused on the needs of residents and fellows in the field of nuclear cardiology.

It has been our pleasure to work on this book with many of our colleagues and fellows. Readers of this book are provided information that allows their optimal use of myocardial perfusion imaging. We are very proud of the results and thank all for their contributions.

CHAPTER 1

Indications for Nuclear Cardiology Procedures: Suspected Coronary Artery Disease

Michael S. Fowler
Gary V. Heller

BACKGROUND

Coronary artery disease (CAD) is still the single greatest cause of death of men and women in the United States, despite a declining total death rate. Using 1998 data (the latest available), over 459,000 deaths were due to CAD—1 of every 5 deaths. There are approximately 2.2 million hospital discharges with CAD as the diagnosis annually. The estimated direct and indirect costs of CAD each year are over \$100 billion.[1] The reduction of the morbidity and mortality due to CAD is thus of primary importance to physicians and patients. This has spurned a great interest in identifying those patients who can benefit from preventive and therapeutic strategies. Stress myocardial perfusion imaging (MPI) has emerged as an important noninvasive means of evaluating patients with suspected CAD, with over 5 million studies performed annually. This chapter will discuss the diagnostic accuracy of stress MPI and how to decide which patients should undergo stress MPI for suspected CAD. Options for the type of stress with MPI and their uses in appropriate patients will also be reviewed. The current recommendations for testing of patients with suspected CAD by the American College of Cardiology (ACC), the American Heart Association (AHA), and the American Society of Nuclear Cardiology (ASNC) are listed in the appendix at the end of this chapter.

Patients with suspected CAD need to be assessed in a stepwise fashion, which includes risk factor analysis, assessment of the risk for significant CAD, and assessment of the risk for having any of the devastating outcomes of CAD, particularly myocardial infarction (MI) and cardiac death.

RISK FACTOR ASSESSMENT

The first step in evaluating patients for CAD involves the assessment of the presence of traditional risk factors. Modifiable risks include hyper-

1

cholesterolemia, tobacco use, hypertension, diabetes mellitus, physical inactivity, and obesity. Nonmodifiable risk factors include a family history of CAD in first-degree relatives under the age of 60, advanced age, and male gender.[2] Clinical prediction models have been developed to stratify patients into low, intermediate, and high risks of CAD and cardiac death based on the presence of these risk factors.[3,4] Recent work has confirmed the value of the gender-specific functions of the Framingham CAD prediction model in whites and blacks, although the model tends to overestimate the risk of cardiac events in other ethnic groups.[5] In the Framingham model, total risk is defined as angina pectoris, recognized and silent MI, unstable angina, and cardiac death. More recent reports from the Framingham study include risk estimates for "hard" CAD, which excludes angina pectoris, but includes unstable angina and silent MI (defined by electrocardiographic findings). Recently, a modified version of the Framingham risk score has been incorporated into the Third Report of the National Cholesterol Education Program Expert Panel on Detection, Evaluation, and Treatment of High Blood Cholesterol in Adults (ATP III).[6] This clinical risk assessment can then be used to divide patients into groups who benefit from noninvasive testing, invasive testing, or no testing for CAD.

ASSESSMENT OF RISK FOR CAD

Once risk factors associated with CAD are evaluated, a patient's risk for having CAD should be assessed. This is often performed by taking symptoms (such as chest pain), age, and gender into account. Symptoms suggestive of CAD, in addition to other risk factors, drive decisions for further testing. The challenge of the physician is to roughly classify patients into categories of risk on the basis of these factors.

An elegant study by Diamond[7] provides a clinically relevant assessment of the probability of angiographically significant CAD based on gender, age, and type of chest pain. Chest pain is classified by three historical characteristics: substernal, precipitation by exertion or emotional stress, and prompt relief by rest or nitroglycerin. Patients are then classified as asymptomatic (0 of 3), nonanginal (1 of 3), atypical angina (2 of 3), or typical angina (all 3 characteristics). The resulting probabilities of significant CAD, after factoring in age and gender, can be seen in Table 1-1. The determination of a patient's risk for CAD using this model allows for stratification of a patient into low, intermediate, or high risk. This allows the appropriate decision for diagnostic testing, as outlined below.

DIAGNOSTIC ACCURACY

Reference Standard for Test Evaluation

Coronary angiography is the gold standard to which diagnostic tests for CAD are compared. However, angiography does have an important limitation—it provides a silhouette view of the vessel, showing luminal irregularities and discrete obstructions, but not actual atherosclerosis in coronary arterial walls. An Italian study of patients with "false-positive" myocardial perfusion imaging (MPI) and angiographically normal coronary arteries revealed angiographically occult atherosclerosis in 95% of patients and relative plaque area of > 40% in 80% of patients as assessed by intravascular ultrasound (IVUS). In addition, Doppler flow velocity revealed abnormal coronary vasodilation capacity in 70% of these patients.[8] This would suggest that MPI might have a greater sensitivity than has been reported.

Another drawback of performing coronary angiography in the assessment of all patients with suspected CAD is the risk of the procedure. In a study of 59,792 patients, mortality occurred in 1 per 1,000 patients and MI occurred in 1 per 2,000 patients. Vascular complications and contrast reactions occurred in approximately 1 per 250 patients, while cerebrovascular accidents occurred in 1 per 1,400 patients.[9] By way of comparison, both death and myocardial infarction are each reported to occur in up to 1 per 2,500 exercise tests.[10] Despite these limitations, coronary

Table 1-1
Probability of Angiographic Coronary Artery Disease

Age (yr)	AS	NA	AA	TA
Women				
35–45	0.007 ± 0.006	0.027 ± 0.024	0.155 ± 0.111	0.454 ± 0.186
45–55	0.021 ± 0.018	0.069 ± 0.051	0.317 ± 0.160	0.677 ± 0.167
55–65	0.054 ± 0.042	0.127 ± 0.080	0.465 ± 0.174	0.839 ± 0.108
65–75	0.115 ± 0.078	0.171 ± 0.097	0.541 ± 0.169	0.947 ± 0.055
Men				
35–45	0.037 ± 0.024	0.105 ± 0.063	0.428 ± 0.144	0.809 ± 0.104
45–55	0.077 ± 0.040	0.206 ± 0.090	0.601 ± 0.129	0.907 ± 0.049
55–65	0.111 ± 0.049	0.282 ± 0.100	0.690 ± 0.106	0.939 ± 0.029
65–75	0.113 ± 0.050	0.282 ± 0.100	0.700 ± 0.103	0.943 ± 0.026

Each estimate is the average probability (± 1 standard deviation) over the indicated age range assuming average levels for the conventional Framingham risk factors. AA = atypical angina; AS = asymptomatic; NA = nonanginal discomfort; TA = typical angina.
Reprinted from Diamond[7] with permission.

angiography remains the best practical reference standard for CAD due to its availability, proven utility, and ability to guide revascularization when required. A stepwise approach using non-invasive testing first, followed by coronary angiography in appropriate patients, has been shown to be cost-effective and clinically useful in identifying at-risk patients.[11]

Predictive Value of a Diagnostic Test

Central to an evaluation of a diagnostic test, one must understand Bayes' theorem of conditional probability. The details of this are explained in Chapter 24. The statistical terms are defined in Figure 1-1. Briefly, sensitivity and specificity define the quality of a test. However, the result of the test cannot be interpreted without knowing the prevalence of disease in the population. This is because the positive predictive accuracy and the negative predictive accuracy rely on the pre-test probability of disease in a population. This idea was outlined in a seminal paper by Diamond and Forrester.[12] As an example, a test with 70%

sensitivity and 90% specificity gives very different information in varying populations. In a patient with a 5% likelihood of disease, a positive test increases this likelihood of CAD to only 27%. In a patient with a 50% likelihood of disease, the same positive test increases the posttest likelihood of CAD to 88%. Similarly, in a patient with a high likelihood of disease, a positive test will make the

Test Result	Presence of Disease	
	Yes	No
Positive	True positive (TP)	False positive (FP)
Negative	False negative (FN)	True negative (TN)

$$\text{Sensitivity} = \frac{TP}{TP + FN} \qquad \text{Specificity} = \frac{TN}{TN + FP}$$

$$\text{Positive Predictive Value (PPV)} = \frac{TP}{TP + FP} \qquad \text{Negative Predictive Value (NPV)} = \frac{TN}{TN + FN}$$

Figure 1-1.   Statistical terms.

likelihood higher, but a negative test will not reduce the likelihood significantly.

The influence of disease prevalence on statistical measures of a diagnostic test also helps to explain the static or declining specificity of MPI even as imaging techniques improve. This phenomenon is known as posttest referral bias.[13] As stress MPI has become more accepted in the risk stratification of patients with suspected CAD, those with abnormal studies tend to be referred for angiography, while those with normal studies are not. Thus, there is a tendency to exclude the patients with "false-negative" MPI studies from angiography, and to catheterize those with false-positive tests. This will cause the measured sensitivity to increase and the measured specificity to decrease. These factors must be kept in mind while evaluating diagnostic strategies that have been studied years or decades apart.

DECIDING ON TESTING PROCEDURES: STRENGTHS AND WEAKNESSES

Exercise Tolerance Test

A cornerstone of the diagnosis of CAD has been exercise tolerance testing (ETT). The exercise tolerance test is safe and easily performed, usually in an office setting. More extensive coverage of ETT can be found in Chapter 9. Briefly, ETT affords the ability to evaluate a patient's symptoms, exercise tolerance (a prognostic factor), hemodynamic response, and electrocardiographic changes during exercise stress. Traditionally, the presence and amount of ST segment depression (≥ 0.1 mV) during or immediately after exercise has been used as an indicator of significant CAD. In general, ETT electrocardiography (ECG) has a sensitivity of 50 to 70%, and a specificity of 60 to 80%.[14] The use of ETT is thus limited by false-positive results (leading to further inappropriate testing) and false-negative results (leading to missed diagnoses). A meta-anlysis of the ETT literature by Gianrossi et al.[15] found a sensitivity of 67% and a specificity of 72% for the diagnosis of

obstructive CAD. These values may be influenced by pretest referral bias.[16] A study by Froelicher et al.[17] minimized referral bias by performing ETT and coronary angiography on all patients, irrespective of indication. In this predominantly male population, the ETT sensitivity was 45% and the specificity was 85%. This suggests that in an unselected population of patients with suspected CAD, a positive result may be very meaningful, but a negative result may be less reassuring.

Multivariate analysis has been performed to investigate the factors that affect the sensitivity and specificity of ETT.[18] A marked reduction in the sensitivity of ETT to detect significant CAD is seen in patients who do not achieve 85% of the maximum predicted heart rate for age. Several different diagnostic indicators have been assessed to make the ETT more predictive, but they do not overcome significant false-positive and false-negative results, and are often cumbersome to use.[14,19–21] These same studies have shown that a patient's inability to do minimal exercise is an independent predictor of poor outcome, but not specifically CAD. Thus, the ETT is very useful in appropriate settings, primarily for patients at low risk of CAD in whom a true-negative test is much more likely than a false-negative test. In patients unable to exercise adequately, other diagnostic tests must be used.

STRESS MYOCARDIAL PERFUSION IMAGING FOR THE DIAGNOSIS OF CAD

Background

A major limitation of the ETT is its diagnostic accuracy for the detection of significant CAD. In patients able to exercise, the diagnostic accuracy of stress MPI is significantly higher than the ETT alone and provides greater risk stratification for predicting future cardiac events. Thus, in a population of patients in which CAD is prevalent, stress MPI is a better choice than ETT alone. Another limitation of the ETT is that the accuracy of the test depends on a patient's ability to reach a predicted maximum heart rate. Patients with medical illness, debilitation, or musculoskeletal problems may be unable to perform an adequate ETT. MPI with pharmachologic stress using vasodilators (dipyridamole and adenosine) or dobutamine can be implemented in such patients. Pharmachologic stress with MPI is most advantageous in older patients who are at the highest risk of CAD, yet are likely to be the population least able to exercise adequately.

Once the decision is made to perform MPI, the physician must choose between exercise or pharmachologic stress. In addition to the choice of stress modality, radionuclide selection can also vary (currently thallium-201 [Tl-201] and technetium-99m [Tc-99m]-based agents). Generally, ETT combined with ECG-gated single photon emission computed tomography (SPECT) with a technetium-99m-based imaging agent is the test of choice for patients able to exercise.

Exercise MPI

Briefly, exercise MPI seeks to uncover areas of infarction or ischemia by comparing the perfusion of the heart at a resting state versus a stressed state. The stress is provided by exercise, generally a treadmill study utilizing the Bruce protocol. At peak stress, the radiopharmaceutical is injected intravenously. The patient is then imaged under a gamma camera to reveal myocardial perfusion at stress. These images are compared with those obtained at rest. Areas that show decreased perfusion at both stress and rest are indicative of MI, whereas areas with normal perfusion at rest but decreased perfusion at stress are indicative of myocardial ischemia. The specific area with a perfusion abnormality indicates the involved coronary artery, and the size of the perfusion abnormality correlates with the severity of CAD.

Radionuclide techniques have evolved considerably in the past 30 years. Early on, radionuclide ventriculography with supine exercise was validated for use in the risk stratification of individuals with known or suspected CAD.[22,23] However, this proved cumbersome and could

not be used with pharmacologic stress. Later, MPI utilizing the radionuclide thallium-201 (Tl-201) was developed. Using exercise as the stress modality, planar Tl-201 MPI has been found to have, on average, 83% sensitivity and 88% specificity for detecting angiographically significant CAD.[24] Today, SPECT has overwhelmingly replaced planar imaging by providing better localization of the vascular territories involved with increased sensitivity (89%) at the expense of specificity (76%).[24] Further refinements of visual analysis have had minimal impact on the performance of Tl-201 MPI.[25–27] As will be explained later, the use of ECG-gated SPECT imaging has increased specificity without sacrificing sensitivity.[28]

The limitations of Tl-201 (including soft tissue attenuation of the low-energy emissions, and poor count statistics) prompted the development of new radionuclides for cardiac imaging.[29] Technetium-99m (Tc-99m) agents have improved imaging characteristics compared to Tl-201 due to higher photon energy and shorter half-life, allowing larger doses. These advantages are somewhat offset by less myocardial extraction, increased uptake in abdominal organs, and lack of redistribution.[29] The different Tc-99m agents include sestamibi, tetrofosmin, teboroxime, furifosmin, and NOET. More detail regarding these agents can be found in Chapter 9. The choice of radiopharmaceutical used with stress MPI is made by the individual laboratory performing the test. Technetium-based agents that are currently available for clinical use include sestamibi (Cardiolite) and tetrofosmin (Myoview).

The sensitivity and specificity of planar Tc-99m exercise MPI has been the subject of several studies. The overall sensitivity and specificity in these trials were 90% and 70%, respectively.[30] Qualitative (visual) and quantitative (computer calculation of relative activity) methods of interpreting planar Tc-99m images after exercise stress have shown similar sensitivity (90%) and specificity (75–80%).[31,32] The introduction of SPECT imaging with Tc-99m agents using exercise has not appreciably improved these measures of test performance. In two studies with a total of 157 patients using both qualitative and quantitative methods, the sensitivity was 85% and the specificity was 79% for the detection of angiographically significant CAD.[33,34] Several other studies have found the sensitivity of exercise Tc-99m MPI to be comparable to that of exercise Tl-201 MPI.[35–38] As stated earlier in this chapter, these equivalent (and occasionally reduced) specificities compared to Tl-201 planar and SPECT imaging may be due to posttest referral bias present in more recent studies. As will be discussed later, the use of functional information provided by gated SPECT acquisition of images allowed by Tc-99m may improve the accuracy of Tc-99m MPI by increasing specificity (reduction of false-positive studies).

A more significant advantage of Tc-99m MPI over standard ETT has been shown by Stratmann and colleagues.[39] The importance of workload achieved on the sensitivity of ETT in the diagnosis of CAD is well known. Their study showed that the sensitivity of Tc-99m sestamibi for angiographic CAD is relatively independent of the peak heart rate achieved in a consecutive series of 250 patients with known CAD by angiography. At all levels of exercise, Tc-99m sestamibi imaging is more sensitive than stress-induced ischemic ST-segment depression. In addition, exercise duration of < 6 minutes is associated with a higher Tc-99m sestamibi abnormality rate than a duration of > 6 minutes, which may indicate the effect of myocardial ischemic burden on exercise ventricular function. This is not a function of age, as the group of patients reaching 85% or more of the age-predicted maximal heart rate was older than the group not achieving this level of exercise (62 ± 9 versus 59 ± 10 years). It should also be noted that SPECT imaging offers advantages in identifying multivessel disease as well as disease in specific vascular territories over planar imagery.

Pharmacologic MPI

One of the important advantages of MPI in assessing patients with suspected CAD is that pa-

tients who are incapable of performing adequate exercise can be studied using pharmacologic stress. It has been estimated that 35 to 40% of all stress MPI is performed with pharmacologic agents.[40] Briefly, dipyridamole and adenosine are potent coronary vasodilators that markedly increase coronary blood flow. This increased flow is less pronounced in arteries that are stenotic (flow restricted) due to atherosclerosis. This causes heterogeneous myocardial perfusion, which can be observed using a tracer that follows coronary blood flow as an alternative to vasodilator stress. Dobutamine works by increasing myocardial oxygen demand (through increased heart rate, systolic blood pressure, and myocardial contractility). This creates increased coronary blood flow, which results in heterogeneous blood flow due to stenotic arteries. As in exercise MPI, scintigraphic images obtained at rest are compared to those obtained during peak pharmacologic stress to distinguish myocardial ischemia from infarction.

Dipyridamole planar scintigraphy has a sensitivity of 90% and a specificity of 70% for detection of significant CAD, similar to exercise MPI.[41] In studies of dipyridamole and exercise Tl-201 planar imaging in the same patients, comparable sensitivity and specificity were observed.[41] The diagnostic accuracy of quantitative dipyridamole Tl-201 SPECT imaging is also comparable.[42] Similar results are seen using adenosine stress.[43]

Dobutamine Tl-201 imaging is used for patients who cannot exercise but have contraindications to vasodilator stress (primarily reversible airway disease). Dobutamine stress using both planar and SPECT imaging has sensitivity and specificity comparable to vasodilators, despite the fact that the increase in coronary blood flow is less pronounced with dobutamine than with the vasodilators.[44,45] However, as with exercise, the accuracy of dobutamine stress is heart-rate dependent.[46] Thus, during dobutamine infusion, atropine and/or arm or leg exercise should be used if an adequate heart rate is not reached.

The diagnostic accuracy of Tc-99m imaging

for angiographically significant CAD has been evaluated in numerous studies. Overall, there has been no significant difference shown between pharmachologic stress and exercise stress when these agents are used, similar to findings with Tl-201. A study using 102 consecutive patients with chest pain and no known history of CAD evaluated four tests (done in random order): ETT, dipyridamole echocardiography, dobutamine echocardiography, and dobutamine Tc-99m sestamibi SPECT imaging.[47] The results can be seen in Figure 1-2. The most sensitive test was dobutamine Tc-99m sestamibi imaging, while the most specific test was dipyridamole echocardiography. Both the positive and negative predictive values of all imaging tests were not significantly different, though the sensitivity and negative predictive value of ETT were inferior to other tests.

Marwick and colleagues studied 97 patients without evidence of previous MI who were referred to coronary angiography for clinical reasons.[48] All patients underwent dobutamine and adenosine echocardiography and Tc-99m sestamibi MPI. The sensitivity, specificity, and diagnostic accuracy are shown in Figure 1-3. This study again demonstrated similar sensitivity and specificity of vasodilator and dobutamine Tc-99m sestamibi MPI.

In general, pharmachologic MPI is superior to the ETT and similar to exercise with MPI for the diagnosis of CAD. In a recent review of the

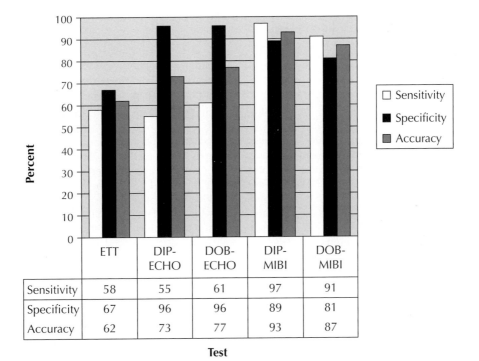

Test	ETT	DIP-ECHO	DOB-ECHO	DIP-MIBI	DOB-MIBI
Sensitivity	58	55	61	97	91
Specificity	67	96	96	89	81
Accuracy	62	73	77	93	87

ETT = Exercise treadmill test
DIP-ECHO = dipyridamole echocardiography
DOB-ECHO = dobutamine echocardiography
DIP-MIBI = dipyridamole myocardial perfusion imaging with Tc-99m sestamibi
DOB-MIBI = dobutamine myocardial perfusion imaging with Tc-99m sestamibi

Figure 1-2. Diagnostic accuracy of various tests for CAD. (Adapted from San Román et al.[47] with permission.)

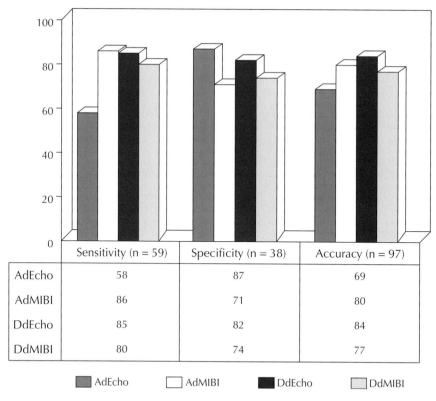

	Sensitivity (n = 59)	Specificity (n = 38)	Accuracy (n = 97)
AdEcho	58	87	69
AdMIBI	86	71	80
DdEcho	85	82	84
DdMIBI	80	74	77

■ AdEcho ☐ AdMIBI ■ DdEcho ☐ DdMIBI

Figure 1-3. Bar graph showing sensitivity, specificity, and accuracy of dobutamine (Db) and adenosine (Ad) stresses, in combination with two-dimensional echocardiography (Echo) (2DE) and methoxyisobutyl isonitrile (MIBI) single photon emission computed tomography (SPECT). The sensitivity of adenosine 2DE was significantly less than adenosine MIBI SPECT ($p = 0.001$), dobutamine 2DE ($p = 0.001$), and dobutamine MIBI SPECT ($p = 0.01$). The accuracy of adenosine 2DE was significantly less than that of adenosine MIBI SPECT ($p < 0.0005$), dobutamine 2DE ($p = 0.001$), and dobutamine MIBI SPECT ($p = 0.005$). The three latter tests did not differ from each other in sensitivity or accuracy; none of the specificities differed significantly. (Reprinted from Marwick et al.[48] with permission.)

literature, Leppo concluded that each test using MPI was diagnostically equivalent (Figure 1-4).[43]

IMPACT OF NEW TECHNOLOGIES FOR TC-99M IMAGING

Electrocardiographic Gating of Image Acquisition

As a result of the higher photon energy available from Tc-99m agents, SPECT imaging can be gated with the ECG and provide good-quality images. Using the same technique as radionuclide ventriculography (RVG), the cardiac cycle is sampled over 8 to 16 frames, capturing an image of the heart at multiple points in the cardiac cycle. The reconstructed images allow displays of myocardial wall thickness, motion, and perfusion simultaneously by connecting the individual frames into a cine loop (similar to animation and motion pictures). Gated SPECT imaging also provides assessment of ventricular volume and ejection fraction.[49]

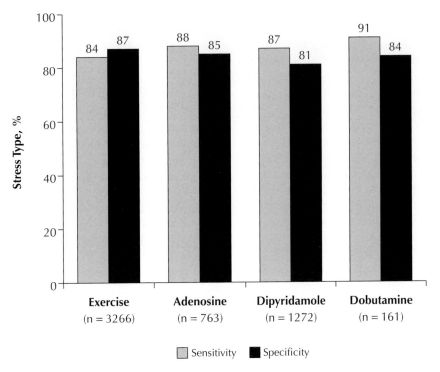

Figure 1-4. Diagnostic accuracy of stress myocardial perfusion imaging. (Adapted from Leppo[43] with permission.)

The accuracy of wall motion assessment and ejection fraction calculation by gated SPECT imaging has compared favorably to other techniques, such as angiography, echocardiography, RVG, and cine-magnetic resonance imaging.[49–51] There are some caveats to the accuracy of gated SPECT MPI. Ababneh and colleagues[52] studied 1,513 patients with suspected CAD and normal ETT results using gated Tc-99m sestamibi and Tl-201 SPECT images. The results using either tracer were equivalent, but both methods consistently reported lower left ventricular (LV) volumes and higher ejection fractions in women versus men. Manrique and colleagues[53] studied 50 patients with a history of MI with Tc-99m gated SPECT MPI, Tl-201 gated SPECT MPI, and equilibrium radionuclide angiography (RNA). The gated SPECT methods used commercially available quantitative gated SPECT (QGS) software. Both tracers similarly and signif-

icantly underestimated the left ventricular ejection fraction (LVEF) in patients with LV dysfunction and large perfusion defects. The proper interpretation of a gated SPECT study thus depends on the knowledge that LVEF may be underestimated when there is a large perfusion defect (by itself a major prognostic factor), and that patients with smaller hearts may have an overestimation of LVEF.

Despite these drawbacks, gated SPECT MPI plays an important role in improving the diagnostic accuracy of MPI. Choi and colleagues[54] studied the impact of gated SPECT MPI on 109 patients who had equivocal fixed defects with perfusion imaging alone. The addition of gated data increased the diagnostic performance, with 66 patients determined disease negative and 25 patients as disease positive. Only 14 readings were still equivocal. The diagnostic accuracy of two readers and their agreement was greater with gated images. Paola and colleagues[55] studied 285 patients and found that the addition of gated data to Tc-99m sestamibi imaging reduced the number of "borderline" interpretations from 89 to 29. More importantly, in the 137 patients with a < 10% pretest likelihood of CAD, the percentage of images designated "normal" increased from 74% to 93%. Similarly, in the 49 patients with previous MI or known coronary artery stenosis of at least 70%, the percentage of "abnormal" image interpretations increased from 78% to 92%. Taillefer and colleagues found that the addition of gated information to myocardial SPECT improved diagnostic accuracy in 85 patients with suspected CAD and 30 normal controls (Figure 1-5).[28] Sharir and colleagues[56] found that functional data provided by gated im-

aging adds further incremental prognostic value in the assessment of severe CAD beyond that of perfusion alone.

Attenuation Correction of SPECT Images

Attenuation correction attempts to increase the specificity and increase the diagnostic accuracy of SPECT imaging. Specificity of MPI is reduced by "false-positive" defects caused by attenuation of photon emission. Breast tissue, the diaphragm, and subdiaphragmatic organs are some of the causes of attenuation. Attenuation correction can be done in several ways. The details will not be discussed here, but some data[57] suggests that attenuation correction can improve the di-

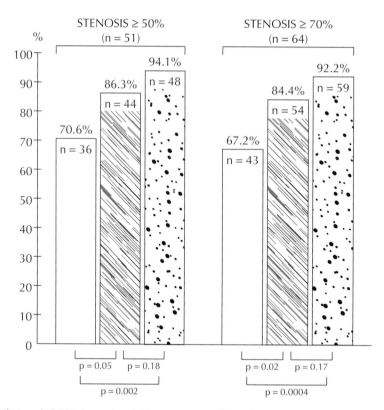

Figure 1-5.   Specificity of Tl-201 (open bars). Tc-99m sestamibi perfusion (striped bars) and Tc-99m sestamibi perfusion and gated SPECT (speckled bars) studies for both patients without CAD and the group of normal volunteers. (Reprinted from Tailleffer et al.[28] with permission.)

agnostic accuracy of cardiac SPECT imaging for the detection and localization of CAD. Detailed information regarding methods of attenuation correction, application, and quality control are contained in a recent position statement from the American Society of Nuclear Cardiology.[58]

RISK STRATIFICATION IN SUSPECTED CAD

Clinical Evaluation of Prognosis

A modified version of the Framingham risk score uses simple clinical variables to assess a patient's absolute risk of total CAD events and hard CAD events over 10 years.[59] This method also provides an estimate of relative risk for CAD. This information can then be used to reduce modifiable risk factors and to initiate appropriate treatment of certain conditions (i.e., diabetes mellitus, hypertension, and hypercholesterolemia). The risk score can also identify patients at low risk, allowing reassurance and avoiding further unnecessary diagnostic testing. Although these data provides prognostic information, more refined risk stratification is possible through the use of noninvasive testing. In recent years, the role of MPI in prognosis of patients with suspected CAD has become more intensively studied than its diagnostic role. This is because normal MPI studies have been shown to indicate an excellent prognosis in patients, even if they have known CAD by coronary angiography.[60] Thus, although the sensitivity and specificity of stress MPI do not appear adequate in the diagnosis of CAD in patients at high risk of disease, there is value in assessing risk for future cardiac events in these same patients using stress MPI. The topic of risk stratification is covered in more depth in Chapter 19.

COST EFFECTIVENESS IN THE DIAGNOSIS OF CAD

It is clear that risk stratification using clinical characteristics is relatively inexpensive, but the method lacks sensitivity. Exercise treadmill testing increases diagnostic accuracy at a modest cost, but still lacks sensitivity compared to other noninvasive methods of diagnosis. Currently, stress MPI appears to be more sensitive for the diagnosis of CAD and more useful for prognosis compared with stress echocardiography.[61,62]

A recent observational assessment[11] directly examined the cost effectiveness of an aggressive (direct coronary angiography) approach versus a conservative approach (stress MPI followed by angiography when indicated) in a group of 11,372 patients. The rates of death or MI during follow-up were similar in both strategies, although the rates of revascularization were higher in the aggressively managed group (Figure 1-6a). The direct and indirect costs of the aggressive strategy were significantly higher in all risk groups (Figure 1-6b).

Another dilemma is whether patients with normal exercise ECGs gain any benefit with MPI. A study by Wackers and colleagues[63] evaluated 313 patients who had normal resting ECGs and underwent exercise MPI. They concluded that patients at low to intermediate risk of CAD per the criteria of Diamond and Forrester[12] gained no benefit and had no adverse events if the exercise ECG was normal. Those with abnormal stress ECGs and those with high pretest risk gained benefit from stress MPI. Furthermore, this "stepwise" strategy resulted in cost savings. Even in the group of low-risk patients with abnormal ETT results, the utility of stress MPI has been questioned. In one study of 4,900 soldiers with a mean age of 43 ± 3 years,[64] the predictive value of an ETT was found to be 21%. Only 6.1% of patients had an abnormal ETT. From this group, 78 men had Tl-201 stress MPI performed, resulting in six abnormal studies (7.7%). Four of these patients underwent coronary angiography, with CAD found in three and hypertrophic cardiomyopathy found in another. The patients with abnormal MPI studies had significantly higher cholesterol levels and a borderline increase in triglyceride levels. All of the patients with total cholesterol under 208 mg/dL and

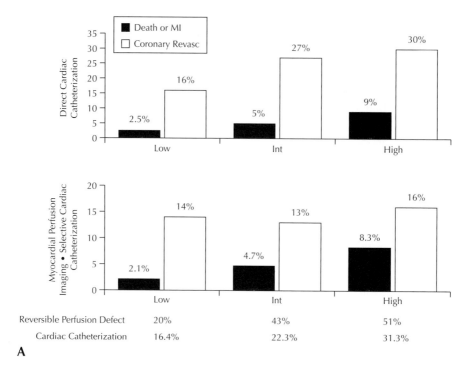

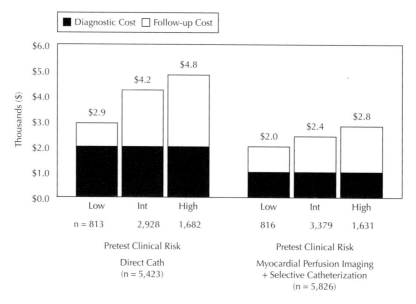

Figure 1-6.   A. Rates of cardiac death or myocardial infarction (MI) and coronary revascularization (Revasc) by pretest clinical risk subsets of low-, intermediate- (Int), and high-risk patients. The rates of ≥ 1 reversible perfusion defect and cardiac catheterization rates for patients undergoing a noninvasive diagnostic strategy are presented for low-, intermediate-, and high-risk patients. **B.** Overall diagnostic and follow-up costs of care for direct catheterization and initial stress perfusion imaging are presented. Diagnostic and follow-up costs of care were 30% to 41% higher for patients undergoing direct cardiac catheterization. **Solid bars** = diagnostic cost; **open bars** = follow-up cost. (Reprinted from Shaw et al.[11] with permission.)

triglycerides under 134 mg/dL had normal MPI studies. The conclusion was that routine exercise testing in young, asymptomatic males for the screening of CAD is ineffective and leads to excess costs. A study by Pilote and colleagues[65] had similar results in a slightly older population.

ORDERING A RADIONUCLIDE MYOCARDIAL PERFUSION IMAGERY TEST FOR SUSPECTED CAD

The preceding sections presented some of the data used to formulate the recommendations for testing that can be found in the appendix to this chapter. What follows is a simplified stepwise approach to the patient suspected of having CAD.

Question 1: Should My Patient Have a Radionuclide Test?

Diagnostic testing is an effort to determine a patient's risk for disease. Tests should be performed only if they significantly alter the probability of disease. This will is the basis of Bayesian analysis. As outlined earlier, patients with an intermediate pretest risk of CAD gain the most benefit from stress MPI. Using simple tools such as those of Diamond (Table 1-1) or the Framingham study[59] helps to assign pretest risk.

This does not mean that patients at high pretest risk of CAD should not undergo stress MPI. Although the probability of angiographically significant CAD is not altered dramatically by MPI in these patients, a negative or minimally abnormal MPI test portends an excellent prognosis in all patients. In high-risk patients (such as older male diabetics with typical angina), coronary angiography may be the best test, as it allows diagnosis and treatment of the culprit lesion(s). However, a patient with a low-risk MPI may wish to avoid the risks of revascularization and seek treatment with maximal medical therapy first.

As there is no clear evidence that patients at low risk for CAD benefit through the use of MPI

for diagnosis of CAD or assessment of prognosis, these patients should undergo ETT alone if there is suspicion of CAD. Radionuclide testing would be appropriate if a patient is unable to exercise, has an uninterpretable ECG, or has an abnormal ETT.

Question 2: Which Type of Stress Should Be Used?

Exercise stress testing provides important diagnostic and prognostic information for patients being assessed for CAD, especially using the Duke treadmill score.[66] Furthermore, MPI provides additive information to the treadmill data.[67] Thus, any patient who can perform exercise should do so. If a patient is not capable of performing adequate stress, then vasodilator stress should be performed if there are no contraindications. In those unable to exercise and with contraindications to vasodilators, dobutamine stress should be considered. Dobutamine is a third-line agent due to the more complicated nature of the test, the relative lack of data compared to other methods, and a relatively high event rate in patients with normal studies.

A newer protocol actually combines the use of exercise and vasodilator stress. This allows a clinician to obtain the prognostic data of exercise while acquiring accurate perfusion data using the pharmacologic MPI. There is evidence that exercise improves the detection of the extent and severity of ischemia in patients with CAD undergoing dipyridamole Tl-201 MPI.[68] In addition, even low-level exercise improves image quality and patient tolerance during adenosine MPI.[69] Further work on these methods is needed.

Question 3: Which Radionuclide Should Be Used?

Historically, the accuracy of MPI is similar using either Tl-201 or Tc-99m imaging agents. Some authorities advocate using Tl-201 for a rest study and Tc-99m for a stress study, which may decrease the total time of the test. However, it is becoming evident that the wealth of data provided by gated SPECT imaging improves diagnostic accuracy and provides important information regarding LV function. To harness the capabilities of ECG-gated imaging, Tc-99m agents are required for good quality images. Thus, these agents are recommended for routine clinical use.

CONCLUSION

This chapter served to introduce the reader to the indications for radionuclide imaging in patients with suspected CAD, compare them to the indications for exercise treadmill testing, and explain the rationale of these guidelines through primary evidence. The starting point in deciding the type of testing is the determination of a patient's risk for having CAD. This then allows the selection of a test with appropriate sensitivity and specificity, and permits accurate interpretation of that test. The goal is to maximize the accuracy of diagnosis without subjecting patients to unneeded and expensive testing.

From the evidence, it is clear that few patients with a low pretest likelihood of CAD benefit from any noninvasive testing. As the Bayesian analysis shows, positive tests do not increase posttest likelihood significantly and negative tests only confirm an already low risk of disease. Conversely, high-risk patients are unlikely to benefit from radionuclide techniques for diagnosis because a negative test still indicates a high posttest probability of CAD. High-risk patients can benefit from radionuclide techniques through their prognostic utility—negative tests indicate a low risk of adverse events even in the setting of known CAD. It is the patient at intermediate risk of CAD who benefits most from radionuclide techniques. The definition of risk depends on the age, gender, and type of pain. Risk is further defined by use of the Framingham risk calculation and by the use of ETT data in the Duke treadmill score. A stepwise use of these methods is able to lead to an appropriate use of radionuclide imaging, providing patients and physicians with valuable information to guide further treatment or diagnostic testing.

APPENDIX

Guidelines for Exercise Testing in Suspected Obstructive CAD[70]

Classification System   Clinical guidelines are presented with evidence to support recommendations. Based on the quality of this evidence, the recommendations are classified as follows[24]:

Class I—usually appropriate and considered useful

Class II—acceptable but usefulness is less well established

Class IIa—weight of evidence in favor of usefulness

Class IIb—can be helpful but not well established by evidence

Class III—generally not appropriate

Diagnosis of CAD

Class I

1. Adult patients (including those with complete right bundle branch block [RBBB] or < 1 mm of resting ST depression) with an intermediate pretest probability of CAD per criteria of Diamond and Forrester[12]

Class IIa

1. Patients with vasospastic angina

Class IIb

1. Patients with a low or high pretest probability of CAD by age symptoms and gender
2. Patients with < 1 mm of baseline ST depression and taking digoxin
3. Patients with ECG criteria for LV hypertrophy and < 1 mm of baseline ST depression

Class III

1. Patients with the following ECG abnormalities:

a. Preexcitation (Wolff–Parkinson–White [WPW]) syndrome
b. Electronically paced ventricular rhythm
c. > 1 mm of resting ST depression
d. Complete left bundle branch block (LBBB)

Risk Assessment and Prognosis in Patients with Symptoms of CAD

Class I

1. Patients undergoing initial evaluation with suspected CAD (exceptions below)
2. Patients with suspected CAD previously evaluated with significant change in clinical status

Class IIb

1. Patients with the following ECG abnormalities:
   a. Preexcitation (WPW) syndrome
   b. Electronically paced ventricular rhythm
   c. > 1 mm of resting ST depression
   d. Complete LBBB
2. Patients with a stable clinical course who undergo periodic monitoring to guide treatment

Class III

1. Patients with severe comorbidity likely to limit life expectancy and/or candidacy for revascularization

Exercise Testing in Asymptomatic Persons without Known CAD

Class I

1. None

Class IIb

1. Evaluation of persons with multiple risk factors [hypercholesterolemia (total cholesterol > 240 mg/dL), hypertension (systolic blood pressure > 140 mm Hg or diastolic blood pressure > 90 mm Hg), smoking, diabetes, and family history of MI or sudden cardiac death in a first-degree relative younger than 60 years, or a Framingham risk score with at least moderate risk of serious cardiac events within 5 years

2. Evaluation of asymptomatic men older than 40 years and asymptomatic women older than 50 years:
   a. Who plan to start vigorous exercise (especially if sedentary)
   b. Who are involved in occupations in which impairment might impact public safety
   c. Who are at high risk of CAD due to other diseases (i.e., chronic renal failure, diabetes mellitus)

Class III

1. Routine screening of asymptomatic men or women

Guidelines for Radionuclide Imaging and Stress Echocardiography of Suspected CAD

Recommendations for Chronic Stable Angina[71]

1. Class I—Diagnosis of symptomatic and selected patients with asymptomatic myocardial ischemia using exercise or pharmacologic MPI, including positron emission tomography (PET) (use of exercise RNA is class IIa)
2. Class I—Assessment of ventricular performance at rest or exercise using RNA (use of gated sestamibi is class IIa)

Recommendations for Cardiac Stress Imaging as the Initial Test in Patients with Chronic Stable Angina Who Are Able to Exercise[72]

Class I

1. Exercise MPI or stress echocardiography in patients with an intermediate pretest

probability of CAD who have one of the following baseline ECG abnormalities:
   a. Preexcitation (WPW) syndrome
   b. > 1 mm of resting ST depression
2. Exercise MPI or echocardiogram in patients with prior revascularization (percutaneous coronary intervention or coronary artery bypass graft [CABG])
3. Adenosine or dipyridamole MPI in patients with an intermediate pretest probability of CAD and either an electronically paced ventricular rhythm or LBBB

Class IIb

1. Exercise MPI or stress echocardiogram in patients with a low or high probability of CAD who have one of the following ECG abnormalities:
   a. Preexcitation (WPW) syndrome
   b. > 1 mm of ST depression
2. Adenosine or dipyridamole MPI in patients with a low or high probability of CAD and 1 of the following ECG abnormalities:
   a. Electronically paced ventricular rhythm
   b. LBBB
3. Exercise MPI or exercise echocardiogram in patients with an intermediate likelihood of CAD and one of the following:
   a. Digoxin use with < 1 mm ST depression on baseline ECG
   b. LV hypertrophy with < 1 mm ST depression on baseline ECG
4. Exercise MPI, exercise echo, adenosine or dipyridamole MPI, or dobutamine echo as the initial stress test in a patient with a normal resting ECG who is not taking digoxin
5. Exercise or dobutamine echo in patients with LBBB

Recommendations for Cardiac Stress Imaging as the Initial Test for Diagnosis of CAD in Patients with Chronic Stable Angina Who Are Unable to Exercise[72]

Class I

1. Adenosine or dipyridamole MPI or dobutamine echo in patients with an intermediate pretest likelihood of CAD
2. The same tests in patients with prior revascularization

Class IIb

1. Adenosine or dipyridamole stress MPI or dobutamine echo in patients with low or high probability of CAD in the absence of electronically paced ventricular rhythm or LBBB
2. Adenosine or dipyridamole stress MPI or dobutamine echo in patients with a low or high probability of CAD and one of the following ECG abnormalities:
   a. Electronically paced ventricular rhythm
   b. LBBB

Recommendations of Cardiac Stress Imaging for Risk Stratification of Patients with Chronic Stable Angina Who Are Able to Exercise[72]

Class I

1. Exercise MPI or echo to identify the extent, severity, and location of ischemia in patients who do not have LBBB or an electronically ventricular paced rhythm and have either an abnormal rest ECG or are using digoxin
2. Dipyridamole or adenosine MPI in patients with LBBB or electronically paced ventricular rhythm

Class IIb

1. Exercise or dobutamine echo in patients with LBBB
2. Exercise, dipyridamole, adenosine MPI, or exercise or dobutamine echo as the initial test in patients who have a normal rest ECG and are not taking digoxin

Class III

1. Exercise MPI in patients with LBBB
2. Exercise, dipyridamole, adenosine MPI, or exercise or dobutamine echo in patients with severe comorbidity likely to limit life expectation or prevent revacularization

Recommendations for Cardiac Stress Imaging as the Initial Test for Risk Stratification of Patients with Chronic Stable Angina Who Are Unable to Exercise[72]

Class I

1. Dipyridamole or adenosine myocardial perfusion imaging or dobutamine echocardiography to identify the extent, severity, and location of ischemia in patients who do not have LBBB or electronically paced rhythm
2. Dipyridamole or adenosine MPI in patients with LBBB or electronically paced ventricular rhythm
3. Dipyridamole or adenosine MPI or dobutamine echo to assess the functional significance of coronary lesions (if not already known) in planning revascularization

Class IIb

1. Dobutamine echo in patients with LBBB

Class III

1. Dipyridamole or adenosine MPI or dobutamine echo in patients with severe comorbidity likely to limit life expectation or prevent revascularization

REFERENCES

1. American Heart Association. *2001 Heart and Stroke Statistical Update*. Dallas, TX: AHA, 2000.
2. Ridker PM, Genest J, Libby P. Risk factors for atherosclerotic disease. In: Braunwald E, Zipes DP, and Libby P, eds. *Heart Disease: A Textbook of Cardiovascular Medicine*, 6th ed. New York: W.B. Saunders Company; 2001:1010–1031.
3. Kannel WB, McGee D, Gordon T. A general cardiovascular risk profile: The Framingham study. *Am J Cardiol* 1976;38:46–51.
4. Pryor DB, Shaw L, McCants CB, et al.: Value of the history and physical in identifying patients at increased risk for coronary artery disease. *Ann Intern Med* 1993;118:81–90.
5. D'Agostino RB, Grundy S, Sullivan LM, et al.: Validation of the Framingham coronary artery disease prediction scores: Results of a multiple ethnic groups investigation. *JAMA* 2001;286:180–187.
6. *Executive Summary of the Third Report of the National Cholesterol Education Panel on Detection, Evaluation, and Treatment of High Blood Cholesterol in Adults* (NIH Pub. No. 01-3096), 2001.
7. Diamond GA. A clinically relevant classification of chest discomfort. *J Am Coll Cardiol* 1983;1:574–575 (letter).
8. Verna E, Ceriani L, Giovanelli L, et al. "False-positive" myocardial perfusion scintigraphy findings in patients with angiographically normal coronary arteries: Insights from intravascular sonography studies. *J Nucl Med* 2000;41:1935–1940.
9. Noto TJ Jr., Johnson LW, Krone R, et al. Cardiac catheterization 1990: A report of the registry of the Society for Cardiac Angiography and Interventions (SCA&I). *Cathet Cardiovasc Diagn* 1991;24:75–83.
10. Stuart RJ, Ellestad MH. National survey of exercise stress testing facilities. *Chest* 1980;77:94–97.
11. Shaw LJ, Hachamovitch R, Berman DS, et al. The economic consequences of available diagnostic and prognostic strategies for the evaluation of stable angina patients: An observational assessment of the value of precatheterization ischemia. *J Am Coll Cardiol* 1999;33:661–669.
12. Diamond GA and Forrester JS. Analysis of probability as an aid in the clinical diagnosis of coronary artery disease. *N Engl J Med* 1979;300:1350–1358.
13. Roger VL, Pellikka PA, Bell MR, et al. Sex and test verification bias: Impact on the diagnostic value of exercise echocardiography. *Circulation* 1997;95:405–410.
14. Koide Y, Masayuki Y, Yoshino H, et al. A new coronary artery disease index of treadmill exercise electrocardiograms based on the step-up diagnostic method. *Am J Cardiol* 2001;87:142–147.
15. Gianrossi R, Detrano R, Lehmann R, et al. Exercise-induced ST depression in the diagnosis of coronary artery disease: A meta-analysis. *Circulation* 1989;80:87–98.
16. Morise A. Are the American College of Cardiology/American Heart Association guidelines for exercise testing for suspected coronary artery disease correct? *Chest* 2000;118:535–541.

17. Froelicher VF, Lehmann KG, Thomas R, et al. The electrocardiographic exercise test in a population with reduced work-up bias: Diagnostic performance, computerized interpretation, and multivariate prediction. *Ann Intern Med* 1998;128:965–974.

18. Hlatky MA, Pryor DB, Harrell FE, et al. Factors affecting sensitivity and specificity of exercise electrocardiography: Multivariable analysis. *Am J Med* 1984;77:64–71.

19. Bonoris PE, Greenberg RS, Castellanet MJ, et al. Significance of changes in R-wave amplitude during treadmill stress testing: Angiographic correlation. *Am J Cardiol* 1978;41:846–852.

20. Elamin MS, Mary DASG, Smith DR, et al. Prediction of severity of coronary artery disease using slope of submaximal ST segment/heart rate relationship. *Cardiovasc Res* 1980;14:681–691.

21. Olein PM, Kligfield P, Milner MR, et al. Heart rate adjustment of ST-segment depression for reduction of false positive electrocardiographic responses to exercise in asymptomatic men screened for coronary artery disease. *Am J Cardiol* 1988;62:1043–1047.

22. Johnson SH, Bigelow C, Lee KL, et al. Prediction of death and myocardial infarction by radionuclide angiocardiography in patients with suspected coronary artery disease. *Am J Cardiol* 1991;67:919–926.

23. Jones RH, Johnson SH, Bigelow C, et al. Exercise radionuclide angiocardiography predicts cardiac death in patients with coronary artery disease. *Circulation* 1991;84(Suppl. I):I-52–I-58.

24. Guidelines for clinical use of cardiac radionuclide imaging: Report of the American College of Cardiology/American Heart Association Task Force on Diagnostic and Therapeutic Cardiovascular Procedures (Committee on Radionuclide Imaging), developed in collaboration with the American Society of Nuclear Cardiology. *J Am Coll Cardiol* 1995;25:521–547.

25. Detrano R, Janosi A, Lyons KP, et al. Factors affecting the sensitivity and specificity of a diagnostic test: The exercise thallium scintigram. *Am J Med* 1988;84:699–710.

26. Faber TL. Tomographic imaging: Methods. In: Gerson MC, ed. *Cardiac Nuclear Medicine,* 3rd ed. New York: McGraw-Hill, 1997:53–80.

27. Mahmarian JJ, Verani MS. Exercise thallium-201 perfusion scintigraphy in the assessment of coronary artery disease. *Am J Cardiol* 1991;67:2D–11D.

28. Tailleffer R, DePuey EG, Udelson JE, et al. Comparative diagnostic accuracy of Tl-201 and Tc-99m sestamibi SPECT imaging (perfusion and ECG-gated SPECT) in detecting coronary artery disease in women. *J Am Coll Cardiol* 1997;29:69–77.

29. Gerson MC, McGoron A, Roszell N, et al. Myocardial perfusion imaging: Radiopharmaceuticals and tracer kinetics. In: Gerson MC, ed. *Cardiac Nuclear Medicine,* 3rd ed. New York: McGraw Hill, 1997:3–27.

30. Gerson MC. Test accuracy, test selection, and test result interpretation in Chronic coronary artery disease. In: Gerson MC, ed. *Cardiac Nuclear Medicine,* 3rd ed. New York: McGraw-Hill, 1997:527–579.

31. Verzibijlbergen JF, van Oudheusden D, Cramer MJ, et al. Quantitative analysis of planar technetium-99m sestamibi myocardial perfusion images. Clinical application of a modified method for the subtraction of tissue crosstalk. *Eur Heart J* 1994;15:1217–1226.

32. Plachcinska A, Kusmierek J, Kosmider M, et al. Quantitative assessment of technetium-99m methoxy isobutylisonitrile planar perfusion heart studies: Application of multivariate analysis to patient classification. *Eur J Nucl Med* 1995;22:193–200.

33. Jamar F, Topcuoglu R, Cauwe F, et al. Exercise gated planar myocardial perfusion imaging using technetium-99m sestamibi for the diagnosis of coronary artery disease: An alternative to exercise tomographic imaging. *Eur J Nucl Med* 1995;22:40–48.

34. Berman DS, Kiat HS, Van Train KF, et al. Myocardial perfusion imaging with technetium-99m sestamibi: Comparative analysis of available imaging protocols. *J Nucl Med* 1994;35:681–688.

35. Maddah J, Kiat H, Van Train KF, et al. Myocardial perfusion imaging with technetium-99m sestamibi SPECT in the evaluation of coronary artery disease. *Am J Cardiol* 1990;66:55E–62E.

36. Sochor H. Technetium-99m sestamibi in chronic coronary artery disease: The European experience. *Am J Cardiol* 1990;66:23E–31E.

37. Najm YC, Maisey MN, Clarke SM, et al. Exercise myocardial perfusion scintigraphy with technetium-99m methoxy isobutylisonitrile: A comparative study with thallium-201. *Int J Cardiol* 1990;26:93–102.

38. Maublant JC, Marcaggi X, Lusson JR, et al. Comparison between thallium-201 and technetium-99m methoxy isobutylisonitrile defect size in single-photon emission computed tomography at rest, exercise, and redistribution in coronary artery disease. *Am J Cardiol* 1992;69:183–187.

39. Stratmann HG, Younis LT, Wittry MD, et al. Effect of the stress level achieved during symptom-limited exercise technetium-99m sestamibi myocardial tomography on the detection of coronary artery disease. *Clin Cardiol* 1996;19:787–792.

40. Thomas GS. Happenings in the private sector. *Am Soc Nucl Cardiol* Newsletter 2001;8(1):5–6.

41. Leppo JA. Dipyridamole-thallium imaging: The lazy man's stress test. *J Nucl Med* 1989;30:281–287.

42. Borges-Neto S, Mahmarian JJ, Jain A, et al. Quantitative thallium-201 single photon emission computed tomography after oral dipyridamole for assessing the presence, anatomic location, and severity of coronary artery disease. *J Am Coll Cardiol* 1988;11:962–969.

43. Leppo JA. Comparison of pharmachologic stress agents. *J Nucl Cardiol* 1996;3:S22–S26.
44. Mason JR, Palac RT, Freeman ML, et al. Thallium scintigraphy during dobutamine infusion: Nonexercise-dependent screening test for coronary artery disease. *Am Heart J* 1984;107:481–485.
45. Hays JT, Mahmarrian JJ, Cochran AJ, et al. Dobutamine-thallium tomography for evaluating patients with suspected coronary artery disease unable to undergo exercise or vasodilator pharmacologic stress. *J Am Coll Cardiol* 1993;21:1583–1590.
46. Shehata AR, Gillam LD, Mascitelli UA, et al. Impact of acute propranolol administration on dobutamine-induced myocardial ischemia as evaluated by myocardial perfusion imaging and echocardiography. *Am J Cardiol* 1997;80:268–272.
47. San Román JA, Vilacosta I, Castillo JA, et al. Selection of the optimal stress test for the diagnosis of coronary artery disease. *Heart* 1998;80:370–376.
48. Marwick T, Willemart B, D'Hondt AM, et al. Selection of the optimal nonexercise stress for the evaluation of ischemic regional myocardial dysfunction and malperfusion. *Circulation* 1993;87:345–354.
49. Wackers FJT, Soufer R, and Zaret BL. Nuclear Cardiology. In: Braunwald E, Zipes DP, and Libby P, eds. *Heart Disease: A Textbook of Cardiovascular Medicine*, 6th ed. New York: WB Saunders, 2001:273–323.
50. Paul AK, Hasegawa S, Yoshioka H, et al. Assessment of left ventricular function by gated myocardial perfusion and gated blood-pool SPECT: Can we use the same reference database? *Ann Nucl Med* 2000;14:75–80.
51. Stollfus JC, Haas F, Matsunari I, et al. Regional myocardial wall thickening and global ejection fraction in patients with low angiographic ejection fraction assessed by visual and quantitative resting ECG-gated 99mTc-tetrofosmin single-photon emission tomography and magnetic resonance imaging. *Eur J Nucl Med* 1998;25:522–530.
52. Ababneh AA, Sciacca RR, Kim B, et al. Normal limits for left ventricular ejection fraction and volumes estimated with gated myocardial perfusion imaging in patients with normal exercise test results: Influence of tracer, gender, and acquisition camera. *J Nucl Cardiol* 2000;7:661–668.
53. Manrique A, Faraggi M, Vera P, et al. Tl-201 and 99mTc-MIBI gated SPECT in patients with large perfusion defects and left ventricular dysfunction: Comparison with equilibrium radionuclide angiography. *J Nucl Med* 1999;40:805–809.
54. Choi JY, Lee KH, Kim SJ, et al. Gating provides improved accuracy for differentiating artifacts from true lesions in equivocal fixed defects on technetium 99m tetrofosmin perfusion SPECT. *J Nucl Cardiol* 1998;5:395–401.
55. Paola E, Smiano P, Watson DD, et al. Value of gating of technetium-99m sestamibi single-photon emission computed tomographic imaging. *J Am Coll Cardiol* 1997;30:1687–1692.
56. Sharir T, Bacher-Stier C, Dhar SL, et al. Identification of severe and extensive coronary artery disease by post-exercise regional wall motion abnormalities in Tc-99m sestamibi gated single photon emission computed tomography. *Am J Cardiol* 2000;86:1171–1175.
57. Ficaro EP, Fessler JA, Shreve PD, et al. Simultaneous transmission/emission myocardial perfusion tomography: Diagnostic accuracy of attenuation-corrected 99mTc-sestamibi single-photon emission computed tomography. *Circulation* 1996;93:463–473.
58. Hendel RC, Corbett JR, Cullom ST, et al. The value and practice of attenuation correction for myocardial perfusion SPECT imaging: A joint position paper from the American Society of Nuclear Cardiology and the Society of Nuclear Medicine. *J Nucl Cardiol* 2002;9:135–143.
59. Grundy SM, Pasternak R, Greenkind P, et al. Assessment of cardiovascular risk by use of multiple-risk-factor assessment equations: A statement for healthcare professionals from the American Heart Association and the American College of Cardiology. *J Am Coll Cardiol* 1999;34:1348–1359.
60. Brown KA. Prognostic value of thallium-201 myocardial perfusion imaging: A diagnostic test comes of age. *Circulation* 1991;83:363–381.
61. Brown KA, Rosman DR, and Dave RM. Stress nuclear myocardial perfusion imaging versus stress echocardiography: Prognostic comparisons. *Prog Cardiovasc Dis* 2000;43:231–244.
62. Mandalupa BP, Amato M, and Stratmann HG. Technetium Tc-99m sestamibi myocardial perfusion imaging: Current role for evaluation of prognosis. *Chest* 1999;33:1684–1694.
63. Mattera JA, Arain SA, Sinusas AJ, et al. Exercise testing with myocardial perfusion imaging in patients with normal baseline electrocardiograms: Cost savings with a stepwise diagnostic strategy. *J Nucl Cardiol* 1998;5:498–506.
64. Livschitz S, Sharabi Y, Yushin J, et al. Limited clinical value of exercise stress test for the screening of coronary artery disease in young, asymptomatic men. *Am J Cardiol* 2000;86:462–464.
65. Pilote L, Pashkow F, Thomas JD, et al. Clinical yield and cost of exercise treadmill testing to screen for coronary artery disease in asymptomatic adults. *Am J Cardiol* 1998;81:219–224.
66. Mark DB, Shaw L, Harrel FE, et al. Prognostic value of a treadmill exercise score in outpatients with suspected coronary artery disease. *N Engl J Med* 1991; 325:849–853.
67. Vanzetto G, Ormezzano O, Fagret D, et al. Long-term additive prognostic value of thallium-201 myocardial perfusion imaging over clinical and exercise stress test in low to intermediate risk patients: Study in 1137 patients

with 6-year follow-up. *Circulation* 1999;
100:1521–1527.

68. Stein L, Burt R, Oppenheim B, et al. Symptom-limited arm exercise increases detection of ischemia during dipyridamole tomographic thallium stress testing in patients with coronary artery disease. *Am J Cardiol* 1995;75:568–572.

69. Thomas GS, Prill NV, Majmundar H, et al. Treadmill exercise during adenosine infusion is safe, results in fewer adverse reactions, and improves myocardial perfusion image quality. *J Nucl Cardiol* 2000; 7:439–446.

70. Gibbons RJ, Balady GJ, Beasley JW, et al. ACC/AHA guidelines for exercise testing: A report of the American College of Cardiology/American Heart Association Task Force on Practice Guidelines (Committee on Exercise Testing). *J Am Coll Cardiol* 1997;30:260–315.

71. Ritchie JL, Bateman TM, Bonow RO, et al. Guidelines for clinical use of radionuclide imaging: Report of the American College of Cardiology/American Heart Association Task Force on Assessment of Diagnostic and Therapeutic Procedures (Committee on Radionuclide Imaging), developed in collaboration with the American Society of Nuclear Cardiology. *J Am Coll Cardiol* 1995;25:521–547.

72. Gibbons RJ, Chatterjee K, Daley J, et al. ACC/AHA/ACP-ASIM guidelines for the management of patients with chronic stable angina: Executive summary and recommendations: A report of the American College of Cardiology/American Heart Association Task Force on Practice Guidelines (Committee on Management of Patients with Chronic Stable Angina). *Circulation* 1999;99:2829–2848.

CHAPTER 2

Known Coronary Artery Disease

Georgios I. Papaioannou
Gary V. Heller

INTRODUCTION: THE CONCEPT OF RISK

Ischemic heart disease and its manifestations remains a major health problem. Despite remarkable achievements in diagnosis and treatment, heart disease remains the single leading cause of death in the United States.[1] Appropriate management of known coronary disease includes assessment of the individual risk of future cardiac events, including death and myocardial infarction (MI). High-risk patients (e.g., those with left main disease and/or three-vessel disease) benefit from an aggressive approach with coronary angiography and revascularization. On the contrary, the vast majority of individuals with low annual risk for cardiac events can be managed conservatively.[2]

Results from stress myocardial perfusion imaging (MPI) (thallium 201 [Tl-201] or technetium 99m [Tc-99m] agents) has the ability to distinguish patients at high risk (> 5% annual incidence of cardiac events) from those at low risk (< 1% annual incidence of cardiac events) and

currently plays an important role in the management of patients with known coronary disease.[3] A normal Tl-201 or Tc-99m sestamibi scan is generally associated with low risk of future cardiac events.[4-6] This low event rate approaches that of a normal age-matched population and also of patients with normal coronary angiograms.[7] The same benign prognosis appears to persist even in patients with strongly positive exercise electrocardiograms (ECGs) or angiographically significant coronary disease.[8-9] The extent and severity of ischemic zones measured by MPI quantify the magnitude of myocardium at risk during exercise or pharmacological stress testing.[10] Studies demonstrating extensive ischemia (> 20% of the left ventricle, defects in > 1 coronary vascular supply region) or reversible ischemia in multiple segments, predict an increased rate of cardiac events.[11] Other parameters, such as transient or persistent left ventricular (LV) cavity dilatation[12] and increased Tl-201 lung uptake[13] play an important role in risk stratification (Table 2-1).[3] All the above variables in-

Table 2-1

Predictors of Stress-Induced Ischemic Extent and Severity with Myocardial Perfusion SPECT

- Number and/or location of reversible defects
- Magnitude (severity and extent) of stress defects
- Tl-201 uptake of isotope[a]
- Transient ischemic left ventricle cavity dilatation after exercise[a]
- Delayed redistribution

---

[a] Best assessed by obtaining a 5-minute poststress and 4-hour redistribution or rest anterior planar scintigram before the initiation of SPECT imaging.
Adapted from Yao and Rozanski[3] with permission.

dependently place patients with known coronary disease at increased risk for future cardiac events.

The introduction of the newer Tc-99m agents and the high count density achieved with them leads to both a higher quality of myocardial perfusion images and stable myocardial distribution with time.[14] By use of electrocardiographic gating during acquisition of tomographic perfusion images, important functional information of the LV is obtained (wall motion, wall thickening, cavity volumes, and ejection fraction). There is growing literature that gated single-photon emission computed tomography (SPECT) gives important additional information beyond MPI alone, with major implications in optimal patient care.[15,16] Patients with an ejection fraction < 45% and mild, moderate, or severe perfusion abnormalities have a high mortality rate, whereas patients with an ejection fraction > 45% have a cardiac death rate of < 1% per year regardless of the degree of the perfusion abnormality.[17]

The use of MPI as a means of risk assessment can be applied to a wide variety of patients, beginning with the initial evaluation of patients without coronary artery disease (CAD). In this chapter the focus will be on patients already diagnosed with CAD and will include subsets such as prior and post revascularization and the role in monitor medical therapy.

MYOCARDIAL PERFUSION IMAGING AND CHRONIC ISCHEMIC HEART DISEASE

Indications for Stress Myocardial Perfusion Imaging

Exercise stress testing alone is an important tool in following patients with known coronary disease, especially whenever there is a change in the frequency or pattern of symptoms. However, several factors may preclude use of exercise stress testing alone as the diagnostic modality to make further decisions. The American College of Cardiology/American Heart Association (ACC/AHA) Guidelines for exercise testing[18] strongly recommend an imaging study as part of the evaluation in patients unable to exercise and in those with baseline ECG abnormalities (preexcitation, paced ventricular rhythm, > 1 mm of resting ST depression, complete left bundle branch block [LBBB]). The use of digoxin, presence of left ventricular hypertrophy (LVH), or any resting ST-segment depression decreases the specificity of exercise testing while sensitivity may remain unaffected.[18] Several other subsets of patients benefit incrementally with the use of radionuclide imaging. Those groups involve patients with previous MI and/or revascularization procedures (coronary artery bypass graft [CABG] or percutaneous transluminal coronary angioplasty [PTCA]), patients with prior angiography demonstrating significant disease (where identification of lesion-causing myocardial ischemia is important), high-risk individuals for future events (e.g., diabetics), and patients with a previous positive nuclear scan.[18–22] A summary of the conditions in which radionuclide perfusion imaging is preferred over conventional exercise stress testing is presented in Table 2-2.[23]

Timing and Follow-Up in Stable Coronary Artery Disease

Millions of patients with CAD undergo stress MPI annually. Stress MPI is indicated in some as part of their initial risk assessment and/or prior

Table 2-2

Indications for the Use of Radionuclide Perfusion Imaging Rather than Exercise Electrocardiography[a]

- Complete left bundle-branch block
- Electronically paced ventricular rhythm
- Preexcitation (Wolff–Parkinson–White) syndrome or other, similar ECG abnormalities
- > 1 mm of ST-segment depression at rest
- Inability to exercise to a level high enough to give meaningful results on routine stress ECG[b]
- Angina and history of revascularization[c]

[a] The Guidelines were developed by the American College of Cardiology, the American Heart Association, the American College of Physicians, and the American Society of Internal Medicine.[1]
[b] Patients with this factor should be considered for pharmacologic stress tests.
[c] In patients with angina and a history of revascularization, characterizing the ischemia, establishing the functional effect of lesions, and determining myocardial viability are important considerations.
Reprinted from Lee and Boucher[23] with permission.

to planning PTCA or CABG, but in the majority as part of their follow-up after an intervention (PTCA or CABG) or medical modification.

The role of stress MPI in stable CAD addresses the concept of risk and is linked to an effort of identifying individuals at higher risk for future cardiac events. Unless cardiac catheterization is indicated, patients with known CAD who present with changing symptoms suggestive of ischemia should first undergo stress testing, with or without MPI, to assess the risk of future events.[1] Furthermore, localization of ischemia, identification of extent and severity of ischemic zones, and assessment of LV performance is desirable for most patients who are being evaluated for intervention or titration of medical therapy[24] (Table 2-3). Routine testing in patients with stable symptoms, and in patients with severe comorbidity that is likely to limit life expectancy or prevent revascularization, is not supported by any evidence.[1]

Although the field of nuclear cardiology has substantial data regarding prognosis and risk stratification, there is a paucity of published evidence regarding the widespread practice of follow-up testing using MPI. Clinical cardiologists and internists must use their best judgment to answer important questions: What constitutes a "definite" change that is outside the limit of reproducibility of the test? What constitutes a "clinically significant" improvement or worsening? What degree of improvement should be expected after medical management or intervention? If the patient does improve on medical therapy, does this mean a favorable prognosis?[25] In the absence of randomized trials, some observational studies try to address this deficiency in the literature. Berman et al.[26] followed a cohort

Table 2-3

Uses of Radionuclide Testing in Assessment of Severity/Prognosis/Risk Stratification of Chronic Ischemic Heart Disease

Indication	Test	Class
1. Assessment of LV performance	Rest or exercise RNA	I
	Gated sestamibi perfusion imaging	IIb
2. Identification of extent and severity of ischemia and localization of ischemia	Exercise or pharmacologic myocardial perfusion imaging	I

LV, left ventricular; RNA, radionuclide angiography.
Reprinted from Rithie et al.[24] with permission.

of 421 patients with abnormal baseline nuclear scans who underwent revascularization or conservative management. Patients had serial MPI with at least a 1-year interval between the two studies. The finding of this study showed that remarkable improvement in reversible ischemia occurred in patients with intermediate and extensive stress defects at baseline. The improvement was greater in those who underwent revascularization. However, it is clear that much more needs to be done. Several randomized trials are already under way that test the hypothesis that the suppression of ischemia with medical therapy is a favorable prognostic indicator that can be used to properly select patients for medical therapy or revascularization. Until results are available, the current literature supports the concept that a low-risk scan has a period of "warranty" of 12 to 18 months and a high-risk scan requires further investigation.[11,27]

MYOCARDIAL PERFUSION IMAGING AND REVASCULARIZATION PROCEDURES

Prior to Revascularization Procedures

Over the years, myocardial perfusion scintigraphy has evolved as an essential tool in the evaluation and assessment of patients prior to coronary revascularization. It has a dual role. Prior to coronary angiography, MPI is extremely useful in documenting ischemia and determining the functional impact of single or multiple lesions identified subsequently. After coronary anatomy is known, and despite some limitations in the setting of multivessel disease,[28] MPI remains the test of choice for identifying the lesion responsible for the ischemic symptoms, or so-called "culprit lesion."[24]

It is now well established that even though the presence of angiographically detected coronary disease increases with age,[29] the prognosis of intermediate lesions in such a population is determined by the extent and severity of re-

versible ischemia.[27] Therefore, in a population with known coronary disease and persistent symptoms despite medical therapy, myocardial perfusion scintigraphy may identify objective evidence of stress-induced ischemia. Although less important prior to CABG, where typically all lesions with ≥ 50% stenosis are bypassed, this is extremely useful for further management decisions with respect to percutaneous interventions.[30] The absence of reversible ischemia in patients with known CAD is an excellent prognostic marker and predicts a low annual event rate.[31] Still in these patients, who represent a considerable proportion of the PTCA population, the decision to perform PTCA is often based on the information obtained by coronary angiography alone, and its benefit is unproven.[32,33]

After Coronary Artery Bypass Surgery (CABG)

Recent figures estimate that 598,000 CABG procedures are performed annually in the United States.[34] The long term effectiveness of this now common procedure is limited by graft stenosis and progression of native disease. Evaluation of post-CABG patients with stress MPI depends on the presence or absence of symptoms as well as timing from the surgical procedure.

Current ACC/AHA Guidelines argue against routine testing of asymptomatic patients but do allow the "assessment of selected symptom-free patients,"[34] such as patients with an abnormal ECG response to exercise or those with resting ECG changes precluding identification of ischemia during exercise. Current literature supports the notion that a cutoff point of 5 years can be applied to patients post-CABG. In patients late post-CABG (> 5 years), irrespective of symptoms, myocardial perfusion single-photon emission computed tomography (SPECT) has been an effective method for risk stratification. Palmas et al.[35] studied 294 patients ≥ 5 years post-CABG. The Tl-201 reversibility score (a global measure of ischemic index) and the presence of increased lung uptake added significant prognostic information to a clinical model. Similarly Zellweger et al.[36] identified 1,765 patients who underwent myocardial perfusion SPECT 7.1 ± 5.0 years post-CABG. Patients > 5 years post-CABG irrespective of symptoms, and symptomatic patients ≤ 5 years post-CABG, benefited from nuclear testing because the assessment of ischemia provided a guide to appropriate therapy. Asymptomatic patients ≤ 5 years post-CABG have a low cardiac death rate (1.3%) and did not benefit from nuclear testing. In both groups, a moderate or severely abnormal summed stress score (based on the interpretation of the stress Tc-99m sestamibi images) predicted a significantly higher annual mortality rate (2.1% and 3.1%, respectively; Figure 2-1).

After Percutaneous Coronary Intervention (PCI)

The explosion of PTCA and stent placement in patients with single- or multivessel disease has created a necessity for early detection of restenosis. A number of clinical studies have documented the usefulness of stress myocardial SPECT for identifying restenosis in patients after coronary angioplasty and/or stent placement.[37,38] One point of controversy is the optimal time of performing SPECT imaging after PTCA. Initial studies[39] reported a high frequency of false-positive transient myocardial perfusion defects when SPECT imaging was performed in the first few weeks after angioplasty. Iskandrian et al.[38] proposed a pharmacologic SPECT strategy early after angioplasty without an increased false-positive rate. Although current consensus is to obtain an exercise myocardial perfusion study 4 to 6 weeks postintervention,[3,24] whenever indicated, the proper timing for use of myocardial perfusion SPECT remains to be determined. Based on existing knowledge about the timing interval of subacute thrombosis[40] (< 4 weeks) and in-stent restenosis[41] (3–6 months), we propose an algorithm (Figure 2-2) as a guide for the management of patients with known CAD after percutaneous coronary intervention (PCI). Asymptomatic patients may be considered for stress MPI 4 to 6 weeks postintervention in order to assess the functional results of PTCA and establish a "new baseline."[24] Subsets of patients that benefit from this approach

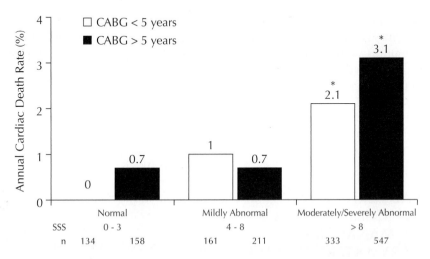

Figure 2-1.   Annual cardiac death (CD) rates as a function of SSS in patients ≤ 5 and > 5 years post-CABG ($n = 1,544$). Statistically significant increase as a function of SSS ($p = 0.049$, 0.005 for ≤ 5 and > 5 years, respectively). CABG = coronary artery bypass graft surgery; SSS = summed stress score. (Reprinted from Zellweger et al.[36] with permission.)

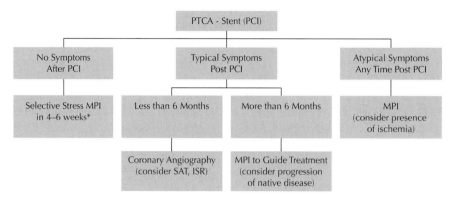

Figure 2-2. Proposed algorithm for management of patients after percutaneous intervention (PCI) with respect to nature and timing of symptoms. ACC/AHA practice guidelines favor selective evaluation in patients considered to be at particular high risk (e.g., patients with decreased LV function, multivessel CAD, proximal left anterior descending disease, previous sudden death, diabetes mellitus, hazardous occupations and suboptimal PCI results).[18] PTCA = percutaneous transluminal coronary angioplasty; PCI = percutaneous intervention; MPI = myocardial perfusion imaging; SAT = subacute thrombosis; ISR = in-stent restenosis.

include those at high risk post PCI (patients with decreased LV function, multivessel disease, proximal left anterior descending disease, previous sudden death, diabetes mellitus, hazardous occupations, and suboptimal PCI results).[18] Stress MPI is also recommended in patients who develop atypical symptoms after PCI and there is necessity to assess whether these symptoms represent ischemia. Patients with symptoms typical of ischemia < 6 months postintervention should proceed with coronary angiography as a first step, unless contraindicated. If angina occurs later (> 6 months post PCI), stress MPI can be used to assess the degree and area of ischemia, since progression of native coronary disease rather than in-stent restenosis is more likely.

MYOCARDIAL PERFUSION IMAGING TO ASSESS EFFICACY OF MEDICAL MANAGEMENT OF CORONARY ARTERY DISEASE

Intensive medical therapy with risk factor modification is essential in the management of patients with coronary artery disease. While high-risk pa-

tients demonstrate a survival benefit from CABG, low and moderate-risk patients have equivalent outcomes with respect to mortality with either approach (medical management or revascularization).[2] The exact definition of what constitutes appropriate medical therapy can be debated, but it would surely include aspirin, beta blockers, lipid-lowering agents and probably angiotensin-converting enzyme (ACE) inhibitors in diabetics or patients with impaired LV function.[42]

Since the degree and extent of ischemia predicts future events,[11] MPI has been used to assess the impact of medical management on the ischemic zones in patients with known coronary disease. In fact, Mahmarian et al.[43] demonstrated that quantitative exercise Tl-201 tomography is highly reproducible and can be used to accurately interpret temporal changes in myocardial perfusion in individual patients.

There are no data or recommendations regarding routine evaluation and follow-up with perfusion imaging of patients with CAD and known myocardial perfusion defects in the absence of symptoms. However, the beneficial impact of various pharmacologic interventions on the natural history of patients with CAD has been well established.[42] This has been linked with improvement in myocardial perfusion defects as a result of either decreased oxygen demand (beta blockers)[44-48] and/or improved coronary blood flow (nitrates, calcium channel blockers, statins).[49,50,51]

Beta Blockers

Among the antianginal medications, beta blockers markedly decrease the amount of exercise-induced ischemia in multiple studies[44-46] and may normalize the test.[46] The impact of 1-week treatment with propranolol on improving myocardial blood flow distribution has been established in men with CAD.[44] Similarly, the effect of acute administration of propranolol was examined in a small series of patients with known reversible perfusion defects who underwent dobutamine MPI.[47] The dobutamine stress test after propranolol was associated with a lower maximum heart rate (83 ± 18 vs. 125 ± 17, $p < 0.001$) and rate pressure product ($14,169 \pm 4,248$ vs. $19,894 \pm 3,985$, $p < 0.001$) despite a higher infusion dose. The SPECT myocardial ischemia score was also lower (6.9 ± 5.8 vs. 10.1 ± 7.1, $p = 0.047$).

Thus, existing data suggest that the antiischemic effect of beta blockers is primarily by decreasing the heart rate and myocardial oxygen demand. Improvement in myocardial ischemia was recorded as early as 1 week after oral treatment, and acutely with intravenous administration of beta blockers.

Calcium Channel Blockers and Nitrates

Although nitrates and calcium channel antagonists are not first-line agents in patients with coronary disease, they do have an impact on existing ischemia. Either in conjunction with beta blockers[48] or alone,[49-50] both of these agents decrease the size of reversible defects (particularly in patients with large ischemic perfusion defects), and appear to have a favorable impact on the deleterious prognostic effect of exercise-induced ischemia. Mahmarian et al.[50] evaluated prospectively whether short-term (6.1 ± 1.8 days) transdermal nitroglycerin patches could limit the extent of exercise-induced LV ischemia as assessed by quantitative Tl-201 tomography. Patients randomized to receive active patch therapy had a significant reduction in their total perfusion defect size ($-8.9 \pm 11.1\%$) compared with placebo-treated patients ($-1.8 \pm 6.1\%$, $p = 0.04$), which was most apparent in those with the largest ($\geq 20\%$) baseline perfusion defects ($-11.4 \pm 13.4\%$ vs. $1.0 \pm 3.6\%$, respectively, $p < 0.02$). Nitrate therapy did not significantly reduce heart rate, blood pressure, or double product, indicating benefit through enhancement of coronary blood flow.

Lipid-Lowering Agents

The impact of lipid-lowering agents in the secondary prevention of coronary disease has been demonstrated in multiple large studies (CARE,[52] 4S,[53] VA-HIT[54]). The mechanism is multifactorial and not solely based on reducing ischemia. Gould et al.[51] showed that there were statistically significant improvements in size and severity of perfusion abnormalities, by rest–dipyridamole positron emission tomography (PET), on comparison of baseline control with perfusion abnormalities after intensive 90-day cholesterol lowering. These results suggested that relatively short-term intensive cholesterol lowering improves myocardial perfusion capacity before anatomic regression of stenosis occurs. Such improvement can be followed noninvasively by dipyridamole PET, reflecting the integrated flow capacity of the entire coronary arterial/arteriolar vascular system affected by diffuse atherosclerosis. Other investigators[55] used SPECT imaging in patients with CAD and hypercholesterolemia, to assess serial changes in myocardial perfusion associated with cholesterol reduction therapy. Following improvement in total cholesterol (pretreatment: 223 ± 51, posttreatment: 147 ± 33, $p < 0.001$), the stress defect score (defined as % LV mass hypoperfused) was significantly improved (pretreatment: 19 ± 16, posttreatment: 9 ± 13, $p = 0.022$). Furthermore, the same investigators studied the effect of short-term (6 weeks) or long-term (6 months) pravastatin in dyslipidemic patients with baseline MPI ischemic defects.[56] Despite a significant reduction of low-density lipoprotein (LDL) at 6 weeks (33%, $p \ll 0.001$), myocardial perfusion scores were reduced only at 6 months (12.6 ± 5.7 at baseline, 9.4 ± 6.2 at 6 months, $p < 0.01$). The time course of reduced perfusion abnormalities paralleled documented clinical benefit[51-53] rather than LDL reduction. Whether stress MPI may identify effective clinical response to statin therapy and facilitate optimal medical and/or revascularization therapy needs to be determined by larger-scale trials in the fututre.[57]

Angiotensin-Converting Enzyme Inhibitors

There is growing evidence that ACE inhibitors exert a beneficial effect in patients with known coronary disease. Since the mechanism is complex (improved endothelial function, vasodilation and reduced afterload, antiplatelet effect, inhibition in neurohormonal activation), there is no large study to examine their direct anti-ischemic mechanism using MPI. In two studies, ACE inhibition was associated with improved epicardial[58] and microvascular blood flow,[59] predominantly endothelium mediated. Using ECG criteria, enalapril increased the timing to 0.1 mV ST-segment depression after 12 weeks of treatment (5.6 ± 1.9 min in the enalapril group vs. 4.4 ± 1.3 min in the placebo group, $p < 0.05$) without affecting the double product.[60] Further studies are needed to elucidate a direct anti-ischemic mechanism and explore the role of MPI in monitoring such an effect.

Lifestyle Modifications

The widespread interest in the noninvasive management of coronary atherosclerosis has brought new attention to the impact of various lifestyle changes on the prognosis of coronary disease. Diet, exercise, and behavioral interventions are generally advised on patients with documented coronary disease. The impact of these changes on the extent of atherosclerosis, as determined by angiography, is modest. However, the size and severity of perfusion abnormalities on rest–dipyridamole PET imaging in an experimental group was decreased (improved) compared to controls, after 5 years of intensive risk factor modification.[61]

CONCLUSIONS

The value of stress MPI has been well established in patients with CAD for both risk stratification and clinical decisions. A normal perfusion scan provides an excellent prognosis. Furthermore, identification and extent of ischemic zones provides information regarding the functional status of single or multiple lesions in patients who are being evaluated for intervention or titration of medical therapy. When coronary anatomy in known, MPI remains the test of choice for identifying the lesion responsible for the ischemic symptoms. After percutaneous coronary interventions, MPI can assist in the diagnosis of in-stent restenosis or establish a "new baseline" in certain high-risk individuals. Recent data suggest that SPECT imaging can be used to assess efficacy of medical treatment (particularly statins) of CAD. Whether this approach may identify individual clinical response to various pharmacologic interventions and facilitate optimal medical and/or revascularization therapy needs to be determined by larger-scale trials in the future.

REFERENCES

1. Gibbons RJ, Chatterjee K, Daley J, et al. ACC/AHA/ACP-ASIM guidelines for the management of patients with chronic stable angina: A report of the American College of Cardiology/American Heart Association Task Force on Practice Guidelines (Committee on Management of Patients with Chronic Stable Angina). *Circulation* 1999;99:2829–2848.
2. Solomon AJ, Gersh BJ. Management of chronic stable angina: Medical therapy, percutaneous transluminal coronary angioplasty, and coronary artery bypass surgery. Lessons from the randomized trials. *Ann Intern Med* 1998;128:216–223.

3. Yao SS, Rozanski A. Principal uses of myocardial perfusion scintigraphy in the management of patients with known or suspected coronary artery disease. *Prog Cardiovasc Dis.* 2001;43:281–302.

4. Heo J, Thompson WO, Iskandrian AS. Prognostic implications of normal exercise thallium images. *Am J Noninvas Cardiol* 1987;1:209–212.

5. Pavin D, Delonca J, Siegenthaler M, et al. Long-term (10 years) prognostic value of a normal thallium-201 myocardial exercise scintigraphy in patients with coronary artery disease documented by angiography. *Eur Heart J* 1997;18:69–77.

6. Raiker K, Sinusas AJ, Wackers FJT, et al. One-year prognosis of patients with normal planar or single-photon emission computed tomographic technetium 99m-labeled sestamibi exercise imaging. *J Nucl Cardiol* 1994;1:905–914.

7. National Center for Health Statistics. *Vital statistics of the United States, 1979: Vol II, Mortality, Part A.* Washington DC: U.S. Government Printing Office, DHHS Publication No. (PHS) 84-1101, 1984.

8. Brown KA, Rowen M. Prognostic value of a normal exercise myocardial perfusion imaging study in patients with angiographically significant coronary artery disease. *Am J Cardiol* 1993;71:865–867.

9. Schalet BD, Kegel JG, Heo J, et al. Prognostic implications of normal exercise SPECT thallium images in patients with strongly positive exercise electrocardiograms. *Am J Cardiol* 1993;72:1201–1203.

10. Ladenheim ML, Pollck BH, Rozanski A, et al. Extent and severity of myocardial hypoperfusion as predictors of prognosis in patients with suspected coronary disease. *J Am Coll Cardiol* 1986;7:464–471.

11. Brown K. Prognostic value of myocardial perfusion imaging: State of the art and new developments. *J Nucl Cardiol* 1996;3:516–537.

12. McClellan J, Travin M, Herman S, et al. Prognostic importance of scintigraphic left ventricular cavity dilatation during intravenous dipyridamole technetium-99m sestamibi myocardial tomographic imaging in predicting coronary events. *Am J Cardiol* 1997;79:600–605.

13. Gill JB, Ruddy TD, Newell JB, et al. Prognostic importance of thallium uptake by the lungs during exercise in coronary artery disease. *N Engl J Med* 1987;317:1485–1489.

14. Acampa W, Cuocolo A, Sullo P, et al. Direct comparison of technetium 99m-sestamibi and technetium 99m-tetrofosmin cardiac single photon emission computed tomography in patients with coronary artery disease. *J Nucl Cardiol* 1998;5:265–274.

15. Bavelaar-Croon C, Pauwels E, Van Der Wall E. Gated single-photon emission computed tomographic myocardial imaging: A new tool in clinical cardiology. *Am Heart J* 2001;141:383–390.

16. Borges-Neto S, Shaw L. The added value of simultaneous myocardial perfusion and left ventricular function. *Curr Opin Cardiol* 1999;14:460–463.

17. Sharir T, Germano G, Kavanagh PB, et al. Incremental prognostic value of post-stress left ventricular ejection fraction and volume by gated myocardial perfusion single photon emission computed tomography. *Circulation* 1999;100:1035–1042.

18. Gibbons RJ, Balady GJ, Beasley JW, et al. ACC/AHA Guidelines for exercise testing: A report of the American College of Cardiology/American Heart Association Task Force on Practice Guidelines (Committee on Exercise Testing). *J Am Coll Cardiol* 1997;30:260–315.

19. Lee T, Boucher C. Noninvasive tests in patients with stable coronary artery disease. *N Engl J Med* 2001;344:1840–1845.

20. Vanzetto G., Halimi S., et al. Prediction of cardiovascular events in clinically selected high-risk NIDDM patients. *Diab Care* 1999; 22: 19–26.

21. Hecht HS, Shaw RE, Chin HL, et al. Silent ischemia after coronary angioplasty: Evaluation of restenosis and extent of ischemia in asymptomatic patients by tomographic thallium-201 exercise imaging and comparison with symptomatic patients. *J Am Coll Cardiol* 1991;17:670–677.

22. Palmas W, Bingham S, Diamond GA, et al. Incremental prognostic value of exercise thallium-201 myocardial single photon emission computed tomography late after coronary bypass surgery. *J Am Coll Cardiol* 1995;25:403–409.

23. Lee T, Boucher C. Noninvasive tests in patients with stable coronary artery disease. *N Engl J Med* 2001;344:1840–1845.

24. Rithie J, Bateman T, Bonow R, et al. ACC/AHA Guidelines for clinical use of cardiac radionuclide imaging: Report of the American College of Cardiology/American Heart Association Task Force on Assessment of Diagnostic and Theurapeutic Cardiovascular Procedures (Committee on Radionuclide Imaging), developed in collaboration with the American Society of Nuclear Cardiology. *J Am Coll Cardiol* 1995;25:521–547.

25. Gibbons R. Follow-up testing: The beginning of an answer (Editorial). *J Nucl Cardiol* 2001;8:520–522.

26. Berman D, Xinping K, Schisterma E, et al. Serial changes on quantitative myocardial perfusion SPECT in patients undergoing revascularization or conservative therapy. *J Nucl Cardiol* 2001;8:428–437.

27. Beller GA, Zaret BL. Contributions of nuclear cardiology to diagnosis and prognosis of patients with coronary artery disease. *Circulation* 2000; 101:1465–1478.

28. Travin MI, Katz MS, Moulton AW, et al. Accuracy of dipyridamole SPECT imaging in identifying individual coronary stenosis and multivessel disease in women versus men. *J Nucl Cardiol* 2000;7:213–220.

29. Maseri A. The variable chronic atherosclerotic background.. In: Maseri A. *Ischemic Heart Disease*. New York, NY: Churchill Livingstone, 1995:193–235.

30. Smith SC, Jr., Dove JT, Jacobs AK, et al. ACC/AHA guidelines for percutaneous coronary intervention: Executive summary and recommendations: A report of the American College of Cardiology/American Heart Association Task Force on Practice Guidelines (Committee to Revise the 1993 Guidelines for Percutaneous Transluminal Coronary Angioplasty). *J Am Coll Cardiol* 2001;37:2215–2238.

31. Gibbons RS. American Society of Nuclear Cardiology project on myocardial perfusion imaging: Measuring outcomes in response to emerging guidelines (Editorial). *J Nucl Cardiol* 1996;3:436–442.

32. Topol EJ, Ellis SG, Delos M, et al. Analysis of coronary PTCA practice in the United States with an insurance-claims data base. *Circulation* 1993;87:1489–1497.

33. Pitt B, Waters D, Brown WV, et al. for the Atorvastatin versus Revascularization Treatment Investigators. Aggressive lipid lowering therapy compared with angioplasty in stable coronary artery disease. *N Engl J Med* 1999;341:70–76.

34. American Heart Association. *2000 Heart and Stroke Statistical Update*. Dallas, TX: American Heart Association, 1999.

35. Palmas W, Bingham S, Diamond GA, et al. Incremental prognostic value of exercise thallium-201 myocardial SPECT late after coronary artery bypass surgery. *J Am Coll Cardiol* 1995;25:403–409.

36. Zellweger M, Lewin H, Shengham L, et al. When to stress patients after coronary artery bypass surgery? *J Am Coll Cardiol* 2001;37:144–152.

37. Hecht HS, Shaw RE, Bruce RT, et al. Usefulness of tomographic thallium-201 imaging for detection of restenosis after percutaneous transluminal angioplasty. *Am J Cardiol* 1990;66:1314–1318.

38. Iskandrian AS, Lemick J, Ogilby JD, et al. Early thallium imaging after percutaneous transluminal coronary angioplasty: Tomographic evaluation during adenosine induced coronary hyperemia. *J Nucl Cardiol* 1992;33:2086–2089.

39. Maryani DE, Knudtson M, Kloiber R, et al. Sequential thallium-201 myocardial perfusion studies after successful percutaneous transluminal coronary angioplasty: Delayed resolution of exercise-induced scintigraphic abnormalities. *Circulation* 1988;77:86–95.

40. Mak K-H, Belli G, Ellis SG et al. Subacute stent thrombosis: evolving issues and current concepts. *J Am Coll Cardiol* 1996;27:494–503.

41. Baim D, Levine MJ, Leon MB, et al. Management of restenosis within the Palmaz–Schatz coronary stent (the U.S. multicenter experience: the U.S. Palmaz–Schatz Stent investigators). *Am J Cardiol* 1993;71:364–366.

42. Blumenthal R, Gregory C, Schulman S. Medical therapy versus coronary angioplasty in stable coronary artery disease: A critical review of the literature. *J Am Coll Cardiol* 2000;36:668–673.

43. Mahmarian J, Moye L, Verani M, et al. High reproducibility of myocardial perfusion defects in patients undergoing serial exercise thallium-201 tomography. *Am J Cardiol* 1995;75:1116–1119.

44. Rainwater J, Steele P, Kirch D, et al. Effect of propranolol on myocardial perfusion images and exercise ejection fraction in men with coronary artery disease. *Circulation* 1982;65:77–81.

45. Steele P, Sklar J, Kirch D et al. Thallium-201 myocardial imaging during maximal and submaximal exercise: Comparison of submaximal exercise with propranolol. *Am Heart J* 1983;106:1353–1357.

46. Hockings B, Saltissi S, Croft DN, et al. Effect of beta adrenergic blockade on thallium-201 myocardial perfusion imaging. *Br Heart J* 1983;49:83–89.

47. Shehata A, Gillam L, Mascitelli V, et al. Impact of acute propranolol administration on dobutamine-induced myocardial ischemia as evaluated by myocardial perfusion imaging and echocardiography. *Am J Cardiol* 1997;80:268–272.

48. Marie P, Danchin N, Branly F, et al. Effects of medical therapy on outcome assessment using exercise thallium-201 SPECT imaging. *J Am Coll Cardiol* 1999;34:113–121.

49. Stegaru B, Loose R, Keller H, et al. Effects of long-term treatment with 120 mg of sustained-release isosorbite dinitrate and 60 mg of sustained-release nifedipine on myocardial perfusion. *Am J Cardiol* 1988;61:74E–77E.

50. Mahmarian J, Fenimore N, Marks G, et al. Transdermal nitroglycerin patch therapy reduces the extent of exercise-induced myocardial ischemia: Results of a double-blind, placebo-controlled trial using quantitative thallium-201 tomography. *J Am Coll Cardiol* 1994;24:25–32.

51. Gould L, Martucci J, Goldberg D, et al. Short-term cholesterol lowering decreases size and severity of perfusion abnormalities by positron emission tomography after dipyridamole in patients with coronary artery disease. *Circulation* 1994;89:1530–1538.

52. Flaker G, Warnica W, Sack F, et al. Pravastatin prevents clinical events in revascularized patients with average cholesterol concentrations. *J Am Coll Cardiol* 1999;34:106–112.

53. Scandinavian Simvastatin Survival Group. Randomized trial of cholesterol lowering in 4444 patients with coronary heart disease. *Lancet* 1994;344:1383–1389.

54. Rubins HB, Robins SJ, Collins D, et al. Gemfibrozil for the secondary prevention of coronary heart disease in men with low levels of high density lipoprotein cholesterol. *N Engl J Med* 1999;341:410–418.

55. Schwartz RG, Kalaria V, Mackin M, et al. Serial quantitative single photon emission computed

tomography monitors improved myocardial perfusion accompanying cholesterol reduction therapy (Abs). *Circulation* 1998;98(Suppl):I-95.

56. Schwartz RG, Pearson T, Williford M, et al. Pravastatin improves stress induced radionuclide myocardial perfusion abnormalities by six months: Coronary artery disease regression SPECT monitoring trial. *J Am Coll Cardiol* 2001;37(Suppl A):424A.

57. Schwartz, RG, Pearson T. Can single photon emission tomography myocardial perfusion imaging monitor the potential benefit of aggressive treatment of hyperlipidemia? *J Nucl Cardiol* 1997;6:555–568.

58. Prasad A, Husain S, Quyyumi A, et al. Abnormal flow-mediated epicardial vasomotion in human coronary arteries is improved by angiotensin-converting enzyme inhibition. *J Am Coll Cardiol* 1999;33:796–804.

59. Schlaifer J, Wargovich T, O'Neil B, et al. Effects of quinapril on coronary blood flow in coronary artery disease patients with endothelial dysfunction. *Am J Cardiol* 1997;80:1594–1597.

60. Van Den Heuvel A, Dunselman P, Kingma T, et al. Reduction of exercise-induced myocardial ischemia during add on treatment with the angiotensin-converting enzyme inhibitor enalapril in patients with normal left ventricular function and optimal beta blockade. *J Am Coll Cardiol* 2001;37:470–474.

61. Gould L, Ornish D, Scherwitz L et al. Changes in myocardial perfusion abnormalities by positron emission tomography after long-term, intense risk factor modification. *JAMA* 1995;274:894–901.

CHAPTER 3

Preoperative Risk Assessment for Noncardiac Surgery

Ahmad Salloum
Gary V. Heller

INTRODUCTION

Background

More than 25 million patients undergo noncardiac surgery in the United States each year. Of these patients, 1 million have diagnosed coronary artery disease (CAD), 2 to 3 million have multiple risk factors for CAD, and 4 million are older than 65 years of age.[1] These patients account for about 80% of the 1 million persons in whom surgery is complicated by perioperative cardiac morbidity and mortality. The associated hospital costs exceed $12 billion annually.[2] Thus, physicians seek ways to identify higher-risk patients prior to surgery in order to reduce perioperative events and costs. An American College of Cardiology/American Hospital Association (ACC/AHA) task force committee developed an extensive discussion about perioperative assessment in 2002.[3] This chapter provides an updated and concise data-driven approach to periopera-

tive assessment, the role of nuclear imaging, and the management of patients once perioperative cardiac risk stratification for is completed.

Goals of Preoperative Evaluation

As a physician evaluates a patient prior to noncardiac surgery, several goals should be kept in mind:

1. Identify the risk of the proposed surgery (Table 3-1).
2. Identify the cohort of patients that are at risk for perioperative cardiac events.
3. Identify patients at risk to develop cardiac events after discharge from the hospital.
4. Develop strategies to decrease risk for short- and long-term events.
5. Follow-up with the patient postoperatively, when most perioperative cardiac events occur.

Table 3-1
Surgery-Specific Cardiac Risk

High-Risk Surgery (reported cardiac risk > 5%)

Emergent major operation (particularly in the elderly)

Aortic and other major vascular

Peripheral vascular

Anticipated prolonged surgical procedures associated with large fluid shifts and/or blood loss

Intermediate-Risk Surgery (reported risk < 5%)

Carotid endarterectomy

Head and neck

Intraperitoneal and intrathoracic

Orthopedic

Prostate

Low-Risk Surgery (reported risk < 1%)

Endoscopic procedures

Superficial procedures

Cataract

Breast

Potential Outcomes of Preoperative Evaluation

1. Modify or cancel the planned procedure.
2. Intervene to reduce perioperative morbidity and mortality.
3. Intervene to reduce long-term cardiovascular morbidity and mortality.

CLINICAL EVALUATION

History (Signs and Symptoms)

The preoperative evaluation begins with a thorough history with special emphasis on the need to identify clinical markers that increase perioperative risk as well as assess functional capacity:

1. Identify clinical markers that increase perioperative risk (refer to criteria for estimating risk). Several different methods to assess risk are discussed below:
   a. Using multivariate analysis, Goldman

et al.[4] identified nine independent predictors of perioperative cardiac events (Table 3-2). Patients in risk class I (0–5 points) had a 0.9% incidence of cardiac death or life-threatening cardiac complications. With increasing class, the complication rate increased incrementally. Class IV patients (> 26 points) had a complication rate of 78%.

Table 3-2
The Goldman Multifactorial Cardiac Risk Index

Criterion	Points, n
History	
Age > 70 years	5
Myocardial infarction in the previous 6 months	10
Physical Examination	
S_3 gallop or jugular venous distention	11
Important aortic valvular stenosis	3
Electrocardiography Results	
Rhythm other than sinus or premature atrial contractions on last preoperative electrocardiography	7
5 premature ventricular contractions per minute documented at any time before surgery	7
General Status	
PO_2 < 60 mm Hg, potassium level < 3.0 mEq/L or bicarbonate level < 20 mEq/L, blood urea nitrogen > 50 or creatinine concentration > 3.0 mg/dL, abnormal serum glutamic-oxaloacetic transaminase, signs of chronic liver disease, or bedridden from noncardiac causes	3
Surgery	
Intraperitoneal, intrathoracic, or aortic surgery	3
Emergency surgery	4
Total	53

Reprinted from Goldman et al.[4] with permission.

b. The applicability of the Goldman risk index for more specific patient subsets and types of surgery has been questioned. Gerson et al.[5] evaluated the predictive value of patient history, physical examination, and rest and exercise radionuclide ventriculography to risk stratify 155 geriatric patients presenting for nonemergency abdominal, thoracic, or aortic surgery. The Goldman risk index was also calculated for each patient. Inability to bicycle 2 minutes to a heart rate > 99 beats per minute was the only significant predictor of a cardiac event.

c. Detsky et al.[6] modified the Goldman's criteria; that is, angina was classified, proximity of the congestive heart failure (CHF) episode to the surgical procedure was added, and the scoring was simplified (Table 3-3). These indices were prospectively validated. However, the Detsky modified risk index was never externally validated. Furthermore, confounding clinical problems and events not included in the risk index may influence the management of individual patients.

d. Eagle et al.[7–8] identified several clinical variables that classified patients into low-, intermediate-, or high-risk categories. These clinical predictors include Q wave on preoperative electrocardiogram (ECG), history of angina, history of ventricular ectopy requiring treatment, diabetes requiring pharmacologic therapy, and age older than 70 years. Analyzing 200 consecutive patients referred for vascular surgery, Eagle et al. identified 64 patients with none of these five clinical predictors (low risk), and only 2 patients (3.1%) experienced postoperative ischemic events. On the other hand, 10 of 20 patients (50%) classified as high risk by having three

Table 3-3

The Modified Multifactorial Cardiac Risk Index

Criterion	Points, n
Coronary Artery Disease	
MI within 6 months	10
MI > 6 months	5
Canadian Heart Association angina	
Class 3	10
Class 4	20
Unstable angina within 3 months	10
Alveolar Pulmonary Edema	
Within 1 week	10
Ever	5
Valvular Disease	
Suspected critical aortic stenosis	20
Arrhythmias	
Sinus plus premature atrial beats or rhythm other than sinus on last preoperative electrocardiography	5
> 5 premature ventricular depolarizations at any time before surgery	5
Poor General Status	
$PO_2 < 60$ mm Hg, $PCO_2 > 50$ mm Hg: potassium level < 3.0 mEq/L or bicarbonate level < 20 mEq/L, blood urea nitrogen ≥ 18 or creatinine concentration > 260 mmol/L; abnormal serum aspartate aminotransferase level, signs of chronic liver disease, or bedridden from noncardiac causes	5
Age older than 70 years	5
Emergency surgery	10

Reprinted from Detsky AS, et al. *J Gen Intern Med* 1986;1:211–219.

or more clinical predictors experienced postoperative ischemic events. Patients with either one or two clinical predictors had an intermediate risk, with 18 ischemic events in 116 patients (15.5%). These findings stimulated investigations to further risk stratify the intermediate-risk group by noninvasive testing.

e. The ACC/AHA task force[3] summarized the available data and classified them according to each variable importance as high-, intermediate-, or low-risk (Table 3-4). This is the most complete approach to assessment based on clinical variables. Identifying a patient's clinical risk and the surgical risk would then lead to whether the patient need further risk assessment with noninvasive or invasive testing.

2. Assess functional capacity (Table 3-5). Poor functional capacity in patients with known CAD or prior myocardial infarction (MI) is associated with an increased risk of subsequent cardiac events.[9] Therefore, multiple investigators studied the importance of functional capacity assessment for preoperative risk stratification.

Carliner et al.[10] prospectively evaluated preoperative exercise testing results in 200 consecutive patients with a mean age of 59 years scheduled for major noncardiac surgery (52% abdominal, 34% vascular, and 14% thoracic). Six patients (3%) had myocardial infarction. However, five of the six had limited maximal exercise capacity of < 5 metabolic equivalents (METs).

Cutler et al.[11] reviewed the results of preoperative treadmill exercise testing in 130 patients who underwent peripheral vascular surgery. Patients who achieved > 75% of MPHR (maximum predicted heart rate) with no ischemia on ECG were at low risk (0 events in 35 patients). In contrast, patients who had ischemia with MPHR < 75% were at high risk (10 events in 26 patients). The intermediate-risk group (6 events in 23 patients) comprised those with ischemia with MPHR of > 75% MPHR.

These and other studies suggest that poor functional status identifies patients at high risk for perioperative complications. Therefore, it is

Table 3-4

Clinical Markers of Increased Perioperative Cardiovascular Risk (MI, CHF, and Death)

Major Predictors

Unstable coronary syndrome

> Recent[a] MI with evidence of important ischemic risk on the basis of clinical symptoms or results of noninvasive studies
>
> Unstable or severe angina[b] (Canadian class 3 or 4)[c]

Decompensated CHF

Marked arrhythmias

> High-grade atrioventricular block
>
> Symptomatic ventricular in the presence of underlying heart disease
>
> Supraventricular arrhythmias with uncontrolled ventricular rate

Severe valvular disease

Intermediate Predictors

Mild angina (Canadian class 3 or 4)

Prior MI (from history or Q waves on ECG)

Prior or compensated CHF

DM

Renal Insufficiency (creatinine ≥ 2.0 mg/dL)

Minor Predictors

Advanced age

Abnormal ECG findings (left ventricular hypertrophy, left bundle branch block, ST-T abnormalities)

Rhythm other than sinus (e.g., atrial fibrillation)

Low functional capacity (< 4 METs)

History of stroke

Uncontrolled hypertension

---

[a] The American College of Cardiology National Database Library defines recent myocardial infarction as having occurred 7 to 30 days before coming to medical attention.
[b] May include stable angina among patients who are usually sedentary.
[c] Campeau L. Grading of angina pectoris. *Circulation* 1976;54:522–523.

Table 3-5
Estimated Energy Requirements
for Various Activities

1 MET

Eat, dress, or use the toilet

Walk indoors around the house

Walk on level ground at 2 mph (3.2 km/hr)

Do light housework such as washing dishes

4 METs

Climb a flight of stairs

Walk on level ground at 4 mph (6.4 km/hr)

Run a short distance

Heavy work such as vacuuming or lifting heavy furniture

Play sports such as golf or double tennis

> 10 METs

Participate in strenuous activities such as swimming, singles tennis, basketball, or skiing

MET = metabolic equivalent.

extremely important to determine the patient's maximal activity during daily activities and assess his or her functional capacity (Table 3-5). This also could be assessed by treadmill exercise stress testing. Patients with poor functional capacity may require further evaluation, including myocardial perfusion testing in multiple clinical situations as detailed later in this chapter.

Physical Examination

Emphasis should be placed on identifying evidence of disease states that might impact on perioperative events, such as severe aortic stenosis, other severe valvular diseases, decompensated heart failure, unstable coronary syndromes, diabetes mellitus, and peripheral vascular disease.

USE OF MYOCARDIAL PERFUSION IMAGING

Thus far, this chapter has dealt with perioperative risk assessment using primarily clinical data and exercise capacity. Despite the value of this information, it has been recognized that further data may be beneficial in selected patients. Landmark studies demonstrated that stress myocardial perfusion imaging (MPI) could stratify patients into low- or high-risk groups. This risk stratification is helpful for both short term (perioperative) and long-term prediction of cardiac events.

Short-Term Prognosis (Perioperative Period)

Clinical variables can define a low-risk group for whom no further testing may be needed and a high-risk group that may need further assessment with the intention for revascularization and/or intensive medical therapy. However, for the majority of the patients in the intermediate-risk group, further assessment with noninvasive testing would be needed. Nuclear imaging has emerged as a useful tool to risk stratify patients undergoing major noncardiac surgeries.

In studies by Eagle et al.,[7-8] both low- and high-risk patients were identified by clinical variables. However, the intermediate-risk group had a 15.5% likelihood of developing perioperative cardiac complication. This group was further classified by dipyridamole thallium into patients with no redistribution (no ischemia) who had a 3.2% perioperative event rate. In contrast, patients with thallium redistribution (evidence of ischemia) had a 29.6% event rate (Figure 3-1). This effectively reclassified the intermediate-risk group into either a low- or a high-risk group.

Further evidence to support selective use of preoperative dipyridamole thallium comes from L'Italien et al.[12] In a multicenter study, they developed a prediction model in 567 patients on the basis of clinical variables (age > 70 years, angina, history of MI, diabetes mellitus, history of CHF, and prior revascularization). A second model was developed from dipyridamole thallium imaging. Model performance, alone and in combination, was evaluated with receiver operating curve (ROC) analysis. The models were then validated in a separate cohort of 514 patients. The observed and predicted cardiac event rates

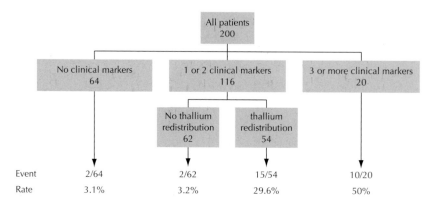

Figure 3-1.   Clinical markers of risk and thallium redistribution. (Reprinted from Eagle KA et al.[7] with permission.)

were similar for both patient sets. The addition of dipyridamole thallium data reclassified more than 80% of the intermediate-risk patients into low-risk (3% event rate) and high-risk (19% event rate) categories. However, it provided no further stratification for patients previously classified as low risk or high risk by the clinical model. In conclusion, clinical markers reliably stratify risk in patients undergoing vascular surgery, and the selective use of myocardial imaging provides additional risk stratification in patients classified as intermediate risk.

The presence of ischemia on MPI identifies patients at higher risk, as noted earlier. The extent of ischemia can further classify this group of patient. Shaw et al.[13] performed a meta-analysis of 15 studies, including peer-reviewed English publications that have available cardiac event rates after vascular surgery. The cardiac events were classified by noninvasive imaging, and these studies were identified by a Medline database search (1985–1994). Ten studies using dipyridamole thallium were identified. A total of 1,994 patients were included. The perioperative event rates (death or MI) were 3% for patients with normal results, 7% for patients with fixed defects, and 9% for patients with reversible defects. Dipyridamole-induced ECG ST-segment depression occurred in 7% of patients and was associated with a cardiac event (death or MI) in 14% of

patients. Furthermore, higher event rates were associated with larger perfusion defects. The event rate was 14% in patients with one or more reversible defects versus 30% in patients with two or more reversible defects. Therefore, patients with larger perfusion defects or evidence of three-vessel ischemia have a worse prognosis.

The predictive value of thallium redistribution for MI or death ranged from 4% to 20% in reports that were selected in the ACC/AHA task force report on preoperative testing.[3] The positive predictive value has decreased over time for thallium redistribution. This has been attributed to appropriate use of thallium redistribution information to guide therapeutic interventions, such as intensive medical therapy or coronary revascularization. Moreover, the results of thallium testing may lead to the performance of less extensive procedures or even cancellation of surgery.[3] Nonetheless, the negative predictive value is very high (approximately 99%), and the prognosis associated with a normal scan is excellent (3). Thus, the physician can feel quite comfortable proceeding with the anticipated surgical procedure with a normal stress MPI.

Historically, most preoperative studies were completed using thalium-201 as the imaging agent. Fewer data are available with technetium-99m (Tc-99m) agents, which are commonly used in laboratories today. Stratmann et al. reported on the value of dipyridamole Tc-99m sestamibi scintigraphy in 285 consecutive patients being considered for major and minor nonvascular surgery[14] and in 229 consecutive patients being considered for vascular surgery.[15] In the first study, 140 major and 89 minor procedures were performed within 4 months of nuclear imaging.[14] Perioperative cardiac events include unstable angina, ischemic pulmonary edema, nonfatal MI, or cardiac death. Twelve events (4%) occurred in the whole cohort with 1/89 minor procedure and 11/140 major procedures. Perioperative cardiac events occurred in 4% of patients with a normal study, 24% with evidence of ischemia, and 37% with a fixed defect. In the second study by Stratmann et al., vascular surgery was performed on 197 patients within 3 months of dipyridamole Tc-99m sestamibi scintigraphy.[15] Only nine events (5%) occurred in this cohort. The event rate was 3% in patients with a normal scan, 5% with an abnormal scan, and 6% with evidence of ischemia. Similar perioperative risk was reported in the group of patients who were identified to have ischemia and had intensive medical therapy or revascularization in comparison to those who had no ischemia. Thus, preoperative evaluation appears equally effective using Tc-99m sestamibi or thallium-201 (Tl-201).

Long-Term Prognosis

It is well recognized that stress has considerable value in predicting cardiac events over a 2- to 3-year period in patients assessed for known or suspected CAD.[16] This is further extended to patients undergoing surgical procedures. Hendel et al. evaluated 360 patients, of whom 327 underwent vascular surgery. A cardiac event (cardiac death or MI) occurred in 14.4% of patients who had transient thallium defects and only in 1% of patients with a normal result.[17] Patients were followed for 31 months after surgery. The late cardiac event rate was 4.9% in those with a normal dipyridamole thallium scan compared with 24% in patients with a fixed perfusion defect. Cox regression analysis showed a fixed perfusion defect on thallium to be the most powerful predictor of

late events and increased the relative risk fivefold. A history of CHF was the only significant clinical variable that contributed additional value to that of a fixed defect alone.

This was further evaluated by the meta-analysis performed by Shaw et al.[13] Late cardiac event rates were largely comparable in patients with fixed or reversible defects, with approximately one third of patients with either defect pattern experiencing a cardiac event 2 to 3 years after vascular surgery. Therefore, it appears that whereas short-term morbidity and mortality may be much greater in patients with a reversible defect, differences in long-term cardiac event rates are indistinguishable between a fixed or reversible thallium defect.[13] This argues toward intensive medical therapy, risk modification, and close follow-up of these patients who have evidence of CAD, whether it is manifested as ischemia or prior MI.

USE OF DOBUTAMINE ECHOCARDIOGRAPHY

Dobutamine echocardiography is also a useful tool for preoperative risk assessment, although fewer data are available in comparison with MPI. In the meta-analysis by Shaw et al., a total of 445 patients were analyzed. Of 173 patients with a dobutamine-induced new or worsening wall motion response, 40 (23%) had a perioperative ischemic event compared with 1 (0.37%) of 270 patients with a normal stress echocardiographic response.[13] The positive predictive value of testing was 13% for cardiac death or MI and 26% for any cardiac event. The negative predictive value of a normal dobutamine echocardiographic response was 99%. The long-term (1 year) cardiac event rate was 2.9% for 69 patients with normal and 15% for 20 patients with abnormal stress echocardiographic result.[13] Summary odds ratios were greater for dobutamine echocardiography (14 to 27) than for dipyridamole thallium (3.7 to 4.0). The wider confidence intervals for dobutamine echocardiography were secondary to smaller sample sizes.[13] The probability of a cardiac event was 13% (95% CI of 7–19%) for dipyridamole thallium imaging and 25% (95% CI of 16–33%) for dobutamine echocardiography.

These data suggest that preoperative evaluation with dobutamine echocardiography is useful when performed by experienced individuals. However, many laboratories do not have the efficiency or skills to perform this test. Furthermore, reproducibility of myocardial perfusion imaging is clearly demonstrated.[18]

WHO SHOULD GET NUCLEAR PERFUSION IMAGING PREOPERATIVELY?

On the basis of current knowledge and the ACC/AHA guidelines,[3] a shortcut approach to noninvasive testing is recommended if two of the three listed factors are true (Table 3-6):

Table 3-6

Shortcut to Noninvasive Testing in Preoperative Patients if Any Two Factors Are Present

---

1. Intermediate clinical predictors are present (Canadian class 1 or 2 angina, prior MI based on history or pathologic Q waves, compensated or prior heart failure, or diabetes)

2. Poor functional capacity (less than 4 METs)

3. High surgical risk procedure (emergency major operations[a]; aortic repair or peripheral vascular surgery; prolonged surgical procedures with large fluid shifts or blood loss)

---

[a] Emergency major operations may require immediately proceeding to surgery without sufficient time for noninvasive testing or preoperative interventions.
HF = heart failure; METs = metabolic equivalents; MI = myocardial infarction.
Modified with permission from: Leppo JA, Dahlberg ST. The question: to test or not to test in preoperative cardiac risk evaluation. *J Nucl Cardiol* 1998;5:332–342. Copyright © 1998 by the American Society of Nuclear Cardiology. This material may not be reproduced, stored in a retrieval system, or transmitted in any form or by any means without the prior permission of the publisher.

WHICH TEST TO ORDER?

The expertise of the local laboratory in identifying advanced coronary disease is probably more important than the particular type of test. Figure 3-2 illustrates an algorithm to help the clinician choose the most appropriate stress test in those various situations.[3]

WHO SHOULD GET CARDIAC ANGIOGRAPHY PREOPERATIVELY?

On the basis of the ACC/AHA guidelines,[3] the indications for coronary angiography are similar to those identified for the nonoperative setting. The following recommendations provide a summary of class I indications for preoperative coronary angiography in patients being evaluated before noncardiac surgery:

1. Evidence for high-risk of adverse outcome based on noninvasive test results

2. Angina unresponsive to medical therapy

3. Unstable angina, particularly when facing intermediate-risk or high-risk surgery

4. Equivocal noninvasive test results in patients at high clinical risk undergoing high-risk surgery

For a complete list including class II and III indications for preoperative coronary angiography in patients being evaluated before noncardiac surgery, please refer to the guidelines.[3] In summary, coronary angiography should be performed in the appropriate clinical context on the basis of noninvasive test results that indicate large zones of ischemia and should not be performed for limited ischemia without other significant clinical findings.

ACC/AHA GUIDELINES STEPWISE APPROACH

On the basis of current knowledge, the ACC/AHA taskforce developed guidelines for cardiac evaluation before noncardiac surgery. A general

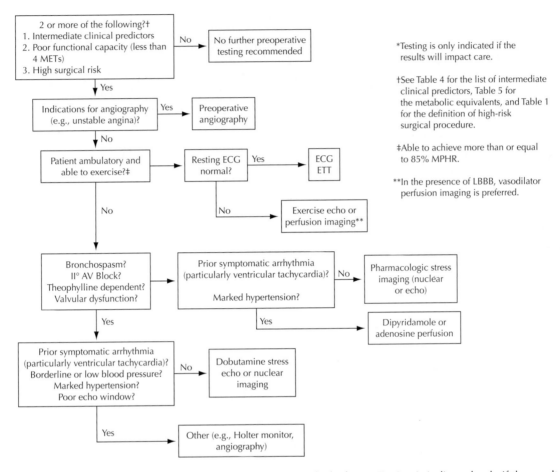

Figure 3-2. Supplemental preoperative evaluation: when and which test. Testing is indicated only if the results will impact care.

strategy for preoperative cardiac risk assessment is summarized in Figure 3-3. A stepwise approach to risk stratification includes the following[3]:

1. Determine the urgency of noncardiac surgery. Preoperative risk assessment may be inappropriate for patients who must undergo emergency surgery.

2. Determine whether the patient has undergone coronary revascularization in the past 5 years. Previous coronary revascularization probably reduces cardiac risk of noncardiac surgery, and if the patient remained with no recurrent

symptoms or signs, there is no need for preoperative noninvasive testing.

3. Determine whether the patient had an adequate, favorable cardiac evaluation in the past 2 years. If there have been no new intercurrent symptoms, repeated testing is not necessary.

4. Determine whether the patient has an unstable coronary syndrome or a major clinical predictor of risk, which usually leads to cancellation or delay of surgery until the problem has been diagnosed and treated.

5. Determine whether the patient has inter-

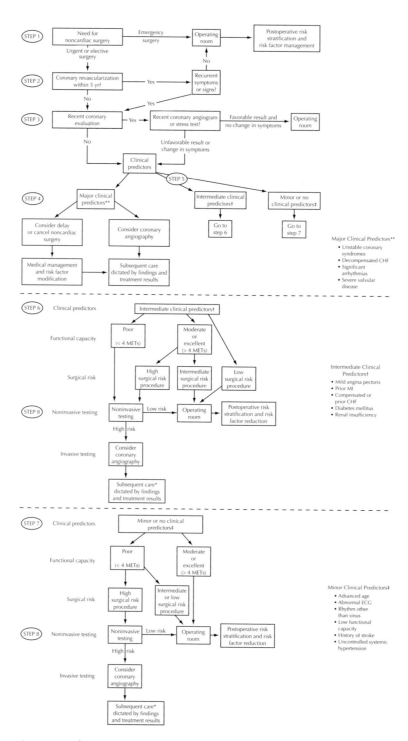

Figure 3-3. Stepwise approach to preoperative cardiac assessment. (Reprinted from Eagle KA, et al.[3] with permission.)

mediate clinical predictors of risk. If so, consider the patient's functional capacity and the surgery-specific risk.

6. Patients with intermediate predictors of cardiac risk and at least moderate functional capacity can generally undergo intermediate-risk surgery with a low probability of perioperative MI or death. On the other hand, patients with poor functional capacity (inability to exercise four METs) or who have multiple markers of risk and who are undergoing higher-risk surgery should undergo noninvasive evaluation to further stratify their risk (see Table 3-6). If the anticipated risk of surgery is high and results of noninvasive testing suggest significant CAD, coronary angiography with the intention to perform coronary revascularization given suitable coronary anatomy should be considered.

7. Cardiac catheterization should be performed for in the appropriate clinical context on the basis of noninvasive test results that indicate large zones of ischemia and should not be performed for patients with limited ischemia without other significant clinical findings.

8. Noncardiac surgery is generally safe for patients with neither major nor intermediate predictors of clinical risk and at least moderate functional capacity.

9. Use results of preoperative evaluation, including noninvasive testing in selected patients, to determine further perioperative management.

10. Use information gained during preoperative evaluation and careful postoperative surveillance to tailor long-term therapy and follow-up.

UTILIZING DECISION ANALYSIS AND COST EFFECTIVENESS METHODOLOGIES

Investigations using decision analysis and cost-effectiveness methodologies have primarily evalu-

ated management strategies involving MPI and coronary angiography in patients undergoing vascular surgery.[19] These studies indicate that selective screening should be performed only in patients with intermediate risk for CAD when the expected risk for surgical death is greater that about 5%.[19] In addition, the expected risk for coronary revascularization should be low ($\leq$ 2–3%). With a selective approach to screening and revascularization, the cost per year of life saved is approximately $20,000.[19] This figure depends on the pretest likelihood of disease and the perioperative risk of an event. With less pretest likelihood of disease, the cost per life saved would be much higher. Although $20,000 is a favorable amount, constantly improving surgical and anesthetic techniques are decreasing the cost-effectiveness of preoperative CAD screening.[19]

RISK REDUCTION

Use of Beta Blockers

Recently, considerable interest has been shown in the medical therapy that might reduce the perioperative cardiac event rate, particularly with beta blockers. Poldermans et al. performed a randomized multicenter trial to assess the effects of perioperative blockade of beta-adrenergic receptors in high-risk patients on the incidence of cardiac death and nonfatal MI within 30 days after major vascular surgery.[22] Of 1,351 patients screened, 846 were found to have one or more of the following cardiac risk factors: age over 70 years, limited exercise capacity, or any of the intermediate-risk predictors (Figure 3-4). Any patient with at least one of these risk factors underwent dobutamine echocardiography. Patients were excluded if they had extensive wall motion abnormalities on dobutamine echocardiography or those with strong evidence during stress testing of left main or three-vessel CAD. A total of 173 of 846 patients (20%) had stress-induced ischemia on dobutamine echocardiography. Of these, 112 patients underwent randomization to a beta-blocking agent (bisoprolol) or no beta-blocking agent. In the bisoprolol group, biso-

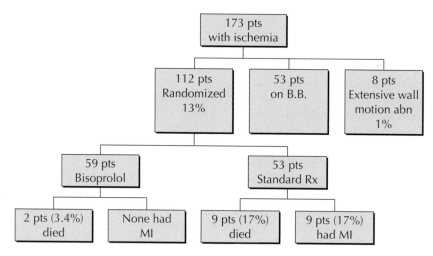

Figure 3-4.   Impact of beta blockers on perioperative death and myocardial infarction. (Reprinted from Poldermans D et al.[22] with permission.)

prolol was started an average of 37 days before surgery and all patients received a bisoprolol orally on the morning of surgery. The day after surgery, beta blockers were administered either orally by nasogastric tube (bisoprolol) in 31 patients and intravenously (metoprolol) in 28 patients. The goal for heart rate was ≤ 60 bpm preoperatively and ≤ 80 bpm postoperatively.

There was a 91% reduction in the risk for death and MI (Figure 3-4). On the basis of these results, Poldermans et al. recommended that high-risk surgical patients receive beta blockers perioperatively, beginning 1 to 2 weeks before surgery. An alternative to this approach would be to omit preoperative noninvasive cardiac testing and prescribe a beta blocker perioperatively for all patients with clinical risk factors who are undergoing intermediate- or high-risk surgery.[22]

This extraordinary 91% reduction in the risk of cardiac events should be looked at cautiously, and perhaps future research will show the benefit to be more modest.[23] However, the findings are consistent with data showing reductions in perioperative ischemia with beta blockers and similar in direction to those of the only other controlled study of beta blockers in patients undergoing

major noncardiac surgery.[23] Patients randomly assigned to receive atenolol had 55% lower mortality over 2 years, but the benefit became apparent only after the hospitalization.[1] In conclusion, beta blockers are very effective in reducing perioperative MI and death and should be initiated preoperatively and continued in the postoperative period.

Use of Coronary Revascularization

Percutaneous Transluminal Coronary Angioplasty (PTCA) and Stent Implantation   The utility of PTCA in the preoperative period has been reported to be "safe" by some investigators,[24–25] but others disagree. Van Norman et al.[26] criticized that neither study is of sufficient size or design to warrant conclusions regarding outcomes in patients who had PTCA versus those who did not. They reported that patients undergoing PTCA < 90 days before noncardiac surgery had twice the rate of perioperative MI compared with patients with uncorrected CAD. Furthermore, 26% of patients undergoing PTCA < 90 days before NCS had adverse cardiac events.[26] Given the limited data, the indications for PTCA in the perioperative setting are identical to those developed by the ACC/AHA task force providing guidelines for the use of PTCA in general.[27]

Coronary stenting within the 2 weeks preceding surgery carries a high risk of complications. Kaluza et al.[28] reported the complication rate with surgery in 40 patients who underwent coronary artery stenting less than six weeks before noncardiac surgery. There were eight deaths, seven MIs, and 11 major bleedings. All deaths and MIs, as well as 8 of 11 bleeding episodes, occurred in patients subjected to surgery < 14 days from stenting. Based on ECG, enzymatic and angiographic evidence, stent thrombosis accounted for most of the fatal events. The time between stenting and surgery appeared to be the main determinant of outcome. They concluded that postponing elective noncardiac surgery for 2 to 4 weeks after coronary stenting should permit completion of the mandatory antiplatelet regimen, thereby reducing the risk of stent thrombosis and bleeding complications.[28]

No randomized trials have evaluated perioperative coronary interventions, and optimal timing of noncardiac surgery after coronary intervention remains poorly defined. Furthermore, the beneficial effects and safety of beta blockers perioperatively are well documented and decrease the need for coronary intervention. In conclusion, one might consider using revascularization with peripheral coronary intervention for patients with extensive ischemia and, if performed, postpone the surgical procedure for at least a week after PTCA and for 2 to 4 weeks after coronary stenting. However, surgery should not be delayed for more than 6 to 8 weeks when restenosis begins to occur (if it is to occur).

Coronary Artery Bypass Grafting (CABG)

Manske et al.[29] reported the results of a randomized trial in which patients with CAD who were scheduled to undergo renal transplantation were assigned to receive CABG surgery or medical therapy. Revascularized patients had a 57% reduction in cardiac events after 1 year compared with the medical therapy group. The value of this study was limited due to small size and loss to follow-up. Retrospective studies revealed a decreased event rate with CABG. However, the recommendations for preoperative CABG are essentially identical to the ACC/AHA task force recommendations for CABG. Examples include patients with the following conditions: acceptable coronary revascularization risk and suitable viable myocardium with left main stenosis, severe three-vessel disease, two-vessel disease involving severe left anterior descending artery obstruction, and intractable coronary ischemia despite maximal medical therapy.[3] As with peripheral coronary intervention, if coronary bypass surgery is performed, the noncardiac surgical procedure may need to be postponed for several weeks.

CONCLUSION

Clinical markers, physical examination, and functional capacity are the most important elements of estimating perioperative risk. Noninvasive testing is helpful in the group of patients estimated to be at intermediate risk, who are being evaluated for high-risk surgery or have limited functional capacity, and in whom the surgical risk is moderate. Coronary angiography should be limited to patients with evidence of unstable coronary disease or evidence of extensive ischemia on noninvasive testing. The remarkable benefit of perioperative beta blockers should make this class of drugs the standard of care for patients who have higher-risk clinical markers. Further research is needed to identify the patient population who would benefit from empiric beta blockers instead of noninvasive testing. However, the perioperative evaluation also represents an opportunity to initiate or modify cardiac care, including primary and secondary preventative measures, which will be beneficial long after the surgical procedure.

REFERENCES

1. Mangano DT, Layug EL, Wallace A. Effect of atenolol on mortality and cardiovascular morbidity after noncardiac surgery. *N Engl J Med* 1996;335:1713–20.

2. Massie BM, Mangano DT: Risk stratification for noncardiac surgery. How (and why)? *Circulation* 1993;87:1752–1755.

3. Eagle KA, et al: ACC/AHA Guideline update on perioperative cardiovascular evaluation for noncardiac surgery. A Report of the American College of Cardiology/American Heart Association Task Force on Practice Guidelines (Committee to Update the 1996 Guidelines on Perioperative Cardiovascular Evaluation for Noncardiac Surgery), *www.acc.org*, 2002.

4. Goldman L, Caldera DL, Nussbaum SR, et al: Multifactorial index of cardiac risk in noncardiac surgical procedures. *N Engl J Med* 1977;297:845–850.

5. Gerson MC, Hurst JM, Hertzberg VS, et al. Cardiac prognosis in noncardiac geriatric surgery. *Ann Intern Med* 1985;103:832–837.

6. Detsky AS, Abrams HB, Fortbath N, et al. Cardiac assessment for patients undergoing noncardiac surgery: A multifactorial clinical risk index. *Arch Intern Med* 1986;146:2131–2134.

7. Eagle KA, Coley CM, Newell JB, et al. Combining clinical and thallium data optimizes preoperative assessment of cardiac risk before major vascular surgery. *Ann Intern Med* 1989;110:859–866.

8. Eagle KA, Singer DE, Brewster DC, et al. Dipyridamole-thallium scanning in patients undergoing vascular surgery. Optimizing preoperative evaluation of cardiac risk. *JAMA* 1987;257:2185–2189.

9. Morris CK, Ueshima K, Kawaguchi T, et al. The prognostic value of exercise capacity: A review of the literature. *Am Heart J* 1991;122:1423–1431.

10. Carliner NH, Fisher ML, Plotnick GD, et al. Routine preoperative exercise testing in patients undergoing major noncardiac surgery. *Am J Cardiol* 1985;56:51–58.

11. Cutler BS, Wheeler HB, Paraskos JA, et al. Applicability and interpretation of electrocardiographic stress testing in patients with peripheral vascular disease. *Am J Surg* 1981;141:501–506.

12. L'Italien GJ, Paul SD, Hendel RC, et al. Development and validation of a Bayesian model for perioperative cardiac risk assessment in a cohort of 1,081 vascular surgical candidates. *J Am Coll Cardiol* 1996; 27:779–786.

13. Shaw LJ, Eagle KA, Gersh BJ, et al. Meta-analysis of intravenous dipyridamole thallium-201 imaging (1985–1994) and dobutamine echocardiography (1991–1994) for risk stratification before vascular surgery. *J Am Coll Cardiol* 1996;27:787–798.

14. Stratmann HG, Younis LT, Wittry MD, et al. Dipyridamole technetium 99m sestamibi myocardial tomography for preoperative cardiac risk stratification before major or minor nonvascular surgery. *Am Heart J* 1996;132:536–541.

15. Stratmann HG, Younis LT, Wittry MD, et al. Dipyridamole technetium 99m sestamibi myocardial tomography in patients evaluated for elective vascular surgery: Prognostic value for perioperative and late cardiac events. *Am Heart J* 1996;131:923–929.

16. Beller GA, Zaret BL. Contributions of nuclear cardiology to diagnosis and prognosis of patients with coronary artery disease. *Circulation* 2000; 101:1465–1478.

17. Hendel RC, Whitfield SS, Villegass BJ, et al. Prediction of late cardiac events by dipyridamole thallium imaging in patients undergoing elective vascular surgery. *Am J Cardiol* 1992;70:1243–1249.

18. Golub RJ, Ahlberg AW, McClellan, et al. Interpretive reproducibility of stress Tc-99m sestamibi tomographic myocardial perfusion imaging. *J Nucl Cardiol* 1999;6:257–269.

19. Cohen MC, Eagle KA: Preoperative risk stratification: an overview. Nuclear Cardiology, state of the art and future directions, 1999.

20. Elliott BM, Robinson JG, Zellner JL, et al. Dobutamine-^{201}Tl Imaging, assessing cardiac risks associated with vascular surgery. *Circulation* 1991;84(Suppl III):III-54–III-60.

21. Van Damme H, Piérard L, Gillain D, et al: Cardiac risk assessment before vascular surgery: a prospective study comparing clinical evaluation, dobutamine stress echocardiography, and dobutamine Tc-99m sestamibi tomoscintigraphy, Cardiovascular Surgery 1997;5:54–64.

22. Poldermans D, Boersma E, Bax JJ, et al. The effect of bisoprolol on perioperative mortality and myocardial infarction in high-risk patients undergoing vascular surgery. *N Engl J Med* 1999;341:1789–1794.

23. Lee TH: Reducing cardiac risk in noncardiac surgery. *N Engl J Med* 1999;341:1838–1840.

24. Huber K, Evans MA, Bresnahan J, et al. Outcome of noncardiac operations in patients with severe coronary artery disease successfully treated with coronary angioplasty. *Mayo Clin Proc* 1992;67:15–21.

25. Elmore JR, Hallett JW, Gibbons R, et al. Myocardial revascularization before abdominal aortic aneurysmorrhaphy: Effect of coronary angioplasty. *Mayo Clin Proc* 1993;68:637–641.

26. Van Norman GA, Posner K. Coronary stenting or percutaneous transluminal coronary angioplasty prior to noncardiac surgery increases adverse perioperative cardiac events: the evidence is mounting. *J Am Coll Cardiol* 36:2351–2352.

27. Smith SC, Jr, et al. ACC/AHA Guidelines for percutaneous coronary intervention: A report of the American College of Cardiology/American Heart Association Task Force on Practice Guidelines (Committee to Revise the 1993 Guidelines Percutaneous Transluminal Coronary Angioplasty). *J Am Coll Cardiol* 2001;27:2215–2238.

28. Kaluza GL, Joseph J, Lee JR, et al. Catastrophic outcomes of non-cardiac surgery soon after coronary stenting. *J Am Coll Cardiol* 35:1288–1294.

29. Manske CL, Wang Y, Rector T, et al. Coronary revascularization in insulin-dependent diabetic patients with chronic renal failure. *Lancet* 1992;340:998–1002.

CHAPTER 4

Evaluation of Myocardial Viability

Asad A. Rizvi
Muthu Velusamy
Gary V. Heller

INTRODUCTION

While there's life, there's hope.
—Terence (c. 190–159 B.C.)

The last four decades have seen tremendous advances in the management of acute coronary syndromes and the chronic management of ischemic heart disease. Mortality from coronary heart disease has more than halved since the early 1960s, and there continues to be a steady decline. This and other factors such as improving therapies aimed at prolonging survival in patients with left ventricular (LV) dysfunction and the aging of the U.S. population, have left an increasing number of people suffering from congestive heart failure (CHF). It is estimated that there are close to 5 million patients with CHF in the United States presently, with an additional 400,000 to 700,000 patients developing the condition annually.[1] According to 2001 figures, over 1 million people were admitted with heart failure as their principal

diagnosis, and in another 2 million admissions the diagnosis was deemed to have contributed.[2] In the year 2000, direct costs alone (not including those accrued from lost productivity) topped $22 billion. Clearly, morbidity and mortality from heart failure are on the ascent, and the condition will pose formidable challenges in the foreseeable future.

In addition to the health and economic burden, the management of patients with coronary artery disease (CAD) and severe LV dysfunction is challenging and complex. A major question that needs to be addressed is what constitutes the best management of such patients: coronary artery bypass surgery, medical management, or medical management followed by orthotopic heart transplantation in a limited few? The data to support bypass surgery are not as robust in this group of patients compared with other subsets of patients with CAD in whom a survival benefit has been clearly shown with surgery over medical therapy. This is due in large part to the

49

fact that the major randomized trials comparing medical versus surgical therapy for patients with CAD conducted in the mid to late 1970s either excluded patients with LV dysfunction (European Coronary Surgery Study) or did not include those with severe dysfunction. The NHLBI sponsored Coronary Artery Surgery Study (CASS),[3] and the VA Cooperative Study demonstrated a survival benefit with surgery over medical therapy in patients with three-vessel disease and moderate depression of LV function (left ventricular ejection fraction [LVEF] > 35%).[4] However, even these studies did not include patients with the most severe LV dysfunction. Therefore, the data supporting any benefit for coronary artery bypass surgery in this group of patients have come mostly from observational studies or registry data.

A number of investigators have demonstrated a survival benefit of coronary bypass surgery over medical therapy in selected patients with CAD and severe LV systolic dysfunction, specifically those whose initial symptom is angina.[5,6] In this specific subgroup, the 3-year mortality was almost 50% lower in the surgically treated group. Of note, patients with the lowest ejection fractions had the most survival benefit (see Figure 4-1). Despite these data, the benefit is offset by a high mortality and perioperative myocardial infarction (MI) rate. In Alderman's study, the mortality rate was 6.9% and the perioperative MI rate was over 10%. Overall, in the surgical literature the reported mortality rate has ranged from 1.6 to 9.7%, and in some series has been as high as 37%.[7–10] Therefore, it is important to identify additional subgroups of patients with severe heart failure who would benefit from surgical revascularization, in addition to those presenting with angina.

One of the purported mechanisms by which patients with CAD and severe LV dysfunction may benefit from coronary bypass surgery is by an improvement of segmental and global ejection fraction post-revascularization.[11] This recovery of function can occur only in patients with reversible myocardial dysfunction or viable myocardium. Thus, the ability to distinguish scar due to prior MI from reversible regional dysfunction due to chronically hypoperfused/hypocontractile ("hibernating") or acute post-ischemic dysfunction ("stunning") would be helpful in determining which patients would benefit from coronary bypass or percutaneous revascularization. This is especially important since resting LVEF is the most important predictor of survival in patients with CAD[12–14] (see Figure 4-2).

Several different approaches have been employed in the evaluation of myocardial viability. These have included assessments of metabolic tracer uptake, resting perfusion and contractile reserve with the use of positron emission tomography (PET), radionuclide imaging with thallium-201 (Tl-201) and technetium-99m (Tc-99m) sestamibi, echocardiography, and magnetic resonance imaging (MRI). This chapter will focus on these available options, describe the rationale for viability testing, and provide a clinically oriented approach to the patient requiring myocardial viability assessment.

Key Points

- The prevalence of heart failure is increasing.
- Contributing causes include (1) better management of acute coronary syndromes and chronic ischemic heart disease, (2) improvement in management of heart failure, and (3) aging of the population.
- CAD remains the number one cause of heart failure.
- Selected patients with CAD and severe heart failure may benefit from surgical revascularization.

DEFINITIONS

The term *viable*, in reference to myocardium, originates from the French and Latin words meaning life. As such, myocardial viability refers to any dysfunctional segment that is still metabolically active and retains the capacity to im-

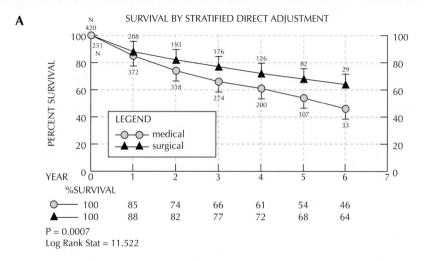

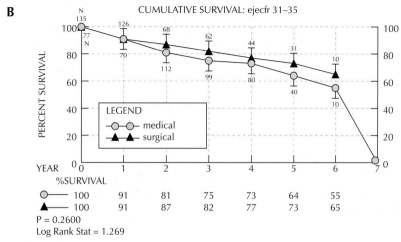

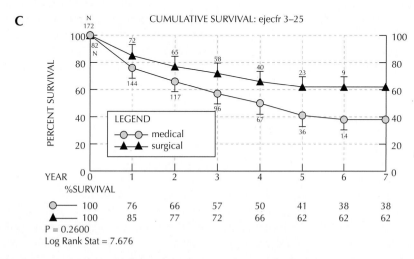

Figure 4-1. Cumulative survival in medically and surgically treated patients with CAD and severe LV dysfunction (LVEF < 35%) whose initial symptom was angina. Note an approximate 50% lower mortality in the surgically treated arm, overall (A). Patients with the lowest LVEFs (3–25%) benefited more than those with relatively higher LVEFs (B & C). (Adapted from Alderman et al. with permission.)

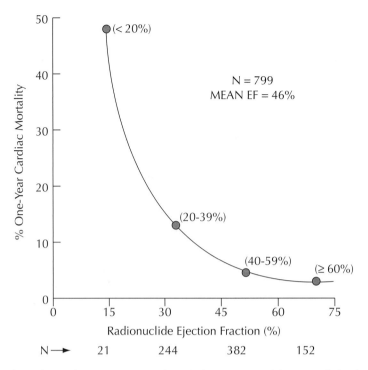

Figure 4-2. Relationship of mortality in patients with CAD having survived myocardial infarction and resting ejection fraction. (Adapted from The Multicenter Postinfarction Research Group.[14] In general, ejection fraction is the most powerful predictor of survival in patients with CAD. (Hammermeister et al.[12]).

prove with the restoration of a more favorable milieu (i.e., improved perfusion). It includes the specific conditions referred to as postischemic stunning and hibernating myocardium.

Postischemic stunning, first described by Braunwald and Kloner in 1982, refers to the delayed recovery of contractile function following an acute ischemic episode.[15] Animal models have demonstrated that with the total occlusion of a coronary artery, wall motion abnormalities begin to occur within 60 seconds corresponding to a depletion in adenosine triphosphate (ATP). Depending on the duration of occlusion, there is a spectrum in the rapidity of recovery. With short periods of ischemia, there is rapid recovery of systolic function. However, within 15 minutes of total coronary occlusion, ultrastructural changes begin to occur that may take up to several days to recover. These changes include widened I-bands indicative of myocardial stretching, de-

pletion of glycogen, clumping of nuclear chromatin, and mild intermyofibrillar and mitochondrial edema.[16–18] These changes persist for several days and completely resolve in about a week. With more prolonged ischemia (> 20 minutes), irreversible changes and necrosis follow. The significance of this phenomenon is that in patients with prolonged myocardial ischemia as occurs with infarction, considerable myocardium may be dysfunctional on the basis of postischemic stunning and may recover function. However, the improvement may not be evident for up to 2 weeks postinfarction.

The term *hibernating* was first used by Diamond et al. to refer to regional left ventricular dysfunction in ischemic, noninfarcted myocardium that was potentially reversible after coronary bypass surgery.[19] The condition was further expounded on by Rahimtoola, who was the first to coin the phrase *hibernating myo-*

cardium, as well as Braunwald and Rutherford.[20] The concept as originally envisioned was that chronically hypoperfused myocardial segments reduce their metabolic and contractile function as a protective and adaptive mechanism against irreversible cellular injury.[11] Features characteristic of the condition include a reduction in myocardial blood flow at rest that is sufficient to cause a reduction in metabolic and contractile function. Despite ischemia, there is no evidence of necrosis. Also, hibernating myocardium demonstrates contractile reserve, which can be elicited by catecholamine infusion. However, an increasing body of evidence suggests that the pathophysiology of the condition is not as simple as originally thought. In addition, whether hibernation represents a truly adaptive versus a pathologic state is also a subject of debate.

Key Points

- Definition of *myocardial viability:* "Any dysfunctional area of myocardium that is still metabolically active and retains the capacity to improve with the restoration of a more favorable milieu (i.e., improved perfusion)."
- Viable myocardium includes potentially reversible dysfunctional areas due to chronically hypoperfused/hypocontractile state (hibernating myocardium) and reversible acute postischemic dysfunction (stunning).

APPROACH TO THE PATIENT REQUIRING VIABILITY ASSESSMENT

Step 1: Indications for Myocardial Viability Testing (Figure 4-3)

In patients with CAD and regional or global LV dysfunction, the differentiation between scar tissue, metabolically active yet mechanically dysfunctional (i.e., viable) myocardium, or a combination of the two is an important distinction. Patients with the latter two may have improvement of function following revascularization as

In patients with CAD and severe LV dysfunction:

- To determine the presence of "hibernating myocardium" (potentially reversible) regional or global dysfunction
- To identify a group of patients with improved prognosis following revascularization

In patients post myocardial infarction:

- To discriminate between scar, viable myocardium, and a combination of the two in the infarct-related artery territory
- To identify patients at high risk for future adverse events if left nonrevascularized

Figure 4-3. Indications for Myocardial Viability Testing

noted above. Clinical variables alone such as the presence of angina pectoris, absence of Q waves, or the severity of asynergy, used alone or in combination, are not sufficient to distinguish between scar and hibernating or stunned myocardium.[21,22] In an electrocardiographic study looking at whether the presence or absence of Q waves could help determine viability compared with PET imaging using perfusion/metabolic tracers, the absence of Q waves did not differentiate viable from scar tissue ("matched" perfusion/metabolic defects).[23] Overall, the presence of Q waves was specific (79%), but not sensitive (41%) for the presence of matched defects representing scar due to prior infarction. Therefore, more sensitive methods have been developed that detect the viability of myocardial tissue more directly through a measure of resting perfusion, function, and metabolism, as well as through the augmentation of perfusion and function.

Numerous studies have shown that preoperative imaging for the evaluation of myocardial viability can help predict recovery of regional function.[24–28] In addition to predicting recovery of regional function, the assessment of viability has been shown to predict improvement in global LV function as well.[29,30] The recovery or improvement in overall LVEF appears to be directly related to the number of viable segments being revascularized[29] (see Figure 4-4).

The presence of myocardial viability on preoperative testing has also been related to outcome.[21,31,32] Patients with viable myocardium who are revascularized do better with a lower incidence of "hard events" (death, cardiac arrest, and nonfatal MI) compared with a strategy of medical management.[21,31] In patients with nonviable tissue, there is no difference in events between either strategy and in addition perioperative events are higher compared with patients with viable myocardium. The presence of viability correlates with improvement in heart failure symptoms and functional class postrevascularization.[31,33] Thus, myocardial viability testing helps guide patient management by identifying

patients who would benefit from revascularization with an improvement in outcome. The lack of viable myocardium selects patients in whom surgical revascularization will not affect prognosis, and for whom the risk of operative or percutaneous techniques may not be justified.

The second group in whom myocardial viability testing is warranted is patients with recent MI. The prognosis of patients having recently survived an MI is related to ejection fraction and extent of jeopardized myocardium in the infarct-related artery territory and remotely.[13,14] Studies have shown that the presence of residual viable myocardium in the infarcted territory that is not revascularized is an independent risk factor for future cardiac events.[21,34–36] Studies have also demonstrated that viability testing helps identify residual viable myocardium in the infarct-related

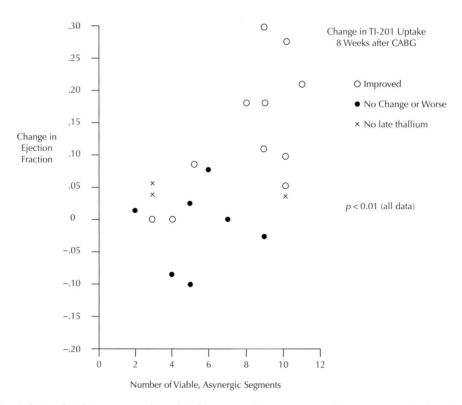

Figure 4-4.   Relationship between number of viable asynergic segments and improvement in function postrevascularization. (Adapted from Ragosta et al.[29] with permission.)

artery territory that may improve postrevascularization, as well as predicting improvement of segments with postischemic stunning.[37]

Step 2: Assess for Ischemia

All patients being considered for myocardial viability assessment should be evaluated by a test that can assess for ischemia provided the patient can tolerate some form of stress. The presence and extent of ischemia demonstrated by myocardial perfusion imaging (MPI) and/or dobutamine echocardiography has been shown to correlate with cardiac mortality and other "hard events" in post-MI patients as well as those with stable CAD.[38–40] Thus, patients with severe heart failure demonstrating ischemia should be offered revascularization.

In addition, the presence of stress-induced ischemia in a dysfunctional segment has been shown to be more predictive of recovery of function compared with mild to moderate fixed defects. Kitsiou et al.[41] studied 24 patients with

pre- and postrevascularization exercise–redistribution–reinjection Tl-201 single photon emission computed tomography (SPECT). A reversible defect was defined as a defect (< 85% max tracer uptake) that increased tracer activity by ≥ 10% on redistribution or reinjection images with final activity being > 50%. Mild to moderate fixed defects were defined as between 50% and 84% maximum uptake of the reference region. There was no difference in the number of segments with abnormal function preoperatively in either group. Postrevascularization, regional function improved in 79% of stress-induced ischemic segments versus 30% of the fixed defects (see Figure 4-5). Final Tl-201 content was greater in ischemic segments that improved postrevascularization, whereas there was no difference in final Tl-201 content between fixed segments that did or did not improve. This is consistent with the dobutamine echocardiographic data, which suggests that a biphasic response (augmentation followed by ischemic

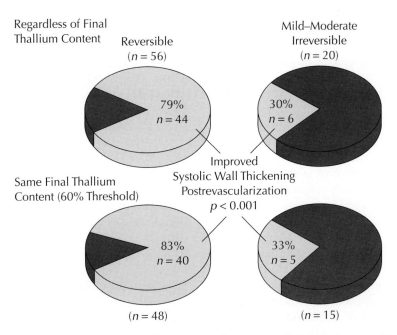

Figure 4-5. Proportion of asynergic segments that improved postrevascularization in reversible and mild to moderate fixed Tl-201 defects. (Adapted from Kitsiou et al.[41] with permission.)

worsening of function) most accurately predicts recovery of function.[42]

Step 3: Knowing the Options Available for Myocardial Viability Testing

Assess Resting Perfusion

Thallium-201 (Tl-201) is the mostly widely used and validated radiolabeled tracer in myocardial viability testing. Tl-201 is a potassium analog that is taken up in proportion to regional blood flow and requires the presence of viable cells with an intact cellular membrane. The first-pass extraction ratio is high (82%) and is not affected by reduced perfusion pressure secondary to critical epicardial stenoses.[43,44] After initial uptake, there is continuous exchange of the tracer between the intracellular and extracellular spaces and the blood pool, giving rise to the phenomenon of redistribution. This results in the disappearance of initial defects obtained after stress or rest injections. However, with rest injections, since the basal level of hypoperfusion remains, the resolution of the defect is more likely related to a delayed washout and thus evidence of viability.

Several different protocols have been used to assess myocardial viability with Tl-201. Commonly, viability evaluation occurs with the injection of tracer at peak stress (either exercise or pharmacologic) or at rest, followed by scanning within 10 to 15 minutes and then after 3 to 4 hours to document redistribution. If a persistent defect remains at the imaging after 3 to 4 hours, an additional dose of tracer is injected at rest and the patient is reimaged (stress–redistribution–reinjection protocol or rest–redistribution–reinjection protocol). Dilsizian et al.[45] demonstrated the benefit of the reinjection technique. In a study of 100 patients with CAD who underwent stress–redistribution imaging, 92 patients were noted to have exercise-induced defects. At redistribution imaging, 85 of 260 defects were noted to be fixed. Following repeat imaging after reinjection at rest, 42 of the 85 (49%) fixed segments

demonstrated either normal or improved uptake, suggesting viability. Rocco et al.[46] similarly demonstrated the benefit of the rest–reinjection technique in a study of 41 patients who underwent exercise–redistribution imaging. Of 141 segments with fixed defects on initial rest imaging, 44 (31%) were found to have redistribution after a second dose of Tl-201 at rest. This approach has been shown to be comparable to F-18 Fluorodeoxyglucose (FDG)–PET imaging. Additional protocols have included delayed redistribution imaging 8 to 72 hours after the initial scan. This has not been shown to improve the accuracy of the test.[47]

Criteria to identify viability with Tl-201 imaging have included the demonstration of redistribution as well as the uptake of tracer > 50 to 65% of maximal tracer uptake. Although this perfusion criteria cutoff to distinguish between viable and nonviable myocardium has been chosen arbitrarily, studies have shown that recovery of function is linearly related to uptake of tracer[29,48] (see Figure 4-6). However, there is little to no chance of recovery with tracer uptake < 30 to 40%. Kitsiou et al.[41] showed that the demonstration of a stress-induced perfusion defect correlated better with improvement postrevascularization compared with resting perfusion criteria alone. Overall, the sensitivity and specificity of myocardial viability testing using the various protocols has been reported as 90% and 54%, respectively, in the literature.[42]

Technetium-99m Agents Tc-99m sestamibi (MIBI) is currently the most widely validated technetium-based tracer employed for myocardial viability testing. Although the use of Tc-99m tetrofosmin as a diagnostic agent is well established, data regarding its use for the assessment of myocardial viability are more limited. Similar to Tl-201, MIBI uptake requires intact cellular membrane and mitochondrial function and reflects regional blood flow. Unlike Tl-201, it does not redistribute and hence criteria for viability are based on tracer uptake alone. Udelson et al.[49] demonstrated concordant regional uptake of MIBI 1 hour after resting injection and Tl-201

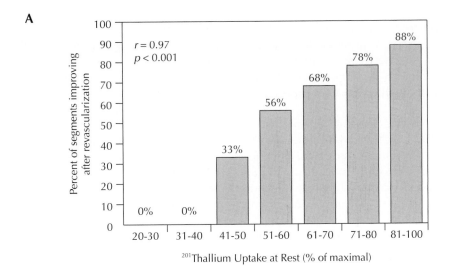

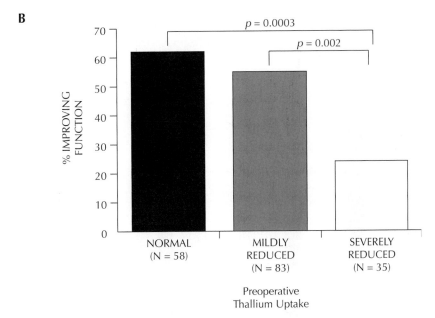

Figure 4-6. **A.** Near linear relationship between percent Tl-201 uptake after rest injection and recovery of function postrevascularization. (Adapted from Perrone-Filardi et al.[48] with permission.) **B.** Bar graph demonstrating relation between preoperative resting Tl-201 uptake and recovery of function in 176 segments with severe regional dysfunction. (Adapted from Ragosta et al.[29] with permission.)

redistribution activity. The mean regional uptake of Tc-99m sestamibi (as expressed as percent of maximum) was 75% ± 9 in areas that had improvement in function postrevascularization compared with 50% ± 8 in those segments without improvement. Similar data were reported by Kauffman et al.[50]

Due to its better imaging characteristics, ECG-gated SPECT Tc-99m MIBI adds the additional benefit of combined assessment of perfusion and function. In a study by Heller et al., 36 patients underwent resting Tc-99m sestamibi gated SPECT imaging preoperatively in addition to 6 weeks postrevascularization.[51] Perfusion criteria alone versus perfusion plus wall motion analysis were compared in the prediction of viability preoperatively. The use of perfusion and wall motion assessment significantly improved the sensitivity and overall accuracy for determination of viability (see Figure 4-7).

The Addition of Nitrates to Augment Resting Perfusion   The administration of nitrates prior to a resting injection of Tl-201, Tc-99m MIBI, or Tc-99m tetrofosmin appears to improve the sensitivity for the detection of viable myocardium.[52] Nitrate augmentation reduced resting Tc-99m MIBI defect size by approximately 29% ± 4. Using a stress–rest imaging protocol with and without administration of nitrates before rest imaging, investigators demonstrated that 52% of previously fixed defects showed reversibility and hence viability. Other investigators have demonstrated the utility of nitrate-augmented MPI in the prediction of postrevascularization recovery of function.[53,54] Nitrates may be administered by either sublingual or intravenous routes.

Assessment of Function and Contractile Reserve   Inotropic stimulation with dobuta-

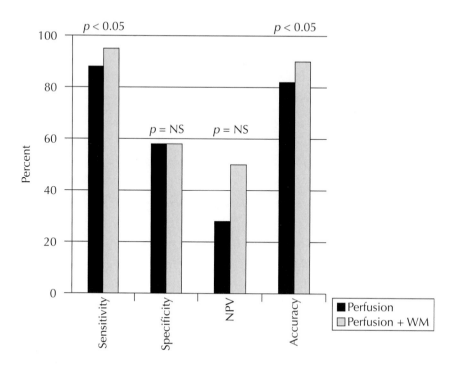

Figure 4-7.   Combined assessment of perfusion and function with Tc-99m sestamibi ECG-gated SPECT myocardial perfusion imaging improves the sensitivity and accuracy for determining viability. (Adapted from Levine et al.[51] with permission.)

mine during echocardiography has been shown to be very useful and is widely used in the assessment of myocardial viability. With inotropic stimulation at initial low doses, there is recruitment of contractile and flow reserve with an enhancement of regional function. This is one of the hallmarks of hibernating myocardium. In the presence of a critical epicardial stenosis and with progressively higher doses of dobutamine, ischemia ensues, with resultant deterioration of function. This biphasic response is highly predictive of recovery of function. In patients with more advanced disease, low-dose dobutamine alone has been used with a dose range of 5 to 15 μg/kg/min, rather than the traditional dose used for dobutamine stress echocardiography (DSE) (5–40 μg/kg/min). Limitations to this technique include the lack of a quantitative method to evaluate change in function. Since the interpretation is based on subjective evaluation, a considerable degree of expertise is required to perform DSE. The overall reported sensitivity, specificity, and accuracy for DSE are 82%, 85%, and 83%, respectively.[42]

More recently, the infusion of low-dose dobutamine (5–10 μg/kg/min) during Tc-99m sestamibi MPI has been shown to be a safe and feasible technique to provide both perfusion data and an assessment of contractile reserve—a unique advantage. Studies have demonstrated an improvement in sensitivity without loss of specificity in predicting postrevascularization recovery of function.[55]

Assessing Myocardial Metabolism: The Role of PET

PET has vast research and potential clinical applications due to the fact that it can assess blood flow, oxygen uptake, autonomic receptor density, and metabolism, including fatty acid uptake and glucose uptake in various organs, including the myocardium.[56] The clinical applications of PET imaging with relation to the heart include the assessment of the impact of stenosis, assessing the impacts of intervention, and the evaluation of myocardial viability. Numerous tracers have been validated for the assessment of perfusion and these include ^{13}N ammonia, ^{15}O-H20, and ^{82}Rubidium. The predominant tracer used to assess metabolism in viability studies with PET is 18-Fluorine 2-fluoro-2-deoxyglucose (^{18}F-FDG). ^{18}F-FDG is a glucose analog that is taken up by myocardial cells via plasma membrane receptors GLUT 1 and GLUT 4. Once in the cell, it is phosphorylated by hexokinase to form ^{18}F-FDG-6-phosphate and hence remains trapped in the myocardial cell. Glucose uptake is increased in ischemic myocardial cells which forms the basis of the determination of viability.

Several different patterns are possible based on flow and FDG uptake. Flow and metabolism can be matched; either both are preserved, as occurs in normal myocardium, or both are reduced, consistent with scar. Conversely, a mismatched pattern with reduced flow and increased uptake of FDG is consistent with viable (i.e., hibernating myocardium). A mismatched pattern with reduced perfusion and normal or mildly reduced FDG uptake can also occur and is usually associated with a combination of viable tissue plus scar.

Two different protocols are used to conduct a PET viability study. The first protocol consists of an oral glucose load of 50 g after an overnight fast. In the fasting state, normal myocardium will be using free fatty acids as the predominant substrate. With the oral glucose load, a hyperinsulinemic response will be elicited, which will help drive FDG into predominantly ischemic but viable cells. Although practical and more sensitive, this protocol may lead to inadequate scans in up to 50% of studies due to a large blood pool. The second protocol consists of creating a hyperinsulinemic euglycemic clamp and produces better quality images through a more standardized technique. Insulin is infused at a rate of 40 U/min/m², and euglycemia is maintained through the infusion of a 20% dextrose solution. During the second hour of the clamp, a steady state is achieved, at which point FDG can be infused.

Tillisch and co-workers[26] were the first to demonstrate that perfusion–metabolic mismatch as demonstrated by PET imaging with ^{13}N ammonia and ^{18}F-fluorodeoxyglucose readily identified viable myocardium from scar with a sensitivity of 85% and specificity of 92% for recovery of function post coronary bypass surgery. In a study of 22 patients with severe regional dysfunction, Tamaki and co-workers[27] showed that preoperative PET imaging with ^{13}N ammonia and ^{18}F-FDG was useful in demonstrating postoperative improvement in regional perfusion and function. Marwick and colleagues[57] showed similar results using $^{82}Rubidium$ and ^{18}F-FDG. Several studies using PET have shown a worse survival in patients with viable myocardium who do not undergo revascularization in terms of hard events (death, cardiac arrest, nonfatal MI, and subsequent revascularization).[31,33]

Newer Techniques

MRI   Cine MRI without tagging has been used to assess contractile reserve during low-dose dobutamine infusion. In post-MI patients, there is considerable concordance between this technique and DSE, with estimated sensitivity, specificity, and accuracy of 91%, 69%, and 79%, respectively. Low-dose dobutamine MRI has also been compared to FDG-PET imaging and found to have comparable results. MRI end-diastolic wall thickness of < 6 mm and wall thickening of < 1 mm were indicative of nonviable myocardium.[58,59]

More recently, contrast-enhanced MRI has been used in the assessment of myocardial viability.[60] In a study of 50 patients with ventricular dysfunction (mean LVEF 43% ± 13) imaged with gadolinium-enhanced cine MRI pre- and postrevascularization, the degree of hyperenhancement correlated with the extent of nonviable tissue and a lack of improvement in regional and global function. In a comparative study of gadolinium-enhanced MRI and PET imaging, contrast-enhanced MRI demonstrated a close correlation with PET imaging for the detection of nonviable tissue.[61]

Key Points

- Myocardial viability testing helps identify those segments with potential for recovery postrevascularization.

- Detection of myocardial viability is related to outcome; nonrevascularized patients with viable myocardium are at high risk for "hard" cardiac events. Revascularization significantly improves this outlook.

- Post-MI viability testing identifies areas of myocardium with residual viable myocardium in the infarct-related artery territory. Nonrevascularization of such tissue results in a worse prognosis for the patient.

- A logical approach to viability testing should include an initial assessment for ischemia. Subsequently, a number of different approaches are available, including evaluation of resting or augmented perfusion with radionuclide imaging, an assessment of contractile reserve with dobutamine echocardiography or ECG-gated SPECT myocardial perfusion imaging, metabolism testing with ^{18}F-FDG and PET, or newer techniques such as cardiac MR (see Figure 4-8).

Step 4: Which Test to Choose

The decision as to which test to choose for an individual patient depends on factors related to the patient as well as the host institution or hospital at which the test will be performed. Patient factors such as clinical instability, the presence of arrhythmia, body habitus, and weight may all influence the decision to order one test over another. For an unstable patient, resting perfusion assessment with radionuclide SPECT imaging offers a reasonable approach. The addition of nitrate enhancement can be particularly helpful in this setting. Inotropic stimulation with low-dose dobutamine during echocardiographic assessment or ECG-gated SPECT MPI would be a reasonable choice in the more stable and arrhythmia-free patient. The ideal test, however, remains a complete stress test in the patient who can tolerate it,

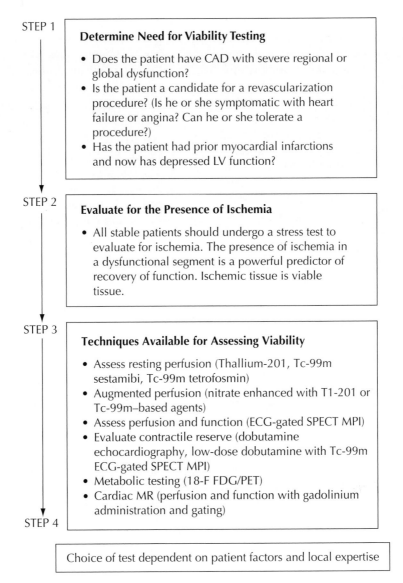

STEP 1

Determine Need for Viability Testing

- Does the patient have CAD with severe regional or global dysfunction?
- Is the patient a candidate for a revascularization procedure? (Is he or she symptomatic with heart failure or angina? Can he or she tolerate a procedure?)
- Has the patient had prior myocardial infarctions and now has depressed LV function?

STEP 2

Evaluate for the Presence of Ischemia

- All stable patients should undergo a stress test to evaluate for ischemia. The presence of ischemia in a dysfunctional segment is a powerful predictor of recovery of function. Ischemic tissue is viable tissue.

STEP 3

Techniques Available for Assessing Viability

- Assess resting perfusion (Thallium-201, Tc-99m sestamibi, Tc-99m tetrofosmin)
- Augmented perfusion (nitrate enhanced with Tl-201 or Tc-99m–based agents)
- Assess perfusion and function (ECG-gated SPECT MPI)
- Evaluate contractile reserve (dobutamine echocardiography, low-dose dobutamine with Tc-99m ECG-gated SPECT MPI)
- Metabolic testing (18-F FDG/PET)
- Cardiac MR (perfusion and function with gadolinium administration and gating)

STEP 4

Choice of test dependent on patient factors and local expertise

Figure 4-8.   Algorithm for the evaluation of myocardial viability.

so that ischemia is not missed. Local expertise at individual hospital departments may also influence the decision to order one modality over another.

Numerous studies have compared the various modalities head to head.[36,42,49,62–66] Bonow and co-workers[67] demonstrated that the predictive accuracy of Tl-201 SPECT stress–redistribu-

tion–reinjection technique (at 4 hrs) was comparable to PET imaging using ^{15}O-H20 and ^{18}F-FDG. Alfieri and co-investigators[62] compared dobutamine echocardiography with rest–redistribution Tl-201 scintigraphy and found comparable sensitivity for both techniques (> 90%) but a lower specificity for Tl-201 imaging (43.7% vs. 78.1%). When delayed imaging was used to assess for late redistribution, the specificity of Tl-201 imaging improved to 64%. In a head-to-head study of exercise–redistribution–reinjection Tl-201 imaging and low-dose dobutamine echocardiography, Vanoverschelde et al.[64] studied 73 patients with CAD and depressed LVEF with regional dysfunction. Using a cutoff value of > 54% uptake of Tl-201, SPECT imaging had a sensitivity of 72%, specificity of 73%, and accuracy of 73%. This compared with 88%, 77%, and 84%, respectively, with low-dose dobutamine echocardiography. In a comparison of rest–redistribution Tl-201 planar imaging, Tc-99m sestamibi rest imaging, and low-dose dobutamine echocardiography, a group of 14 patients with regional dysfunction were studied for evidence of viability.[63] The investigators found a strong correlation between response to dobutamine and percent uptake of Tl-201 and Tc-99m MIBI. Only delayed redistribution of Tl-201 and response to dobutamine, however, appeared to predict recovery of function accurately. In contrast, Udelson and co-workers[49] demonstrated a comparable predictive accuracy of rest–redistribution Tl-201 imaging and resting Tc-99m MIBI uptake 1 hour after injection with positive predictive and negative predictive accuracy of 80% and 96%, respectively, for Tc-99m MIBI.

Two other studies have reported similar results to those above when comparing Tl-201 rest–redistribution imaging and dobutamine echocardiography.[65,66] In general, Tl-201 imaging is associated with a comparable or slightly higher sensitivity but lower specificity compared with dobutamine echocardiography. Sciagra compared rest–redistribution Tl-201 imaging with nitrate-enhanced Tc-99m SPECT imaging and found comparable results with both techniques.[36]

Key Points

- PET imaging has a slightly higher sensitivity than Tl-201 SPECT imaging in the assessment of viability. However, due to lower cost and more accessibility, Tl-201 is the most widely used radionuclide test for assessing viability.

- The two most commonly used tests compare favorably with each other—Tl-201 has a higher sensitivity and marginally lower specificity compared with dobutamine echocardiography.

- Tc-99m sestamibi uptake has a high concordance with rest–redistribution Tl-201 activity and can be used readily in place of Tl-201 with no loss in accuracy.

- The decision as to which test to choose for myocardial viability assessment depends on patient factors and local expertise in individual hospital departments.

CONCLUSION

Myocardial viability testing has evolved into an integral part of the evaluation of patients with CAD and severe LV dysfunction. The recognition that LV dysfunction in patients with chronic CAD or after MI may be reversible with revascularization has led to techniques to try and predict recovery. Studies have demonstrated that the presence of viability, as detected by any of the modalities discussed in this chapter, helps identify those patients most likely to have recovery of regional and global function, alleviation of symptoms, and improvement in outcome postrevascularization. Conversely, in patients with no evidence of viable myocardium, the excessive risk of revascularization would not be justified, and for such patients a treatment strategy of optimal medical therapy would be the best approach.

REFERENCES

1. Morbidity & Mortality: 2002 ChartBook on Cardiovascular, Lung, and Blood Diseases. National Center of Health Statistics. *www.nhlbi.nih.gov/index.html*.
2. Healthcare Cost and Utilization Project (HCUP) Nationwide Inpatient Sample 2001. Agency for Healthcare Research & Quality (AHRQ). *http://hcup.ahrq.gov/HCUP*.
3. Killip T, Passamani E, Davis K, et al. Coronary artery surgery study (CASS): A randomized trial of coronary bypass surgery. Eight years follow up and survival in

patients with reduced ejection fraction. *Circulation* 1985;72(Suppl V):V102–V109.

4. Passamani E, Davis K, Gillespie MJ, Killip T, et al. A randomized trial of coronary artery bypass surgery survival of patients with a low ejection fraction. *N Engl J Med* 1985;312:1665–1671.

5. Alderman EL, Fisher LD, Litwin P, et al. Results of coronary artery surgery in patients with poor left ventricular function (CASS). *Circulation* 1983;68:785–795.

6. Pigott JD, Kouchoukos NT, Oberman A, Cutter GR. Late results of surgical and medical therapy for patients with coronary artery disease and depressed left ventricular function. *J Am Coll Cardiol* 1985;5:1036–1045.

7. Dreyfus GD, Duboc D, Blasco A, et al. Myocardial viability assessment in ischemic cardiomyopathy: Benefits of coronary revascularization. *Ann Thorac Surg* 1994;57:1402–1408.

8. Cosgrove DM, Loop FD, Lytle BW, et al. Primary myocardial revascularization: Trends in surgical mortality. *J Thorac Cardiovasc Surg* 1984;88:673–684.

9. Guyton RA, Arcidi JM, Langford DA, et al. Emergency coronary bypass for cardiogenic shock. *Circulation* 1987;88:673–684.

10. Hochberg MS, Parsonnet V, Gielchinsky I, Hussain SM. Coronary artery bypass grafting in patients with ejection fractions below forty percent: Early and late results in 466 patients. *J Thorac Cardiovasc Surg* 1983;86:519–527.

11. Rahimtoola SH. The hibernating myocardium. *Am Heart J* 1989;117:211–221.

12. Hammermeister KE, DeRouen TA, Dodge HT. Variables predictive of survival in patients with coronary disease: Selection by univariate and multivariate analyses from the clinical, electrocardiographic, exercise, arteriographic, and quantitative angiographic evaluations. *Circulation* 1979;59:421–430.

13. De Feyter PJ, Van Eenige MJ, Dighton DH, et al. Prognostic value of exercise testing, coronary angiography, and left ventriculography after myocardial infarction. *Circulation* 1982;66:527–536.

14. The Multicenter Postinfarction Study Group. Risk stratification and survival after myocardial infarction. *N Engl J Med* 1983;309:331–336.

15. Braunwald E, Kloner RA. The stunned myocardium: Prolonged, post-ischemic dysfunction. *Circulation* 1982;66:1146–1149.

16. Heyndrickx GR, Baig H, Nellers P, et al. Depression of regional blood flow and wall thickening after brief coronary occlusions. *Am J Physiol* 1973;234:H653.

17. Weiner JM, Apstein CS, Arthur JH, et al. Persistence of myocardial injury following brief periods of coronary occlusion. *Cardiovasc Res* 1976;10:678–680.

18. Wood JM, Hanley HG, Entman ML, et al. Biochemical and morphologic correlates of acute myocardial ischemia in the dog. *Circ Res* 1979;44:52–56.

19. Diamond GA, Forrester JS, deLuz PL, et al. Post-extrasystolic potentiation of ischemic myocardium by atrial stimulation. *Am Heart J* 1978;l95:204–209.

20. Vanoverschelde JJ, Wijns W, Borgers M, et al. Chronic myocardial hibernation in humans: From bedside to bench. *Circulation* 1997;95:1961–1971.

21. Pagley PR, Beller GA, Watson DD, et al. Improved outcome after coronary bypass surgery in patients with ischemic cardiomyopathy and residual myocardial viability. *Circulation* 1997;96:793–800.

22. Braunwald E, Rutherford J. Reversible ischemic left ventricular dysfunction: Evidence for the "hibernating myocardium." *J Am Coll Cardiol* 1986;8:1467–1470.

23. Al-Mohammad A, Norton MY, Mahy IR, et al. Can the surface electrocardiogram be used to predict myocardial viability. *Heart* 1999;82:663–667.

24. Rozanski A, Berman DS, Gray R, et al. Use of thallium-201 redistribution scintigraphy in the preoperative differentiation of reversible and nonreversible myocardial asynergy. *Circulation* 1981;64:936–944.

25. Iskandrian AM, Hakki AH, Kane S, et al. Rest and redistribution thallium-201 myocardial scintigraphy to predict improvement in left ventricular function after coronary arterial bypass grafting. *Am J Cardiol* 1983;51:1312–1316.

26. Tillisch J, Brunken R, Marshall R, et al. Reversibility of cardiac wall motion abnormalities predicted by positron tomography. *N Engl J Med* 1986;314:884–888.

27. Tamaki N, Yonekura Y, Yamashita K, et al. Positron emission tomography using fluorine-18 deoxyglucose in evaluation of coronary artery bypass grafting. *Am J Cardiol* 1989;64:860–865.

28. Mori T, Minamiji K, Kurogane H, et al. Rest-injected thallium 201 imaging for assessing viability of severe asynergic regions. *Journal of Nuclear Medicine* 1991;32:1718–1724.

29. Ragosta M, Beller GA, Watson DD, et al. Quantitative planar rest–redistribution 201-thallium imaging in detection of myocardial viability and prediction of improvement in left ventricular function after coronary bypass surgery in patients with severely depressed left ventricular function. *Circulation* 1993;87:1630–1641.

30. Cornel JH, Bax JJ, Elhendy A, et al. Biphasic response to dobutamine predicts improvement of global left ventricular function after surgical revascularization in patients with stable coronary artery disease: Implications of time course of recovery on diagnostic accuracy. *J Am Coll Cardiol* 1998;31:1002–1010.

31. Eitzman D, Al-Aouar Z, Kanter HL, et al. Clinical outcome of patients with advanced coronary artery disease after viability studies with positron emission tomography. *J Am Coll Cardiol* 1992;20:559–565.

32. Senior R, Kaul S, Lahiri A. Myocardial viability on echocardiography predicts long-term survival after revascularization in patients with ischemic congestive heart failure. *J Am Coll Cardiol* 1999;33:1848–1854.

33. Di Carli MF, Asgarzadie F, Schelbert HR, et al. Quantitative relation between myocardial viability and improvement in heart failure symptoms after revascularization in patients with ischemic cardiomyopathy. *Circulation* 1995;92:3436–3444.

34. Lee KS, Marwick TH, Cook SA, et al. Prognosis of patients with left ventricular dysfunction, with and without viable myocardium after myocardial infarction: Relative efficacy of medical therapy and revascularization. *Circulation* 1994;90:2687–2694.

35. Tamaki N, Kawamoto M, Takahashi N, et al. Prognostic value of an increase in fluorine-18 deoxyglucose uptake in patients with myocardial infarction: Comparison with stress thallium imaging. *J Am Coll Cardiol* 1993;22:1621–1627.

36. Sciagra R, Bisi G, Santoro GM, et al. Comparison of baseline-nitrate technetium 99m sestamibi with rest–redistribution thallium 201 tomography in detecting viable hibernating myocardium and predicting post-revascularization recovery. *J Am Coll Cardiol* 1997;30:384–391.

37. Schwaiger M, Brunken R, Grover-McKay M, et al. Regional myocardial metabolism in patients with acute myocardial infarction assessed by positron emission tomography. *J Am Coll Cardiol* 1986;8:800–808.

38. Brown K, Heller GV, Landin RS, et al. Early dipyridamole ^{99m}Tc-sestamibi single photon emission computed tomographic imaging 2 to 4 days after acute myocardial infarction predicts in-hospital and postdischarge cardiac events: Comparison with submaximal exercise imaging. *Circulation* 1999;100:2060–2066.

39. Sicari R, Picano E, Landi P, et al. EDIC: Echo Dobutamine International Cooperative Study. The prognostic value of dobutamine–atropine stress echocardiography early after acute myocardial infarction. *J Am Coll Cardiol* 1997;29:254–260.

40. Brown KA. Prognostic value of myocardial perfusion imaging: State of the art and new developments. *J Nucl Cardiol* 1996;3:516–37.

41. Kitsiou AN, Srinivasan G, Quyyumi AA, et al. Stress-induced reversible and mild to moderate irreversible thallium defects: Are they equally accurate for predicting recovery of regional left ventricular function after revascularization? *Circulation* 1998;98:501–508.

42. Bax JJ, Wijns W, Cornel JH, et al. Accuracy of currently available techniques for prediction of functional recovery after revascularization in patients with left ventricular dysfunction due to chronic coronary artery disease: Comparison of pooled data. *J Am Coll Cardiol* 1997;30:1451–1460.

43. Perrone-Filardi P, Chiariello M. The identification of myocardial hibernation in patients with ischemic heart failure by echocardiography and radionuclide studies. *Progr Cardiovasc Dis* 2001;43:419–432.

44. Iskandrian AS, Verani MS (Eds.) *Nuclear Cardiac Imaging: Principles and Application*, 2nd ed. Philadelphia: FA Davis, 1996.

45. Dilsizian V, Rocco TP, Freedman NMT, et al. Enhanced detection of ischemic but viable myocardium by the reinjection of thallium after stress–redistribution imaging. *N Engl J Med* 1990;323:141–146.

46. Rocco TP, Dilsizian V, McKusick KA, et al. Comparison of thallium redistribution with rest "reinjection" imaging for the detection of viable myocardium. *Am J Cardiol* 1990;66:158–163.

47. Dilsizian V, Smeltzer WR, Freedman NMT, et al. Thallium reinjection after stress–redistribution imaging: Does 24 hour delayed imaging after reinjection enhance detection of viable myocardium? *Circulation* 1991;83:1247–1255.

48. Perrone-Filardi P, Pace L, Prastaro M, et al. Dobutamine echocardiography predicts improvement of hypoperfused dysfunctional myocardium after revascularization in patients with coronary artery disease. *Circulation* 1995;91:2556–2565.

49. Udelson JE, Coleman PS, Metherall J, et al. Predicting recovery of severe regional ventricular dysfunction: Comparison of resting scintigraphy with 201-Tl and 99m TC-sestamibi. *Circulation* 1994;89:2552–2561.

50. Kauffman GJ, Boyne TS, Watson DD, et al. Comparison of rest thallium-201 imaging and rest technetium-99m sestamibi imaging for assessment of myocardial viability in patients with coronary artery disease and severe left ventricular dysfunction. *J Am Coll Cardiol* 1996;27:1592–1597.

51. Levine M, McGill C, Ahlberg A, Heller GV, et al. Functional assessment with electrocardiographic gated single-photon emission computed tomography improves the ability of technetium-99m sestamibi myocardial perfusion imaging to predict myocardial viability in patients undergoing revascularization. *Am J Cardiol* 1999;83:1–5.

52. He ZX, Verani MS. Evaluation of myocardial viability by myocardial perfusion imaging: Should nitrates be used? *J Nucl Cardiol* 1998;5:527–532.

53. Sciagra R, Leoncini M, Marcucci G, et al. Technetium-99m sestamibi imaging to predict left ventricular ejection fraction outcome after revascularization in patients with chronic coronary artery disease and left ventricular dysfunction: Comparison between baseline and nitrate-enhanced imaging. *Eur J Nucl Med* 2001;28:680–687.

54. Basu S, Senior R, Raval U, Lahiri A. Superiority of nitrate enhanced ^{201}Tl over conventional redistribution ^{201}Tl imaging for prognostic evaluation after myocardial

infarction and thrombolysis. *Circulation* 1997;
96:2932–2937.

55. Rizvi A, Ahlberg A, Heller GV, et al. Prediction of
myocardial viability using regional and global assessment
models during low dose dobutamine enhanced Tc-99m
sestamibi gated single photon emission computed
tomography imaging. *Circulation* 2001;104:II-719
(Abstract).

56. Dutka DP, Camici PG. The contribution of positron
emission tomography to the study of ischemic heart
failure. *Progr Cardiovasc Dis* 2001;43:399–418.

57. Marwick TH, MacIntyre WJ, Lafont A, et al. Metabolic
responses of hibernating and infarcted myocardium to
revascularization: A follow up study of regional
perfusion, function and metabolism. *Circulation*
1992;85:1347–1353.

58. Kramer CM. Imaging of function. Chapter 30. In:
Pohost GM, O'Rourke RA, Berman DA, Shah PM.
(Eds.), *Imaging in Cardiovascular Disease*. Philadelphia:
Lippincott Williams & Wilkins, 2000.

59. Fuisz AR, Pohost GM. Myocardial perfusion and
magnetic resonance imaging. Chapter 31. In: Pohost
GM, O'Rourke RA, Berman DA, Shah PM (Eds.),
Imaging in Cardiovascular Disease. Philadelphia:
Lippincott Williams & Wilkins, 2000.

60. Kim RJ, Wu E, Rafael A, et al. The use of contrast-
enhanced magnetic resonance imaging to identify
reversible myocardial dysfunction. *N Engl J Med*
2000;343:1445–1453.

61. Klein C, Nekolla SG, Bengel FM, et al. Assessment of
myocardial viability with contrast-enhanced magnetic
resonance imaging: Comparison with positron emission
tomography. *Circulation* 2002;105:162–167.

62. Alfieri O, La Canna G, Giubbini R, et al. Recovery of
myocardial function. The ultimate target of
revascularization. *Eur J Cardio-Thorac Surg*
1993;7:325–330.

63. Marzullo P, Parodi O, Reisenhofer B, et al. Value of rest
thallium-201/technetium 99m sestamibi scans and
dobutamine echocardiography for detecting myocardial
viability. *Am J Cardiol* 1993;71:166–172.

64. Vanoverschelde JL, D'Hondt AM, Marwick T, et al.
Head to head comparison of exercise–redistribution–
reinjection thallium single photon emission computed
tomography and low dose dobutamine
echocardiography for prediction of reversibility of
chronic left ventricular ischemic dysfunction. *J Am Coll
Cardiol* 1996;28:432–442.

65. Perrone-Filardi P, Pace L, Prastaro M, et al. Assessment
of myocardial viability in patients with chronic coronary
artery disease. Rest–4-Hour 24 Hour 201-Tl
tomography versus dobutamine echocardiography.
Circulation 1996;94:2712–2719.

66. Qureshi U, Nagueh SF, Afridi I, et al. Dobutamine
echocardiography and quantitative rest–redistribution
201-Tl tomography in myocardial hibernation: Relation
of contractile reserve to 201-Tl uptake and comparative
prediction of recovery of function. *Circulation*
1997;95:626–635.

67. Bonow RO, Dilsizian V, Cuocolo A, Bacharach SL.
Identification of viable myocardium in patients with
chronic coronary artery disease and left ventricular
dysfunction: Comparison of thallium scintigraphy with
reinjection and PET imaging with 18-F
fluorodeoxyglucose. *Circulation* 1991;83:26–37.

CHAPTER 5

Role of Myocardial Perfusion Imaging in the Assessment of the Diabetic Patient

Mohammed I. Awaad

Gary V. Heller

INTRODUCTION

Cardiovascular disease is the leading cause of mortality and morbidity among patients with type 1 and type 2 diabetes, and accounts for half of diabetic patients.[1,2] Diabetes mellitus constitutes a complex clinical problem that will grow in importance in the future. According to a Centers for Disease Control and Prevention report, the prevalence of diabetes has increased from 4.9% in 1990 to 6.5% in 1998 and to 6.9% in 1999.[3,4] The increase in the number of cases of diabetes has closely paralleled the changes in the incidence of obesity. The aging of the population has contributed to a greater number of cases.

The complications of diabetes have a considerable impact on patient survival and quality of life, especially with respect to cardiovascular disease (CVD). Several forms of CVD have increased in diabetes. The overall prevalence of CAD has been estimated to be as high as 55% in diabetic patients versus 2 to 4% in the general population. Diabetes mellitus has added another new dimension to the usual risk factors of CAD.[5] Approximately 20 to 25% of patients presenting with acute coronary syndromes or with percutaneous interventions have diabetes.[6] Because CAD risk can be modified by intervention, it is important not to underestimate the effect of diabetes in the development of CAD, as these patients may benefit by appropriate screening and aggressive intervention.

Not only do diabetic patients have a high incidence of CAD, they also suffer from an increased risk of cardiovascular complications. Myocardial ischemia is frequently silent or asymptomatic in patients with diabetes.[7] Not only is the likelihood of diabetic patients having CAD high, but also the outcome of those patients is worse than in comparable nondiabetic patients. Examples are numerous: Following acute myocardial infarction (MI), both in-hospital and 1-year mortality are twice that of nondiabetic patients with or without primary coronary intervention (PCI).[8] Patients with hyperlipidemia have significantly higher event rates than nondiabetic patients at the same cholesterol levels.

Many patients are debilitated by symptoms of congestive heart failure (CHF) or angina. Patients with type 2 diabetes usually have other associated risk factors such as hypertension or hyperlipidemia. This further increases their cardiovascular risk. Diabetic women have increased risk of cardiovascular death up to 7.5 times that of women without diabetes. They lose the premenopausal protection seen in their healthy counterparts.[2,9,10] Diabetic patients suffering from MI have a higher chance of dying from their event or of subsequent heart failure. Thrombolytic therapy may be less beneficial in diabetic patients.[10–12] Surgical and percutaneous revascularization are associated with greater long-term mortality in diabetic patients.[13–17] Therefore, early diagnosis of CAD and risk stratification are essential to improve the prognosis in this high-risk population.

DIAGNOSIS OF CAD IN DIABETIC PATIENTS

Clinical Evaluation

Diabetes mellitus is considered an important risk factor for CAD. The American Diabetes Association (ADA) recommends annual risk factor assessment, including symptoms of angina, a 12-lead electrocardiogram (ECG), evaluation of associated risk factors as hypertension, smoking, and hyperlipidemia.[18] Current guidelines emphasize blood pressure of < 130/85 and low-density lipoprotein (LDL) cholesterol < 130 mg/dL.[19] ECG abnormalities are associated with increased risk of previously undetected CAD. The presence of significant Q waves suggests a history of a silent MI. In type 1 diabetes, early onset of the disease in the third or fourth decade suggests a worsened outcome. It has been recommended that screening for CAD should start as early as age 30 to 40 because of possible 35% mortality by age 55 in type 1 diabetes.[20]

The presence of peripheral vascular disease (PVD) is associated with a worsened cardiovascular mortality and morbidity in a diabetic patient.[18,21] Lower-extremity PVD represents an increased risk for any surgical interventional procedure and is an independent risk factor for mortality in diabetic patients with similar severity of CAD.[9] In such patients, the limitation of the lower extremity on physical activity may mask their pain expression. In a study evaluating 30 patients with PVD but without known CAD, stress radioisotope perfusion imaging revealed evidence of ischemia or infarction in 57% of patients.[7] This suggests that stress testing with an imaging modality is an invaluable tool in their evaluation.

Noninvasive Evaluation of Diabetic Patients with Suspected CAD

Diabetic patients who develop symptoms or other indications suggestive of CAD need further evaluation. The ADA recommendations are listed in Figures 5-1 and 5-2 and Table 5-1. Indications include symptoms as well as multiple risk factors, abnormal ECG, evidence of peripheral vascular disease and others. The type of stress testing is not specific.

Exercise tolerance testing alone as a means of evaluating diabetic patients meeting ADA criteria (Table 5-2) may not be adequate. The sensitivity and specificity is low (see Chapter 1), and many patients who also manifest peripheral arterial disease will not be able to complete an adequate degree of exercise for diagnosis.[22,23]

Role of Stress Myocardial Perfusion Imaging in Symptomatic Patients

Stress myocardial perfusion imaging (MPI) in symptomatic diabetic patients can be very beneficial in providing the appropriate diagnosis and risk stratification. Although somewhat limited, several studies point to similar diagnostic accuracy between diabetic and nondiabetic patients. In a prospective study, Paillole et al.[24] reported the sensitivity of dipyridamole thallium to be

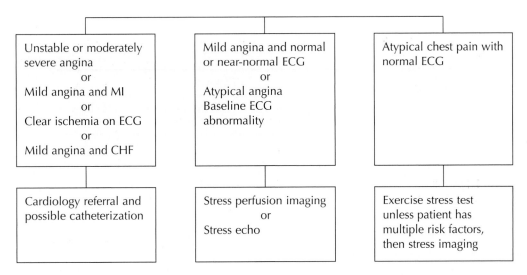

Figure 5-1.   ADA guidelines for symptomatic diabetic patients.

80%, with a specificity of 87% in diabetic patients. Similarly, Boudreau et al.[25] reported a sensitivity and specificity of 86% and 79%, respectively, in patients with type 1 diabetes in the presence of end-stage renal disease. Other investigators[26] reported a retrospective review of diabetic patients who had a myocardial perfusion study followed by cardiac catheterization within a year. They reported a sensitivity of 97% and positive predictive value of 88%. In a more recent study, Kang and colleagues[27] reported overall sensitivity and specificity of single photon emission computed tomography (SPECT) technetium-99m (Tc-99m) sestamibi imaging for de-

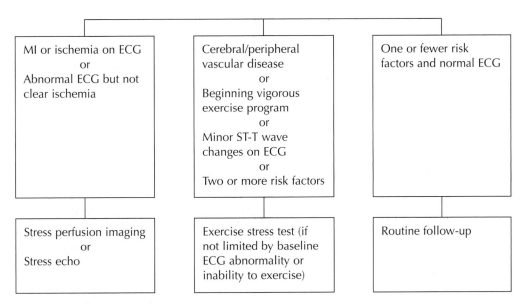

Figure 5-2.   ADA guidelines for asymptomatic diabetic patients.

Table 5-1

ADA Guidelines for Follow-up After Screening Exercise Treadmill Test (ETT)

		ETT Results		
Pretest Risk	Normal	Mildly Positive	Moderately Positive	Markedly Positive
High	++	+++	++++	++++
4–5 risk factors				
Moderate	+	+++	+++	++++
2–3 risk factors				
Low	+	+++	+++	++++
0–1 risk factors				

+ = routine follow-up; ++ = close follow-up; +++ = imaging; ++++ = cardiology referral/possible catheterization.

Table 5-2

American Diabetes Association Indications for Cardiac Evaluation

Number	Indication
1.	Typical or atypical cardiac symptoms
2.	Resting electrocardiogram suggestive of ischemia or infarction
3.	Peripheral or carotid occlusive arterial disease
4.	Plans to begin a vigorous exercise program, sedentary lifestyle, age ≥ 35 years
5.	Two or more of the risk factors listed below in addition to diabetes:
	(a) Total cholesterol ≥ 240 mg/dL, LDL cholesterol ≥ 160 mg/dL, or HDL cholesterol < mg/dL
	(b) Blood pressure > 140/90 mm Hg
	(c) Family history of premature CAD
	(d) Positive micro/macroalbuminuria test

tecting CAD with the criterion of ≥ 50% diameter stenosis to be 86% and 56% in diabetic patients, and 86% and 46% in nondiabetic patients (p = nonsignificant), respectively. The normalcy rate for low-likelihood patients was 89% in diabetics and 90% in nondiabetics (p = not significant). The sensitivity and specificity for individual vessel detection were also similar in patients with or without diabetes, except for a lower sensitivity and higher specificity for detecting LAD disease in the diabetic group ($p < 0.05$).

In total, these studies demonstrate considerable value in using stress SPECT imaging to evaluate symptoms or other conditions suggested by the ADA to be worthy of testing for CAD. Data are available for both exercise or pharmacological stress. Thus, the physician can choose the mode of stress for his or her diabetic patient based on previously described indications (Chapters A1, B1).

Risk Stratification in Diabetic Patients with Stress SPECT Imaging

Previous chapters have demonstrated the value of risk stratification in the general population with over 20 years of data. (Chapters E2, E1). The concept of management based on imaging results appears solid and is often used. Data are now emerging for the diabetic patients as well. One of the first studies was reported by Felsher et al.[28] They studied 123 diabetic patients and demonstrated that abnormal stress thallium studies were clearly associated with greater cardiac events than those with normal results. Further evaluation was not possible because of limited numbers of patients.

More recent data including a greater number of patients has demonstrated that risk stratification in diabetic patients can be performed successfully. In a single center study of 1,271 consecutively registered diabetic patients and 5,862 without diabetes, Kang et al.[29] evaluated risk stratification according to defect size and extent (Figures 5-3 and 5-4). As with studies in the general population, the greater the defect extent, the greater the risk for coronary events (cardiac death, nonfatal MI). Patients with moderately to severely abnormal images had a > 7% annual event rate. By multivariate analysis, the greatest prediction of cardiac events was defect size.

More recent data from a multicenter analysis corroborates these findings. Using data from six centers, Giri et al.[30] examined whether the nuclear perfusion study could contribute to risk stratification beyond the presence of diabetes using the incremental chi-square approach (Figures 5-5 and 5-6). Indeed, for both prediction of cardiac death alone or as a combined end point with nonfatal MI, the perfusion imaging data was a substantially and significantly better predictor of cardiac events than the presence of diabetes in combination with clinical risk. These data demonstrate the utility of stress perfusion imaging in diabetic patients. This study also demonstrates value in female diabetic patients, which have been shown to be at even greater risk for poor outcome than diabetic men. In this study, the presence of multivessel perfusion defects was the best predictor of cardiac events, not gender. These data demonstrate stress SPECT imaging is useful in both genders.

Management Decisions Based on Imaging Results

The previous sections have demonstrated the diagnostic and prognostic value of stress MPI. Thus,

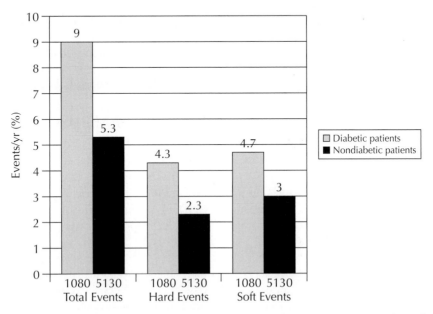

Figure 5-3. Total, hard, and soft event rates among patients with diabetes and patients without diabetes. Reprinted from Kang et al.[27] with permission.

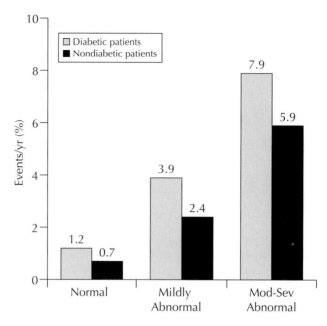

Figure 5-4. Hard event rates among patients with diabetes and patients without diabetes as a function of stress defect extent and severity. Reprinted from Kang et al.[27] with permission.

results of the nuclear cardiology study can be used for management decisions in patients with diabetes. The following scenario is suggested:

1. In patients with diabetes, those with a low risk of events (mild abnormalities) may be managed with aggressive risk factor modification and medical management. With further increase of risk, more aggressive management may be needed, including catheterization and revascularization (moderate to severe abnormality).

2. In diabetic patients with a normal stress image result, the same principles using risk data applies as with the nondiabetic population. It should be cautioned that the degree of risk based on a normal imaging appearance tends to be slightly higher (1–2%) according to Kang et al.[29] However, using Kaplan–Meier evaluation of cardiac cath risk over time, Giri et al.[31] demonstrated similar low risk over approximately 1 year as with nondiabetic

subjects (Figure 5-7). After that, the curves diverged significantly ($p < 0.001$), although the risk was still quite low. These data suggest that earlier retesting in diabetic patients may be warranted. This may also be true in those managed medically with abnormal studies.

Evaluation of the Asymptomatic Diabetic Patient

The dilemma of which asymptomatic diabetic patient to evaluate for CAD is difficult. On the other hand, it is known that the incidence of CAD in asymptomatic diabetic patients is 8 to 10%. As important, the first manifestation of CAD may be acute MI or sudden cardiac death. On the other hand, screening every asymptomatic diabetic patient for CAD is not practical or cost-effective. Very few guidelines on viability are not based on hard data.

A recent ADA consensus panel[18] assumed that asymptomatic diabetic patients recognized as hav-

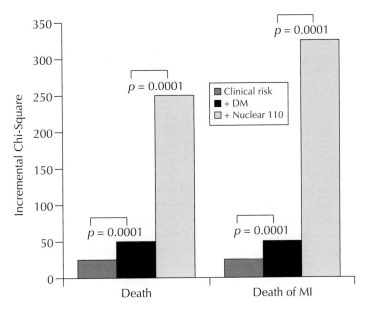

Figure 5-5. Incremental chi-squared value of nuclear and clinical variables to the total model chi-squared value for prediction of cardiac death or cardiac death/MI in diabetic (DM) patients. Reprinted from Giri et al.[30] with permission.

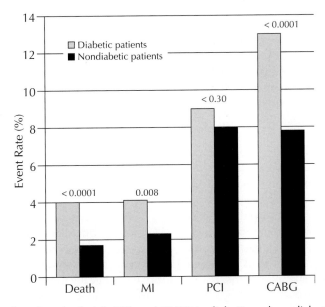

Figure 5-6. Outcomes of cardiac death, MI, PCI, and CABG in diabetic and nondiabetic patients. Reprinted from Giri et al.[30] with permission.

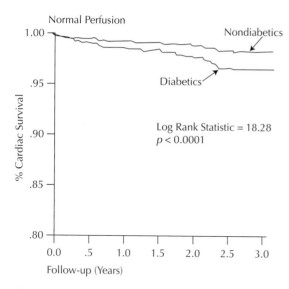

Figure 5-7. Kaplan–Meier survival curves comparing the subset of diabetic and nondiabetic patients with normal stress MPI. Reprinted from Giri et al.[30] with permission.

ing CAD by noninvasive testing were at substantial cardiac risk. Framingham Study Data suggest that even asymptomatic diabetic patients with multiple risk factors have a 3% year incidence of cardiac events, as would be expected with the high incidence of silent ischemia. In February 1998, the ADA published a consensus statement on the diagnosis of CAD in people with diabetes mellitus.[18] It was recommended (Figure 5-2) that asymptomatic diabetic patients with two or more risk factors for CAD or those beginning an exercise program should undergo an exercise stress testing. It was stated that asymptomatic diabetic patients with 1 or fewer risk factors don't need cardiac testing. However, these recommendations were based on the clinical judgment of a panel of experts rather than on data. Partial justification comes from Stamler et al.,[1] who demonstrated significant cardiac mortality in diabetic patients with two or more risk factors.

Annual follow-up (Table 5-1) is suggested to monitor the development or progression of risk

factors that would indicate the need for cardiac testing. If risk increases or symptoms change, reevaluation should be considered. Reevaluations should be considered every 2 to 3 years, depending on the actual annual risk of events.

Role of Stress Myocardial Perfusion Imaging in Asymptomatic Diabetic Patients

The value of stress MPI in asymptomatic patients is not established. Recent data presented by Miller et al.[31] from the Mayo Clinic suggested a high incidence of positive studies, including high-risk scans in 22%. However, the study is retrospective, and many patients may not have been completely asymptomatic. An important prospective study is being conducted at the time of this writing. The Detection of Ischemia in Asymptomatic Diabetics (DIAD)[32] is a multicenter prospective trial, Wackers, MD/PhD, Principal Investigator, in which 1,000 asymptomatic diabetic patients will be enrolled. An extensive history and battery of tests will be performed. The patients will be randomized to adenosine sestamibi SPECT imaging or usual care with a 2-year follow-up. This study will provide invaluable assistance in identifying which asymptomatic patients should be studied.

SUMMARY

Diabetes mellitus is associated with an increased risk of cardiovascular events. In this population, CAD often can be silent and more advanced at the time of diagnosis and may be associated with an unfavorable prognosis. Early intervention is important to prevent progression of disease and decrease the risk.

MPI and gated SPECT imaging provide perfusion and cardiac function data that have been of great value in the diagnosis and risk stratification of those patients. Prognosis has been validated clinically in diabetic patients. This information provided by MPI and gated SPECT has helped to direct patients to medical versus surgical intervention.

REFERENCES

1. Stamler J, Vaccaro O, Neaton JD, Wentworth D. Diabetes, other risk factors, and 12-year cardiovascular mortality for men screened in the multiple risk factor intervention trial. *Diabetes Care* 1993;16:434–444.
2. Uusitupa MI, Niskanen LK, Siitonen O, et al. Ten-year cardiovascular mortality in relation to risk factors and abnormalities in lipoprotein composition in type 2 (non-insulin-dependent) diabetic and non-diabetic subjects. *Diabetologia* 1993;36:1175–1184.
3. Mokdad AH, Ford ES, Bowman BA, et al. Diabetes trends in the U.S.: 1990–1998 [see comments]. *Diabetes Care* 2000;23(9):1278–1283.
4. Mokdad AH, Ford ES, Bowman BA, et al. The continuing increase of diabetes in the U.S. [letter; comment]. *Diabetes Care* 2001;24(2):412.
5. Hammond T, Tanguay JF, Bourassa MG. Management of coronary artery disease: Therapeutic options in patients with diabetes [Review] [144 refs]. *J Am Coll Cardiol* 2000;36(2):355–365.
6. Braunwald E, Antman EM, Beasley JW, et al. ACC/AHA guidelines for the management of patients with unstable angina and non-ST-segment elevation myocardial infarction. A report of the American College of Cardiology/American Heart Association Task Force on Practice Guidelines (Committee on the Management of Patients with Unstable Angina) [erratum appears in *J Am Coll Cardiol* 2001;38(1):294–295]. *J Am Coll Cardiol* 2000;36(3):970–1062.
7. Nesto RW, Phillips RT, Kett KG, et al. Angina and exertional myocardial ischemia in diabetic and nondiabetic patients: Assessment by exercise thallium scintigraphy [erratum appears in *Ann Intern Med* 1988;108(4):646]. *Ann Intern Med* 1988;108(2):170–175.
8. Laskey WK, Selzer F, Vlachos HA, et al. Comparison of in-hospital and one-year outcomes in patients with and without diabetes mellitus undergoing percutaneous catheter intervention. *Am J Cardiol* 2002;90:1062–1067.
9. Sniderman A, Michel C, Racine N. Heart disease in patients with diabetes mellitus [Review] [144 refs]. *J Clin Epidemiol* 1992;45(12):1357–1370.
10. Zuanetti G, Latini R, Maggioni AP, et al. Influence of diabetes on mortality in acute myocardial infarction: Data from the GISSI-2 study. *J Am Coll Cardiol* 1993;22(7):1788–1794.
11. Fava S, Azzopardi J, Muscat HA, Fenech FF. Factors that influence outcome in diabetic subjects with myocardial infarction. *Diabetes Care* 1993;16(12):1615–1618.
12. Gray RP, Yudkin JS, Patterson DL. Enzymatic evidence of impaired reperfusion in diabetic patients after thrombolytic therapy for acute myocardial infarction: A

13. role for plasminogen activator inhibitor? *Br Heart J* 1993;70(6):530–536.
13. Orlander PR, Goff DC, Morrissey M, et al. The relation of diabetes to the severity of acute myocardial infarction and post-myocardial infarction survival in Mexican–Americans and non-Hispanic whites. The Corpus Christi Heart Project. *Diabetes* 1994;43(7)897–902.
14. Stein B, Weintraub WS, Gebhart SP, et al. Influence of diabetes mellitus on early and late outcome after percutaneous transluminal coronary angioplasty. *Circulation* 1995;91(4):979–989.
15. Barsness GW, Peterson ED, Ohman EM, et al. Relationship between diabetes mellitus and long-term survival after coronary bypass and angioplasty. *Circulation* 1997;96(8):2551–2556.
16. The BARI Investigators. Influence of diabetes on 5-year mortality and morbidity in a randomized trial comparing CABG and PTCA in patients with multivessel disease: The Bypass Angioplasty Revascularization Investigation (BARI) [see comments]. *Circulation* 1997;96(6):1761–1769.
17. The BARI Investigators. Comparison of coronary bypass surgery with angioplasty in patients with multivessel disease. The Bypass Angioplasty Revascularization Investigation (BARI) Investigators [see comments] [erratum appears in *N Engl J Med* 1997;336(2):147]. *N Engl J Med* 1996;335(4):217–225.
18. American Diabetes Association. Consensus development conference on the diagnosis of coronary heart disease in people with diabetes. *Diabetes Care* 1998;21:1551–1559.
19. American Diabetes Association. Standards of medical care for patients with diabetes mellitus. *Diabetes Care* 1998;21:S23–S39.
20. Krolewski AS, Kosinski EJ, Warram JH, et al. Magnitude and determinants of coronary artery disease in juvenile-onset, insulin-dependent diabetes mellitus. *Am J Cardiol* 1987;59:750–755.
21. Janka HU. Increased cardiovascular morbidity and mortality in diabetes mellitus: Identification of the high risk patient [Review] [24 refs]. *Diabetes Res Clin Pract* 1996;30(Suppl):85–88.
22. Iskandrian AS, Heo J, Kong B, Lyons E. Effect of exercise level on the ability of thallium-201 tomographic imaging in detecting coronary artery disease: Analysis of 461 patients [see comments]. *J Am Coll Cardiol* 1989;14(6):1477–1486.
23. Heller GV, Ahmed I, Tilkemeier PL, et al. Influence of exercise intensity on the presence, distribution, and size of thallium-201 defects. *Am Heart J* 1992;123(4 Pt 1):909–916.
24. Paillole C, Ruiz J, Juliard JM, et al. Detection of coronary artery disease in diabetic patients. *Diabetologia* 1995;38(6):726–731.

25. Boudreau RJ, Strony JT, duCret RP, et al. Perfusion thallium imaging of type I diabetes patients with end stage renal disease: Comparison of oral and intravenous dipyridamole administration. *Radiology* 1990;175(1):103–105.

26. Bell DS, Yumuk VD. Low incidence of false-positive exercise thallium-201 scintigraphy in a diabetic population. *Diabetes Care* 1996;19(2):185–186.

27. Kang X, Berman DS, Lewin H, et al. Comparative ability of myocardial perfusion single-photon emission computed tomography to detect coronary artery disease in patients with and without diabetes mellitus. *Am Heart J* 1999;137(5):949–957.

28. Felsher J, Meissner MD, Hakki AH, et al. Exercise thallium imaging in patients with diabetes mellitus: Prognostic implications. *Arch Intern Med* 1987;147(2):313–317.

29. Kang X, Berman DS, Lewin HC, et al. Incremental prognostic value of myocardial perfusion single photon emission computed tomography in patients with diabetes mellitus. *Am Heart J* 1999;138(6 Pt 1):1025–1032.

30. Giri S, Shaw LJ, Murthy DR, et al. Impact of diabetes on the risk stratification using stress single-photon emission computed tomography myocardial perfusion imaging in patients with symptoms suggestive of coronary artery disease [see comments]. *Circulation* 2002;105(1):32–40.

31. Miller TD, Rajagopalan N, Hodge DO, et al. The yield of screening stress myocardial perfusion imaging in asymptomatic diabetics. *J Am Coll Cardiol* 2002 March: 163A.

32. Wackers FJ, Chyun DA, Inucchi SE, et al. Detection of Ischemia in Asymptomatic Diabetes (The DIAD Study) investigators. *J Am Coll Cardiol* 2003;76:411A.

CHAPTER 6

Assessment of Women

Andrea Fossati
Laura Ford-Mukkamala
Gary V. Heller

INTRODUCTION

Cardiovascular disease, including coronary artery disease (CAD) and stroke, is the leading cause of death in both men and women in the United States, with comparable morbidity and mortality. More women die from cardiovascular disease than from all cancers combined. CAD alone is the primary cause of death among American women, and accounts for over 250,000 deaths, or almost one third of all deaths per year.[1] The detection of heart disease in women presents an important challenge to the clinician.

THE PROFILE OF WOMEN WITH HEART DISEASE

There are well-described differences in the presentation of women and men with heart disease. Women develop angina 10 years later and sustain their first myocardial infarction (MI) 20 years later than men.[2] The incidence of CAD in women is age-related, and in the postmenopausal state approximates that of men.[3] This may reflect the loss of a cardioprotective effect of estrogen.[4,5]

Women share the major cardiac risk factors of hypertension, diabetes, high cholesterol, smoking, and family history with men, although their risk factor profiles differ.[4–7] At presentation, women have a greater number of risk factors and comorbid conditions. Fewer women survive their initial MI than men, with higher 30-day and 1-year mortality rates.[8,9] Women are more likely to sustain non-Q-wave and silent MIs and have a higher rate of reinfarction as well as heart failure post-MI.[8–10]

Differences have been demonstrated in referral patterns for women with suspected CAD. The greatest difference in referral rates is in the initial screening for CAD.[11,12] Pope et al.[13] performed a prospective emergency room study analyzing the factors that contribute to inappropriate discharges. Gender was one factor that was analyzed. Women < 55 years old tended to be discharged compared with men of the same age. This was attributed to the atypical symptoms that women commonly possess. Roger et al.[14] demonstrated differences in referral patterns when men and women presented to the emergency room for the first time with chest pain and were diagnosed with unstable angina. Unstable angina was defined as chest pain for ≥ 20 minutes, new exertional angina (Canadian Cardiovascular Society Class 3 or more), variant angina, or post-MI angina. Women were less likely to be referred to cardiac procedures in general, and less likely to be sent to cardiac catheterization. Women were found to have more atypical chest pain and were referred to gastrointestinal procedures more frequently than men (see Tables 6-1 and 6-2). From the point of a completed stress test, there is literature that supports no gender bias with referral to appropriate intervention following a positive stress imaging test.[15-17] As already demonstrated, women undergo fewer cardiac tests.

However, they are treated equally when the diagnosis of ischemia or acute MI is confirmed by noninvasive and invasive testing.

DIAGNOSTIC TESTING IN WOMEN

The first challenge in diagnosing heart disease in women is determining who to screen and how. Premenopausal women have a high prevalence of noncardiac chest pain.[18-19] In the Coronary Artery Surgery Study (CASS), 50% of women referred for coronary catheterization for chest pain had no significant coronary obstruction.[20,21] Women are more likely to have atypical symptoms of stable angina and acute coronary syndromes.[22] Table 6-3 illustrates criteria that are helpful in determining the likelihood of cardiac disease in these women, and Table 6-4 stratifies the likeli-

Table 6-1

Use of Cardiac Procedures Within 90 Days After Emergency Department Visit for Unstable Angina

Procedure	Men, %[a] (n = 1306)	Women, %[a] (n = 965)	Crude Relative Risk (95% CI) [b]	P Value	Adjusted Relative Risk (95% CI)[b]
Noninvasive Diagnostic Tests					
Any noninvasive test	74	62	1.27 (1.14–1.40)	< 0.001	1.21 (1.09–1.35)
Echocardiography and other resting tests[c]	35	36	0.96 (0.84–1.10)	0.57	1.06 (0.91–1.22)
Stress test	58	38	1.68 (1.48–1.90)	< 0.001	1.43 (1.26–1.63)
Noninvasive diagnostic tests only	34	39	0.84 (0.73–0.96)	0.01	0.85 (0.74–0.98)
Stress test only	21	18	1.17 (0.96–1.42)	0.11	1.01 (0.83–1.24)
Invasive Diagnostic Procedures					
Coronary angiography	50	33	1.72 (1.51–1.97)	< 0.001	1.59 (1.38–1.82)
Coronary angiography only	11	11	1.02 (0.79–1.31)	0.88	0.93 (0.72–1.21)
Noninvasive Test and Angiography					
	39	22	1.92 (1.64–2.26)	< 0.001	1.80 (1.53–2.12)

[a] Data presented as percentage of men and women who undergo the corresponding procedure.
[b] Relative risk is for men vs women; the adjusted relative risks are adjusted for age and Agency for Health Care Policy and Research risk category. CI indicates confidence interval.
[c] Other resting tests include resting radionuclide angiography, sestamibi study, and ultrafast computed tomography.

Table 6-2

Predictors of the Use of Any Cardiac Procedure Within 90 Days After Emergency Department Visit[a]

Variable	Crude Relative Risk (95% CI)[b]	P Value	Adjusted Relative Risk (95% CI)[b]	P Value
Male sex	1.34 (1.22–1.47)	< 0.001	1.24 (1.11–1.37)	< 0.001
Age	0.99 (0.989–0.994)	< 0.001	0.99 (0.986–0.992)	< 0.001
Typical chest pain	1.21 (1.08–1.36)	0.001	1.23 (1.09–1.38)	< 0.001
ST-segment depression	1.29 (1.08–1.55)	0.005	1.25 (1.03–1.52)	0.02
Elevated CPK	1.44 (1.28–1.61)	< 0.001	1.49 (1.32–1.69)	< 0.001
AHCPR Intermediate risk	1.08 (0.93–1.25)	0.31	1.18 (1.00–1.38)	0.049
AHCPR high risk	1.13 (0.95–1.34)	0.16	1.22 (1.01–1.48)	0.045

[a] CI indicates confidence interval; CPK, creatine phosphokinase; and AHCPR, Agency for Health Care Policy and Research (the low-risk category is the reference level).
[b] Relative risk is for men vs women; the adjusted relative risks are adjusted for all variables listed in the first column.

Table 6-3

Determinants of Coronary Heart Disease in Women with Chest Pain

Major

Typical angina pectoris

Postmenopausal status without hormone replacement

Diabetes mellitus

Peripheral vascular disease

Intermediate

Hypertension

Smoking

Lipoprotein abnormalities, especially low HDL cholesterol levels

Minor

Age > 65 years

Obesity, especially central obesity

Sedentary lifestyle

Family history of coronary heart disease

Other risk factors for coronary heart disease (e.g., psychosocial or hemostatic)

hood of disease based on the presence of criteria. The prevalence of coronary disease in these women has been shown to increase with age and presence of classic features of angina[18] (Figure 6-1). Due to the combination of atypical angina and the low prevalence of CAD in premenopausal women, angina alone is a poor predictor of heart disease in women, but becomes of increasing importance with age and the presence of risk factors.

Exercise stress testing is the most common screening test used to detect CAD. Table 6-5 summarizes the low sensitivity and specificity of this modality in women.[19,23–29] Women have a high rate of false-positive responses during exercise testing.[24,25,29,30] This may be attributed to the lower pretest likelihood of heart disease in premenopausal women, altered exercise capacity, and more comorbid conditions at the time of presentation, as well as baseline gender differences in the normal physiologic response to exercise.[30,31] Women are more likely to have single-vessel disease, which is less detectable by stress testing than the multiple-vessel or left main disease found more commonly in men.[18–19,32]

Although a positive stress test is a poor predictor of coronary disease in women, the nega-

Table 6-4

Use of Diagnostic Tests in Women with Chest Pain

Likelihood of Coronary Heart Disease	Initial Test	Subsequent Test
Low (< 20%)	None indicated	None indicated
No major and ≤ 1 intermediate or ≤ 2 minor determinants		
Moderate (20–80%)	Routine ETT	
One major or multiple intermediate and minor determinants	Negative	None indicated
	Inconclusive	Further testing indicated; selection must be individualized
	Positive	Imaging test or catheterization
	Imaging ETT	
	Negative	None indicated
	Inconclusive	Catheterization
	Positive	Catheterization
High (> 80%)	Routine ETT	
≥ 2 Major or 1 major plus > 1 intermediate and minor determinants	Negative	None indicated; observe patient carefully
	Inconclusive	Catheterization
	Positive	Catheterization
	Imaging ETT	None indicated

ETT = exercise tolerance test.

tive predictive value of a normal exercise test is high.[28] Therefore, exercise stress testing may be used to exclude the presence of CAD in women who achieve target heart rate with normal electrocardiographic (ECG) and blood pressure responses, particularly in a low likelihood cohort.

RADIONUCLIDE STRESS IMAGING IN WOMEN

Radionuclide perfusion imaging is an important technique to improve the diagnostic accuracy of stress testing in men and women. It allows assessment of perfusion, viability, and ventricular function and provides prognostic information regarding future events and patient outcomes. The addition of radionuclide imaging improves the sensitivity and specificity in the detection of

coronary disease compared to exercise testing alone.[19,25,33–36] The higher specificity is particularly useful in identifying women with false-positive exercise tests[19] (see Figure 6-2). The highest accuracy for exercise radionuclide stress testing has been found in women with multiple-vessel disease compared to those with single-vessel disease, although radionuclide imaging does have a higher sensitivity than exercise stress testing in the detection of single-vessel disease.[19,37]

The use of pharmacologic stress instead of exercise is an important alternative in imaging women with limited exercise capacities. Both dipyridamole and adenosine stress have been found to be comparable to exercise imaging in primarily male populations.[38,39] In a prospective study of 201 women, adenosine SPECT imaging had a 95% sensitivity, 66% specificity, and 85%

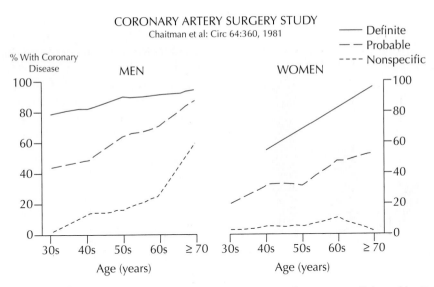

Figure 6-1. Prevalence of coronary disease according to age, sex, and symptoms. (Adapted by D. Waters, MD, from Coronary Artery Surgery Study (CASS) data in Chaitman et al.[18] with permission.

accuracy in the detection of coronary stenosis > 70% regardless of presenting symptoms, prior history of MI, or pretest probability of coronary disease.[39] Dobutamine imaging has been reported to have a slightly lower overall sensitivity of 82% and specificity of 73%.[39]

Table 6-5

Women and Heart Disease Ex Test

Study, year	Women (n =)	Men (n =)	Angiographic endpoint (degree of stenosis)	Sensitivity (%)	Specificity (%)
Detry et al., 1979	47	231	≥ 50	80 in women / 87 in men	63 in women / 74 in men
Weiner et al., 1979	580	1465	≥ 70 or ≥ 50 left main	76 in women / 80 in men	64 in women / 74 in men
Barolsky et al., 1979	92	85	≥ 75	60 in women / 65 in men	68 in women / 89 in men
Friedman et al., 1982	60	NA	≥ 70	32	41
Guiteras et al., 1982	112	NA	≥ 70	79	66
Hung et al., 1984	92	NA	≥ 70 or ≥ 50 left main	73	59
Morise et al., 1995*	284	504	≥ 50	47 ± 5 in women / 56 ± 3 in men	73 ± 3 in women / 81 ± 3 in men
Miller et al., 2001*	205	838	≥ 70 or ≥ 50 left main	53 in women / 63 in men	69 in women / 74 in men

*subgroup analysis

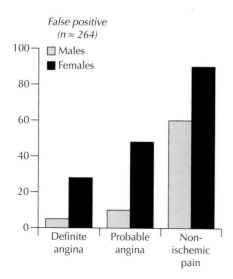

CHALLENGES OF RADIONUCLIDE STRESS IMAGING IN WOMEN

The quality of radionuclide imaging is affected by factors that are well documented.[42–45] Two factors prevalent in women are breast attenuation and small heart size.

Breast attenuation occurs in approximately 25% of female patients undergoing myocardial perfusion imaging (MPI).[19,25,34,40–44] Radionuclide imaging is performed with low-energy radioactivity. As a result, any tissue between the heart and the camera will result in fewer counts. If this soft tissue artifact is breast, it can appear as a defect in the heart in a patient without CAD. This reduces the specificity of the procedure.

Several methods have been proposed to minimize breast attenuation defects.[40,43,44] We have found that the most practical approach is to begin with a review of the unprocessed photon images. These raw images resemble a ghost image

of the patient and may be used to assess body shape, including the size and location of breast tissue relative to the heart. Following this, standard image interpretation is performed. If the defect correlates with an area of soft tissue on the raw images and the wall motion is normal with gated single photon emission computed tomography (SPECT), then it is determined to be artifact and not CAD. In centers using a technetium-based imaging agent, gated images are used to evaluate the wall motion of that area and are helpful in determining presence or absence of disease. The use of technetium-99 imaging agents and ECG gating has been found to increase the accuracy of detection of coronary disease in women.[45,46]

Heart size (specifically, left ventricular chamber size) has been found to affect the accuracy of thallium-201 SPECT myocardial perfusion imaging. In a prospective study of 323 patients (127 women and 196 men), 67% of women and only 20% of men had small chamber sizes. The higher accuracy of imaging in men appeared to be due to their larger heart size, with no gender differences reported for similar-size hearts.[47] This study introduced smaller heart size as a factor affecting thallium-201 stress imaging in women; the effect of heart size on technetium-99m stress imaging is under current investigation.

OUTCOMES AND MANAGEMENT OF WOMEN FOLLOWING STRESS IMAGING

Men and women are both benefited by MPI. There is improved accuracy in diagnosis as well as prognostication for future events.[48,49–54] This is covered in great depth in Chapter 19.

In addition, cost-effectiveness is an issue when comparing genders. An ischemic approach using MPI outweighs an anatomic approach in women with an intermediate probability. The presence of a significant reversible defect with progression to coronary angiography would be most cost-effective given the atypical features of women and the decreased incidence in the first five decades compared to men.[55]

CONCLUSION

In summary, women should be approached clinically with reference to their likelihood of CAD. Low likelihood is not appropriate for stress testing, whereas intermediate and high likelihood are appropriate for diagnostic and prognostic evaluation, respectively. Exercise tolerance testing by itself is helpful if the study is negative, but can be misleading when it is positive in women with atypical symptoms. MPI improves the sensitivity as well as the specificity in diagnosing CAD, and represents an important adjunct in the screening process. If exercise is not feasible, then pharmacologic stress is an appropriate alternative. Breast attenuation poses a unique problem in interpreting images in women. However, review of the whole study as well as new software currently being instituted will decrease the number of false-positive tests due to soft tissue attenuation.

REFERENCES

1. Harvard Medical School. Coronary heart disease, *Women's Health Watch* 1994;1:6.
2. Kannel WB, Feinleib M. Natural history of angina pectoris in the Framingham study: Prognosis and survival. *Am J Cardiol* 1972;29:154–163.
3. Castelli WP. Cardiovascular disease in women. *Am J Obstet Gynecol* 1988;158:1553–1560.
4. Eaker ED, et al. AHA medical/scientific statement: Cardiovascular disease in women. *Circulation* 1993;88(4):1999–2009.
5. Rich-Edwards JW, et al. The primary prevention of coronary heart disease in women. *N Engl J Med* 1995;332(26):1758–1766.
6. American Heart Association. *Heart and Stroke Facts: 1996 Statistical Supplement.* Dallas: American Heart Association, 1996.
7. Wenger NK. Coronary heart disease in women: An overview (myths, misperceptions, and missed opportunities). *Cardiovasc Rev Rep* 1993;14:24–41.
8. Kannel WB, Sorlie P, McNamara. Prognosis after initial myocardial infarction: The Framingham study. *Am J Cardiol* 1979;44:53–59.
9. Lerner DJ, Kannel WB. Patterns of coronary heart disease morbidity and mortality in the sexes: A 26-year follow-up of the Framingham population. *Am Heart J* 1986;111(2):383–390.
10. Tofler GH, et al. Effects of gender and race on prognosis after myocardial infarction: Adverse prognosis for women, particularly black women. *J Am Coll Cardiol* 1987;9(3):473–482.
11. Shaw LJ, et al. Gender differences in the noninvasive evaluation and management of patients with suspected coronary artery disease. *Ann Intern Med* 1994; 120(7):559–566.
12. Steingart RM, et al. Sex differences in the management of coronary artery disease. *N Engl J Med* 1991; 325(4):226–230.
13. Pope J, Aufderheide T, Ruthazer R, et al. Missed diagnoses of acute cardiac ischemia in the emergency department. *N Engl J Med* 2000;342(16).
14. Roger V, Farkouh M, Weston S, et al. Sex differences in evaluation and outcome of unstable angina. *JAMA* 2000;283(5).
15. Hachamovitch R, et al. Gender-related differences in clinical management after exercise nuclear testing. *J Am Coll Cardiol* 1995;26(6):1457–1464.
16. Lauer MS, et al. Gender and referral for coronary angiography after treadmill thallium testing. *Am J Cardiol* 1996;78:278–283.
17. Travin MI, et al. Relationship of gender to physician use of test results and to the prognostic value of stress technetium-99m sestamibi myocardial SPECT scintigraphy. *Am Heart J* 1997;134(1):73–82.
18. Chaitman BR, et al. Angiographic prevalence of high-risk coronary artery disease in patient subsets (CASS). *Circulation* 1981;64(2):360–367.
19. Hung J, et al. Noninvasive diagnostic test choices for the evaluation of coronary artery disease in women: A multivariate comparison of cardiac fluoroscopy, exercise electrocardiography and exercise thallium myocardial perfusion scintigraphy. *J Am Coll Cardiol* 1984; 4(1):8–16.
20. Kennedy JW, et al. The clinical spectrum of coronary artery disease and its surgical and medical management, 1974–1979, the Coronary Artery Surgery Study. *Circulation* 1982;66(Suppl III):16–23.
21. Wenger NK. Coronary heart disease in women: An overview (myths, misperceptions, and missed opportunities). *Cardiovasc Rev Rep* 1993;14:24–41.
22. Douglas PS, Ginsburg GS. The evaluation of chest pain in women. *N Engl J Med* 1996;334(20):1311–1315.
23. Barolsky SM, et al. Differences in electrocardiographic response to exercise of women and men: A non-Bayesian factor. *Circulation* 1979;60(5):1021–1027.
24. Detry JM, et al. Diagnostic value of history and maximal exercise electrocardiography in men and women suspected of coronary heart disease. *Circulation* 1977;56(5):756–761.
25. Friedman TD, et al. Exercise thallium-201 myocardial scintigraphy in women: Correlation with coronary arteriography. *Am J Cardiol* 1982;49:1632–1637.
26. Gordon EE. Noninvasive diagnosis of coronary artery disease in women. *Cardio* 1992 December: pp. 29–32, 37–39, 58.
27. Guiteras P, et al. Diagnostic accuracy of exercise ECG lead systems in clinical subsets of women. *Circulation* 1982;65(7):1465–1474.

28. Sketch MH, et al. Significant sex differences in the correlation of electrocardiographic exercise testing and coronary arteriograms. *Am J Cardiol* 1975;36(2):169–173.

29. Wenger NK. Coronary heart disease: diagnostic decision making. In Douglas P (ed.). *Cardiovascular Health and Disease in Women.* Philadelphia: WB Saunders, 1993: 25–42.

30. Gibbons RJ, et al. Ejection fraction response to exercise in patients with chest pain and normal coronary arteriograms. *Circulation* 1981;64(5):952–957.

31. Higginbotham MB, et al. Sex-related differences in the normal cardiac response to upright exercise. *Circulation* 1984;70(3):357–366.

32. Hlatky MA, et al. Factors affecting sensitivity and specificity of exercise electrocardiography. *Am J Med* 1984;77:64–71.

33. Bailey IK, et al. Thallium-201 myocardial perfusion imaging at rest and during exercise. *Circulation* 1977;55(1):79–87.

34. Goodgold HM, et al. Improved interpretation of exercise Tl-201 myocardial perfusion scintigraphy in women: Characterization of breast attenuation artifacts. *Radiology* 1987;165(2):361–366.

35. Melin JA, et al. Alternative diagnostic strategies for coronary artery disease in women: demonstration of the usefulness and efficiency of probability analysis. *Circulation* 1985;71(3):535–542.

36. Okada RD, et al. Exercise radionuclide imaging approaches to coronary artery disease. *Am J Cardiol* 1980;46:1188–1204.

37. Kaul S, et al. Comparison of exercise electrocardiography and quantitative thallium imaging for one-vessel coronary artery disease. *Am J Cardiol* 1985;56:257–261.

38. Gupta NC, et al. Comparison of adenosine and exercise thallium-201 single photon emission computed tomography (SPECT) myocardial perfusion imaging. *J Am Coll Cardiol* 1992;19(2):248–257.

39. Mahmarian JJ, Verani MS. Myocardial perfusion imaging during pharmacologic stress testing. *Cardiology Clinics* 1994;12(2):223–245.

40. DePuey EG, Garcia EV: Optimal specificity of thallium-201 SPECT through recognition of imaging artifacts. *J Nucl Med* 1989;30(4):441–449.

41. Dunn RF, et al. The inconsistent pattern of thallium defects: A clue to the false positive perfusion scintigram. *Am J Cardiol* 1981;48:224–232.

42. Wackers FJ. Artifacts in planar SPECT myocardial perfusion imaging. *Am J Cardiac Imaging* 1992;6(1):42–58.

43. Wackers FJ. Diagnostic pitfalls of myocardial perfusion imaging in women. *J Myocardial Ischemia* 1992;4(10):23–37.

44. Johnstone DE, et al. Effect of patient positioning on left lateral thallium-201 myocardial images. *J Nucl Med* 1979;20(3):183–188.

45. DePuey EG, Rozanski A: Using gated technetium-99m-sestamibi SPECT to characterize fixed myocardial defects as infarct or artifact. *J Nucl Med* 1995; 36(6):952–955.

46. Taillefer R, et al. Comparative diagnostic accuracy of thallium-201 and Tc-99m sestamibi SPECT imaging (perfusion and ECG-gated SPECT) in detecting coronary artery disease in women. *J Am Coll Cardiol* 1997;29:69–77.

47. Hansen CL, Crabbe D, Rubin S: Lower diagnostic accuracy of thallium-201 SPECT myocardial perfusion imaging in women: An effect of smaller chamber size. *J Am Coll Cardiol* 1996;28(5):1214–1219.

48. Amanullah AM, et al. Adenosine technetium-99m sestamibi myocardial perfusion SPECT in women: Diagnostic efficacy in detection of coronary artery disease. *J Am Coll Cardiol* 1996;27(4):803–809.

49. Chae SC, et al. Identification of extensive coronary artery disease in women by exercise single-photon emission computed tomographic (SPECT) thallium imaging. *J Am Coll Cardiol* 1993;21(6):1305–1311.

50. Fintel DJ, et al. Improved diagnostic performance of exercise thallium-201 single photon emission computed tomography over planar imaging in the diagnosis of coronary artery disease: a receiver operating characteristic analysis. *J Am Coll Cardiol* 1989;13(3):600–612.

51. Geleijnse ML, et al. Prognostic significance of normal dobutamine–atropine stress sestamibi scintigraphy in women with chest pain. *Am J Cardiol* 1996;77:1057–1061.

52. Hachamovitch R, et al. Effective risk stratification using exercise myocardial perfusion SPECT in women: Gender-related differences in prognostic nuclear testing. *J Am Coll Cardiol* 1996;28(1):24–44.

53. Heller GV, Brown KA: Prognosis of acute and chronic coronary artery disease by myocardial perfusion imaging. *Cardiol Clin* 1994;12(2):271–287.

54. Travin MI, Katz MS, et al. Accuracy of dipyridamole SPECT imaging in identifying individual coronary stenoses and multivessel disease in women versus men. *J Nucl Cardiol* 2000;7:213–220.

55. Miller DD, et al. Cost analysis of stress myocardial perfusion imaging in 4,638 women with stable angina: Comparison to a strategy of direct coronary angiography. *J Nucl Med* 1996 June; 264 (Abstract).

CHAPTER 7

Acute Rest Myocardial Perfusion Imaging in the Emergency Department

Muthu Velusamy

Asad Rizvi

Gary V. Heller

INTRODUCTION

It has been estimated that over 7 million patients present annually to the emergency department (ED) with symptoms suggestive of coronary artery disease (CAD).[1] In those patients without CAD, admission to the hospital is not necessary and may strain bed resources for the patients in need of acute care. On the other hand, patients with acute coronary syndrome (ACS) have a high morbidity and mortality. If the symptoms are classic and accompanied by diagnostic electrocardiographic (ECG) changes (new ST-segment elevation, ST-segment depression, etc.), the identification of ACS is straightforward and admission and therapy is warranted. However, in the absence of diagnostic ECG changes either with or without classic symptoms, the decision to admit or discharge the patient is far more difficult and complex. The clinical history and ECG itself (if nondiagnostic) do not serve as sufficient discriminators for optimal clinical decision making. Thus, many patients who do not have ACS

are hospitalized unnecessarily and those with ACS are discharged inappropriately. Recently, the use of acute rest myocardial perfusion imaging (ARMPI) has been developed to assist in the triage decision. This chapter will evaluate the role of ARMPI in the management of ED patients.

BACKGROUND

Pathophysiology of Acute Coronary Syndrome

ACS comprises a spectrum of presentations, including ST elevation myocardial infarction (MI), non-ST elevation MI, and unstable angina (UA). The hallmark of ACS is the rupture or erosion of vulnerable atherosclerotic plaque(s) with associated occlusive or nonocclusive thrombus formation, with resultant myocardial ischemia and/or injury. The evolution is very complex, with interaction of the vessel wall, coagulation system, and inflammatory agents, culminating in ACS.[2-4] The clinical result is quite variable from spontaneous resolution of the thrombus and healing of the plaque to extensive MI, cardiogenic shock, and sudden cardiac death.

Clinical Presentation and Triage

Of all the patients presenting to the ED with chest pain, about 95% do not have ECG evidence of evolving Q-wave myocardial infarction, and only about 20% will ultimately have evidence of unstable angina or non-Q-wave myocardial infarction.[5] The initial triage of these patients involves three important goals, as prioritized in Figure 7-1. The primary goal is to identify ACS for admission and appropriate therapy. The second goal is to identify patients with CAD, at high risk for short-term cardiac events, who should be admitted. The third goal is to identify patients suitable for discharge and outpatient evaluation, and a large percentage of patients actually fall in this category. If myocardial ischemia is considered to be unlikely, patients should be evaluated for nonischemic cardiac conditions causing chest pain for appropriate therapy or discharge from the ED. Clinical indicators and ECGs are useful when they identify patients with acute myocardial infarction (AMI) and UA, but a large number of patients have nondiagnostic ECG[6] and clinical features resulting in unnecessary admissions and escalation of cost. Poor accuracy in the clinical diagnosis of noncardiac chest pain in the ED, inability of initial cardiac enzyme markers to identify all ACS, high morbidity and mortality associated with the missed diagnosis, and discharge of patients with ACS coupled with the litigation risks have led to a low threshold for admission of these patients. The majority of the admitted patients with chest pain do not have evidence for AMI, or ischemia (in a study by Pope et al.,[6] only 17% of the 10,689 patients suspected to have ACS ultimately met the criteria for acute cardiac ischemia and up to 6% of patients discharged from ED have missed myocardial infarctions.[7–9] Patients with AMI who are mistakenly discharged from the ED have a very high short-term mortality rate of about 25%,[8] and the risk-adjusted mortality was twice that of hospitalized patients.[6] Hence, additional tools are required for risk stratification to avoid unnecessary admission and inappropriate discharge.

Diagnostic Tools

Figure 7-2 illustrates the potential and evolving diagnostic tests (many of them not validated for

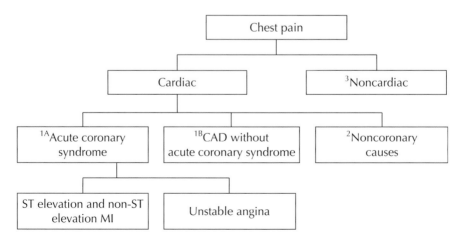

Figure 7-1.   Evaluation of chest pain: Goals of initial triage in the ED. Nontraumatic chest pain.
ED = emergency department; CAD = coronary artery disease; MI = myocardial infarction. Serial numbers signify the priority in triaging the patients with chest pain in the ED.

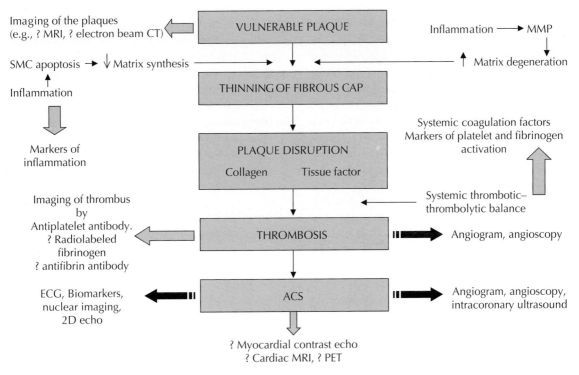

Figure 7-2. Potential diagnostic tools in ACS. ACS = acute coronary syndrome; MRI = magnetic resonance imaging; CT = computed tomography; SMC = smooth muscle cell; MMP = matrix metalloproteinases; PET = positron emission tomography.

➡ Ideal/potential diagnostic tool based on the pathophysiology

➡ Practically available tests

clinical use) based on the ideal pathophysiologic approach for an earlier diagnosis of ACS. A variety of methods are utilized currently, including clinical risk stratification models, rapid laboratory and bedside biomarker assays,[10,11] two-dimensional echocardiography (ECHO), ARMPI, comprehensive diagnostic 9-hour evaluation (Heart ER Program),[12] rapid rule out protocol in the ED,[13] chest pain centers with accelerated protocols,[14] and a comprehensive clinical strategy (Acute Cardiac Team Strategy, which involves assigning five levels of risk categories and utilizing ARMPI in low- and moderate-risk groups) for the evaluation and triage of the patient with chest pain.[15]

Many of these methods have significant limitations in the accurate diagnosis of the etiology of the chest pain.[16] Several clinical risk stratification models[17–19] aid in initial triage, but they have not gained wide acceptance in the decision-making process. While serial ECG performed over 2 to 3 days has a better accuracy in diagnosing AMI, a single ECG at the initial presentation is less sensitive, as only 35 to 60% of patients with AMI have diagnostic changes.[20,21] Although serial cardiac enzymes show excellent sensitivity in the diagnosis of AMI, the use of single measurement as a guide to triage is not reliable except in those who had prolonged (> 8–10 hours) symptoms before presentation. Elevated troponin levels in suspected ACS identify short-term adverse cardiovascular events,[22] but the cardiac enzymes have inherent limitations in diagnosing all acute coronary syndromes and CAD not accompanied by ongoing or recent myocyte injury, and only 22 to 36% of patients with unstable angina have elevated troponin, limiting its application to all patients with chest pain.[10] Hence, the indiscriminate use of troponin in all patients with suspected ACS has been challenged.[23]

Echocardiographic imaging for chest pain evaluation in the ED is promising, but it is limited by the need for active chest pain at the time of imaging and the need for 24-hour availability of highly trained technical staff.[24,25] The presence of wall motion abnormalities due to prior MI, as well as conduction abnormalities (bundle branch block and pacemaker) and poor echocardiographic windows in some patients due to body habitus, are limitations of this procedure. While newer technologies such as harmonic imaging and contrast echocardiography will improve

some of the limitations, these resources are not available in the majority of the facilities.

Accelerated chest pain unit protocols and early exercise stress testing[26] have been validated, but the timely evaluation of these patients is restricted by the need for documentation of no myocardial necrosis, inability to perform adequate exercise by a certain proportion of patients, and personnel availability. A conceptual model depicting the practical role of diagnostic modalities in the spectrum of chest pain syndrome is shown in Figure 7-3.

Rationale for ARMPI

In the ischemic cascade,[27] myocardial perfusion heterogeneity occurs before the development of left ventricular dysfunction, ECG changes, chest pain, and myocardial necrosis. Therefore, nuclear imaging can identify areas of myocardial ischemia and infarction long before biochemical markers of myocardial necrosis appear in serum. Consequently, ARMPI is increasingly used for an early and accurate diagnosis of myocardial ischemia in

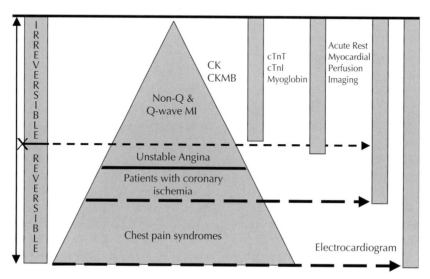

Use of markers and ECG in the spectrum of chest pain. CK = creatine kinase, cTnT = cardiac troponin T, cTnI = Cardiac troponin I.

Figure 7-3.   Diagnostic modalities in chest pain syndromes. Modified from Duca et al.[61] with permission.

patients presenting to the ED with chest pain and nondiagnostic ECG changes.

Current Approach Using ARMPI

The current practice in the evaluation of chest pain with suspected myocardial ischemia is to use the ECG to choose the initial management pathway.[28] When diagnostic changes are present, the patient is admitted and therapy begun. If the ECG is nondiagnostic with ongoing chest pain or the patient has a pain-free interval of less than 2 hours, ARMPI will be adjunctive in diagnosing the etiology of the chest pain with the biomarkers serving a complementary role. If the study is abnormal, consistent with either UA or AMI, the patient is admitted. If the study is normal, patients can often be safely discharged because of a very high negative predictive value.

ACUTE REST MYOCARDIAL PERFUSION IMAGING

History

Nuclear imaging was first used in the detection of MI more than 30 years ago by using various isotopes including rubidium and cesium.[29–31] Thallium 201 (Tl-201) was applied for the noninvasive identification of AMI by Wackers et al. in 1975[32] and subsequently reported a sensitivity of 96%.[33] Maseri et al.[34] demonstrated the perfusion defects with Tl-201 in variant angina when injected during ST elevation, following which Wackers et al. also identified Tl-201 imaging to be clinically useful in the evaluation of unstable angina. Tl-201 was shown to identify patients likely to have a complicated hospital course, as well as its capability to risk stratify patients with nondiagnostic ECG, admitted to exclude MI.[35] Other studies have confirmed the utility of Tl-201 in AMI as well as UA (Table 7-1).[36–39]

Imaging with Technetium Agents

Although pioneering studies demonstrated the value of ARMPI in ACS decades earlier, the interest and implementation increased in the last several years because of the pressure to decrease unnecessary admissions in an increasingly cost-conscious medical environment. However, a serious limitation of Tl-201 is the characteristic of redistribution; because of this, imaging must be begun immediately or ischemia is missed. Thus, technetium-based imaging agents (sestamibi, tetrofosmin) that do not have clinically significant redistribution are preferred. Consequently, imaging can be performed up to several hours after technetium 99m (Tc-99m) administration, allowing patient stabilization without the loss of sensitivity. Tc-99m with its higher energy profile and less attenuation also has the advantage of higher-quality images compared with Tl-201. A clinical example of sestamibi perfusion images from a 60-year-old male with atypical chest pain, injected during symptoms, is shown in Figure 7-4. He had persistent symptoms over 3 hours, despite a nondiagnostic ECG, and negative enzymes. The images revealed a defect in the anterolateral and anteroapical areas consistent with acute ischemia, which was subsequently confirmed by coronary angiography. Several investigations demonstrating the utility of Tc-99m sestamibi or tetrofosmin in ACS have been published and are listed in Table 7-2.[15,20,40–45]

Clinical Trials

In 1991, Bilodeau et al.[20] were the first to report one of the most important perfusion studies for the diagnostic ability of Tc-99m sestamibi single photon emission computed tomography (SPECT) imaging for CAD in 45 high-risk patients hospitalized with the clinical suspicion of UA without a history of prior MI. The SPECT studies obtained after injection of 25 to 30 mCi Tc-99m sestamibi during an episode of spontaneous chest pain showed a sensitivity of 96% and a specificity of 79% for the detection of CAD defined as ≥ 50% luminal diameter reduction by coronary angiography performed between 1 and 9 days of the initial evaluation. These findings were vastly superior to the clinical and ECG

Table 7-1

Acute Rest Myocardial Perfusion: Studies with Thallium-201

Study	Year	No	Cardiac event rates %		Normal	Abnormal	Criteria/Patient Population
			Sensi- tivity %	Speci- ficity %			
Myocardial Infarction							
Wackers et al.[32]	1975	10	100	—	—	—	2–5 days from MI
Wackers et al.[33]	1976	200	100	—	—	—	< 6 hours of symptom onset
Ritchie et al.[36]	1978	145	85		—		Three centers, mean 5.4 days
Unstable Angina							
Maseri et al.[34]	1976	6	100	—	—	—	Patients with variant angina, injected during ST elevation
Wackers et al.[37]	1978	56	50	—	—	—	Total of 98 patients injected 0–18 hours, 50% sensitivity for those injected within 6 hours of last angina
Brown et al.[38]	1983	31	100	—	—	—	Patients with unstable angina
		34	12	—	—	—	Patients with stable angina
Freeman et al.[39]	1989	66	82	—	32	61	Patients with unstable angina, mean 5.6 hours from last angina. Coronary artery stenosis ≥ 50%

data, the latter of which is illustrated in Figure 7-5. With the patient in the pain-free state, the radionuclide study had a lowered sensitivity of 65% but a similar specificity of 84%. Thus, ARMPI is feasible, is superior to clinical and ECG data, and has a high diagnostic accuracy for detecting and localizing CAD in patients with spontaneous chest pain, if injection is made during symptoms.

A more common presentation in the ED is patients with chest pain but normal or nondiagnostic ECG changes. Varetto et al.[40] evaluated 64 patients with chest pain lasting ≥ 30 minutes within 12 hours of ED presentation. All 30 patients with abnormal perfusion images underwent angiography, and of the 34 patients with normal images, 64% underwent catheterization and the remaining 36% had stress sestamibi after

48 hours of admission. With end points of CAD or MI, the results revealed a sensitivity of 100%, a specificity of 92%, and a negative predictive value of 100% for ARMPI. All the patients with negative perfusion images remained event free for up to 18 months after discharge. The authors concluded that this is a powerful technique to identify patients with ischemic chest pain, with important implications on short- and long-term patient management.

In a similar study, Hilton et al.[41] evaluated the practicality and short-term predictive value of ARMPI in 102 ED patients with typical angina and normal or nondiagnostic ECG changes. However, all patients were injected during symptoms and the hospital course was followed for cardiac death, nonfatal MI, coronary angioplasty,

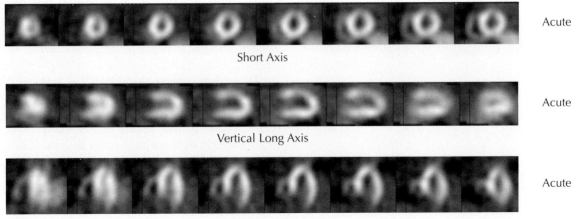

Short Axis

Acute

Vertical Long Axis

Acute

Horizontal Long Axis

Acute

Figure 7-4. Acute rest images. A 60-year-old male with atypical chest pain, persistent over 3 hours, nondiagnostic ECG, negative enzymes, injected during symptoms. Anterior, anteroapical, and anterolateral defects are seen.

Table 7-2

Acute Rest Myocardial Perfusion: Studies with Technetium Agents

Study	Year	No	Tracer	Sensi-tivity %	Speci-ficity %	NPV %	Normal D/MI%	Normal Revasc %	Abnormal D/MI%	Abnormal Revasc %	End Point
Bilodeau[20]	1991	45	Tc Mibi	96	79	94					Cath
Varetto[40]	1993	64	Tc Mibi	100	92	100	0	0	43	17	Cath
Hilton[41]	1994	102	Tc Mibi	94	83	99	0	1	71[a]		Clinical
Varetto[42]	1994	27	Tc Mibi	100	93	99					Cath
Hilton[b,43]	1996	150	Tc Mibi	100	78	99	0	0.01	53	34	Clinical
Kontos[44]	1997	532	Tc Mibi	93	71	99	0.6	3	15	27	Clinical
Tatum[15]	1997	438	Tc Mibi	100	78	100	0	3	7	32	Clinical
Heller[45]	1998	357	Tc Tetro	90	60	99	0.9	5	12	16	Clinical

Cath = coronary angiogram; D/MI = death or myocardial infarction; Revasc = coronary revascularization; Nu = number of patients studied; NPV = negative predictive value; Tc Mibi = technetium 99m sestamibi; Tc Tetro = technetium-99m tetrofosmin.
Table modified from Duncan & Heller[49] with permission.
[a] Combined end point D/MI/Revasc.
[b] Using MI as only end point.

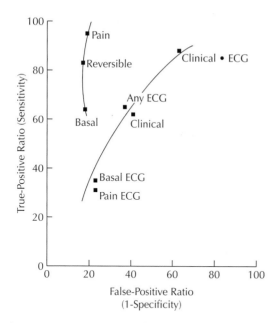

Figure 7-5. Comparison of ARMPI to clinical risks and ECG. Demonstrates high sensitivity for ARMPI compared to clinical criteria and ECG for the diagnosis of significant coronary artery disease, particularly when injected during pain, and it also has a high specificity. Basal = sestamibi SPECT during pain-free state; Pain = sestamibi SPECT during chest pain; Reversible = presence of reversible sestamibi SPECT defect; Clinical = clinical criteria; Pain ECG = electrocardiogram during pain; Basal ECG = electrocardiogram between episodes of pain; Any ECG = any electrocardiographic changes. Reprinted from Bilodeau[20] with permission.

coronary surgery, or coronary thrombolysis. The ECG was classified as normal or nondiagnostic, and the clinical risks were categorized into low-, intermediate-, and high-risk groups. When the predictive ability of ARMPI results were compared with ECG variables alone or combined clinical and ECG risk status, the imaging group had the best risk stratification. The normal scan identified a very low event rate of 2% compared to a very high event rate of 71% for an abnormal scan, as demonstrated in Figure 7-6. The sensitivity, specificity, and overall accuracy for the ab-

normal scan for predicting cardiac events are 94%, 83%, and 85%. With only MI as an end point, an abnormal scan the sensitivity rose to 100%, yielding a negative predictive value of 99.8%.

These data suggest that ARMPI is a practical technique to distinguish among low-, intermediate-, and very high-adverse cardiac events in ED patients with typical angina and nondiagnostic ECG. Patients with normal images are candidates for early ED discharge based on the negative predictive value of 99%.

Kontos et al.[44] evaluated 532 consecutive patients presenting to the ED with chest pain and nondiagnostic ECG for the prediction of adverse cardiac events by ARMPI with gating. Positive image, defined as perfusion defect associated with wall motion abnormality, was the only multivariate predictor of MI ($p < 0.001$, odds ratio − 33) and the most important independent predictor of subsequent revascularization/MI ($p < 0.0001$, odds ratio − 14). The sensitivity of 93% and negative predictive value of 99% for AMI was quite similar to previously published trials, but with a much greater patient base.

In a multicenter trial, Heller et al.[45] evaluated the clinical use and cost-effectiveness of ARMPI using Tc-99m tetrofosmin in 357 patients presenting to six EDs with chest pain and nondiagnostic ECG. Patients were injected during active chest pain, or within 6 hours of chest pain, and then followed in hospital and 30 days after discharge. Twenty patients had MI, 18 of whom had abnormal studies yielding a sensitivity of 90%, with a negative predictive value of 99%. Data comparing traditional triage markers with nuclear imaging identified the abnormal image as the best predictor of MI. The very high negative predictive value of multiple studies demonstrated that ARMPI can substantially and safely reduce the number of unnecessary hospital admissions.

In a recent large, prospective, randomized, multicenter trial Udelson et al.[46] evaluated the actual impact of ARMPI in the initial ED triage of suspected acute cardiac ischemia (ACI). Patients without a prior history of MI, presenting

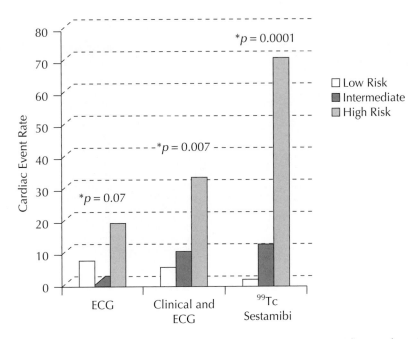

Figure 7-6.   ED risk stratification using Tc-99m sestamibi SPECT acute imaging. Risk status based on: (1) ECG results (normal versus abnormal but nondiagnostic), (2) a combination of clinical and ECG variables, and (3) the results of the Tc-99m sestamibi scan (normal, [low risk, solid bars], versus abnormal [high risk, hatched bars]). Tc-99m imaging identifies both lower (< 2%) and higher (> 70%) risk groups than the ECG alone or in combination with clinical variables. Reprinted from Hilton et al.[41] with permission.

with chest pain or other symptoms suggestive of ACI and nondiagnostic ECG ($n = 2,475$), were randomized to ARMPI ($n = 1,215$) or usual care ($n = 1,260$). Gated SPECT imaging was performed after the injection of sestamibi either during the symptoms or within 3 hours of cessation of pain, and the results were called to the ED physician for incorporation into triage decision. To confirm or refute the diagnosis of ACI, both the admitted patients and discharged patients were followed for the results of serial ECGs, enzymes, follow-up stress test with imaging, and 30-day follow-up for cardiac events. The data revealed that incorporation of ARMPI in the ED evaluation reduced unnecessary admissions among patients without ACI, thereby improving the overall clinical effectiveness of the ED triage process.

Diagnostic Accuracy and Incremental Value

Several studies have confirmed that ARMPI when employed in the evaluation of chest pain in the ED has a good sensitivity and a very high negative predictive value, for the diagnosis of both AMI and UA. However, in a group of patients with suspected ACS, it has only a moderate specificity for the diagnosis of AMI, as it is also able to identify patients with myocardial ischemia without necrosis.[33,40,41,43] ARMPI has incremental diagnostic value for cardiac events when added to clinical variables such as age and gender, three or more risk factors for CAD, and normal or nondiagnostic ECG with chest pain, as shown by Heller et al.[45] in their study using Tc-99m tetrofosmin (Figure 7-7).

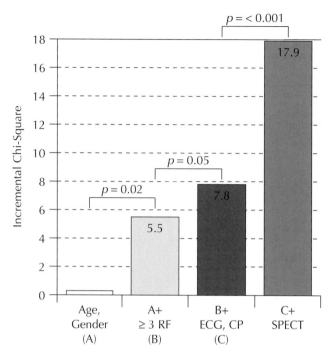

Figure 7-7. Incremental value of acute rest myocardial perfusion imaging: Comparison with clinical data. The incremental value of acute rest imaging in the prediction of cardiac events when compared to clinical risks. A = age and gender; B = A + three coronary artery disease risk factors; C = B + normal or nondiagnostic ECG with chest pain; C + SPECT = acute rest images combined with C. Reprinted from Heller et al.[45] with permission.

Risk Stratification

Early perfusion imaging allows rapid and accurate risk stratification of ED patients with possible cardiac ischemia and nondiagnostic ECGs. Patients with normal perfusion images have very high negative predictive values for both AMI and symptomatic ischemia, as the patients have been shown to be cardiac event free up to 18 months.[40] Figure 7-8 illustrates the negative predictive values for AMI (ranging from 99% to 100%) from four studies, and this is of considerable clinical importance as patients with normal ARMPI have a very low risk of MI in the ensuing days, enabling them to be discharged from the ED safely.

When cardiac death alone was considered as the endpoint, the negative predictive value of

ARMPI extended up to 3 years, as demonstrated by Miller et al.[47] in a study involving 111 patients with spontaneous chest pain, a normal or nondiagnostic ECG, no enzymatic evidence of MI and nonischemic quantitative Tc-99m sestamibi images. The 3-year survival free of cardiac death was 100%, emphasizing the very high negative predictive value. Thus, it is reasonable that a majority of patients with normal images could be discharged from the ED, with a plan to have an expedited cardiac evaluation. It should be specially emphasized that although cardiac event rates may be low with normal ARMPI, 2 to 5% of patients with normal images have required subsequent revascularization in the short and intermediate term (30 days to 12 months),[15,45] a very small but important stable CAD not diagnosed by rest imaging. Subsequent care of the

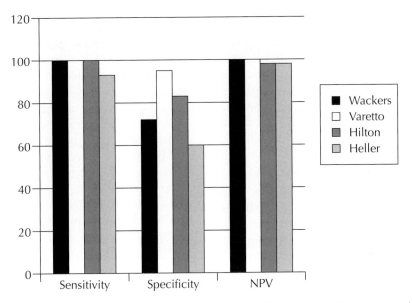

Figure 7-8. Diagnostic accuracy of acute rest imaging for myocardial infarction. Comparison of accuracy for four trials. High sensitivity and negative predictive values are seen in all the studies shown. Data from Wackers et al.,[33] Varetto et al.,[40] Hilton et al.,[41] and Heller et al.[45]

patient with normal acute rest imaging should therefore be based on the remaining suspicion of CAD. Despite the lower specificity for AMI, perfusion defects have been associated with a worse prognosis, both in the near and intermediate term, many times higher than patients with normal perfusion images.[15,44] Figure 7-9 demonstrates the prognostic ability of abnormal images for an intermediate period of 12 months compared to normal images. Multivariate regression analysis comparing clinical history, cardiac risk factors, patient age, history of previous AMI, and presence of a perfusion defect identified only a perfusion defect as a predictor of subsequent AMI or cardiac events. As illustrated in Figure 7-6, the ARMPI had the best risk stratification, with the normal images identifying a very low risk of < 2% and the abnormal images identifying the very high risk status of > 70% for cardiac events up to 90 days.[41]

Because patients are injected at rest, it is assumed that only the immediate risk is assessed; however, several studies have assessed the ability

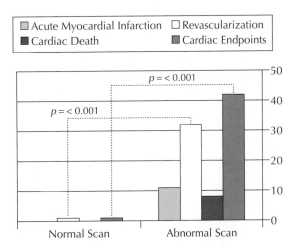

Figure 7-9. Risk stratification with ARMPI. Cardiac outcomes between 1 and 12 months after initial evaluation. Abnormal images portend a much worse prognosis compared to normal images in the intermediate term (as well as short term, which is not shown here). Data from Tatum et al.[15]

of ARMPI to predict risk after discharge. Using Tc-99m sestamibi, Hilton et al.[43] evaluated ($n = 150$) patients with typical chest pain who were then followed for 90 days ($n = 140$) after discharge. At follow-up, none of the 87 patients with normal MPI had an adverse coronary event defined as cardiac death, nonfatal MI, or readmission due to chest pain. Patients with abnormal studies had an event rate of 8% ($p = 0.008$).

Timing of Radionuclide Injection

The timing of the injection in relation to symptoms is an important issue in the successful use of ARMPI in ACS. It is well known that as the time after pain resolution increases, the size and the incidence of the perfusion defects decrease as shown by serial imaging studies with thallium from the prethrombolytic era.[37,48] Wackers et al.[37] showed when the imaging was performed within 6 hours of pain in AMI, the incidence of perfusion abnormality was 84%, which decreased to 19% at 12 to 18 hours after the last episode of pain.

Varetto et al.[40] noted that of the 14 patients with defined CAD and no MI, 11 were injected 2 to 8 hours (mean = 4.7 ± 2.13 hours) after cessation of pain. Despite this delay, all patients showed perfusion defects that subsequently normalized in 12 patients, leaving less extensive residual defects in two patients at control imaging 24 and 48 hours after onset of chest pain. However, Kontos et al.[42] found that sensitivity did not significantly differ between patients who were and who were not experiencing pain at the time of injection. Although the exact time of injection was not reported, none of the patients were injected more than 6 hours after the last episode of the pain. In the study by Bilodeau,[20] patients hospitalized with the suspicion of UA were injected during chest pain at presentation (five patients) or during in-hospital recurrence of chest pain (40 patients), and imaging was repeated ≤ 4 hours after cessation of chest pain. Normalization of a perfusion defect in a pain-free state was evident in eight patients who had a defect during pain and defined CAD. Thirteen

other patients had at least one grade improvement in defect severity in a pain-free state. Persistence of the defect in the pain-free state was associated with a larger initial defect, and complete recovery was possible if the initial defect was smaller with a score < 5, suggesting the sensitivity of radionuclide imaging would be optimal when injected during chest pain. Figure 7-10 demonstrates the highest sensitivity (96%) for ARMPI for the detection of CAD when the radionuclide was injected during pain.

The available data are not conclusive but suggest a reduced diagnostic accuracy for the detection of CAD when patients are injected after the resolution of pain. A review by Duncan and Heller[49] on this topic recommended a cut-off time of 2 hours for ARMPI to optimally exclude unstable angina.

Comparison to Clinical and ECG

History, physical examination, and ECG are the most important aspects of the initial management of any patient with suspected ACS. Various clinical prediction models have attempted to risk stratify these patients to characterize the short-term risk for adverse cardiac events including nonfatal MI and cardiac death.[19,50–53]

Clinical risk stratification efforts have concentrated on high-risk clinical indicators and ECG findings, although with significant limitations.[54] Normal or nonischemic ECG does not exclude acute myocardial ischemia,[55] and the sensitivity of ECG for the diagnosis of cardiac events is low (35–40%).[20,56] When the ECG was compared to ARMPI for the diagnosis of symptomatic CAD in the suspected UA population, the diagnostic accuracy for the imaging was vastly superior to ECG both during chest pain and at least 4 hours after cessation of the pain, as illustrated in Figure 7-10.

In a study by Young et al.,[57] 44% of patients with MI showed no changes from the previous ECG, including patients with an initial normal ECG. Thus, negative predictive value of ECG for MI is very poor, resulting in an unacceptable rate of missed MIs with its potential adverse consequences.

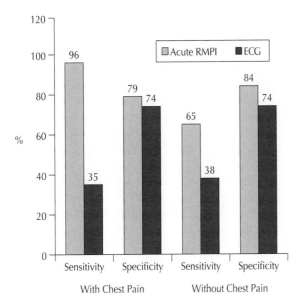

Figure 7-10. Diagnostic accuracy of ECG compared to sestamibi in symptomatic CAD. Shows vastly superior sensitivity of 96%, and a specificity of 79% for ARMPI in detecting CAD, compared to the electrocardiographic data during symptoms with a far lower sensitivity of 38% and a specificity of 59%. Acute RMPI = acute rest myocardial perfusion imaging; ECG = electrocardiogram; CAD = coronary artery disease. Data from Bilodeau et al.[20]

Comparison to Serum Markers

Serum markers of myocyte injury, both cardiac troponin T (cTnT) and I (cTnI), have helped to identify low-risk patients presenting with chest pain and provide independent prognostic information with regard to cardiac death and AMI.[10,11,57] However, the use of troponin (early at presentation) for a reliable diagnosis of ACS is hampered by its low sensitivity. Polanczyk et al.[59] reported a sensitivity and specificity of 40% and 95%, respectively, for AMI from their prospective study involving 1,047 patients with acute chest pain from a lower risk heterogeneous group.

Similarly, Kontos et al.[60] found a sensitivity of 35% for initial cTnI levels, showing the need for serial testing to achieve adequate sensitivity to diagnose ACS. When the diagnostic ability of

ARMPI was compared with serial TnI in 620 patients, ARMPI had a significantly higher sensitivity over initial cTnI for the diagnosis of MI and significant CAD and prediction of revascularization, as illustrated in Figure 7-11. The specificity for all end points for the initial as well as serial troponin was higher than ARMPI, and the sensitivity for the diagnosis of AMI for the serial troponin equaled ARMPI.

Duca et al.[61] evaluated ARMPI in 75 patients presenting to the ED with chest pain and nondiagnostic ECG and compared to serum markers of myocardial injury drawn at admission and at 8 to 24 hours later. ARMPI was demonstrated to have the highest sensitivity of 73% and similar specificity for patients with objective evidence of CAD when compared with the serum markers creatine kinase (CK), CK-MB fraction, cTnT, cTnI, and myoglobin both at the time of presentation and at the time of subsequent analyses (see Figure 7-12). Serum markers had very low sensitivities at early and late time points ranging from 3% to 33%. For the diagnosis of AMI, the ARMPI had a sensitivity and negative predictive value of 100%, and the sensitivities for the initial serum markers were quite low, ranging from 11% to 33%, but with a higher specificity, ranging from 92% to 100%. The diagnostic ability of serial markers improved with a sensitivity of 100% for cTnI at 24 hours.

Troponin is useful in the diagnosis of AMI as it detects myocyte necrosis undetectable by other conventional markers and has an equal or higher specificity than ARMPI, but timely diagnosis is hampered by the need for serial testing. Troponin has a role in risk stratification of UA but has a limited reliance in identifying all UA patients as studies have shown only 22 to 36% of patients have positive results. In summary, serum markers of injury have a very high specificity but a low specificity for AMI in the initial evaluation of chest pain. Further, the detection of UA without AMI is severely limited.

Comparison to Echocardiography

There is a lack of information from large, prospective, randomized clinical trials comparing

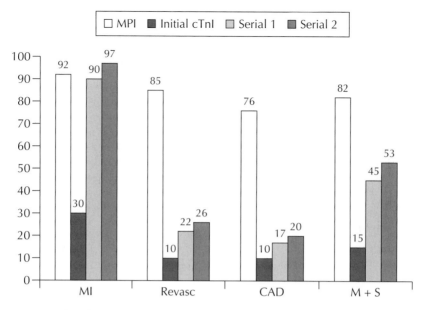

Figure 7-11. Sensitivity of perfusion imaging and cTnI for identifying cardiac end points. Shows much higher sensitivities for all end points for MPI compared to the initial cTnI. cTnI = cardiac troponin I; MPI = myocardial perfusion imaging; MI = myocardial infarction; Revasc = revascularization; CAD = coronary artery disease; M + S = myocardial infarction + significant coronary artery disease. Data from Kontos et al.[60]

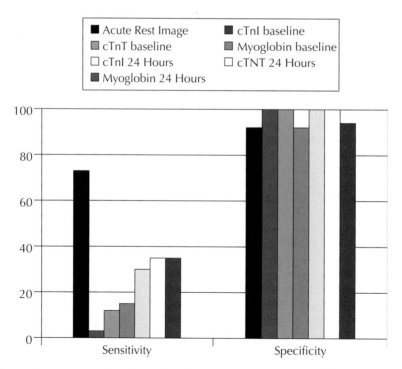

Figure 7-12. Diagnostic accuracy of markers at baseline vs. acute rest imaging for detecting symptomatic ischemia. Acute rest MPI had the highest sensitivity (73%) for detecting symptomatic CAD. Serum markers had very low sensitivities at early and late time points ranging from 3% to 33%. Data from Duca et al.[61]

both nuclear and echocardiography for the diagnosis of chest pain in the ED setting. Available data on the diagnostic ability of ECHO is variable, with sensitivities ranging between 42% and 94%, and the specificities from 46% to 100%.[56,62]

ECHO and ARMPI were compared in a study by Kontos et al.,[63] involving 185 patients in the ED, for predicting cardiac events and significant CAD, who were assessed to be at low or moderate risk for myocardial ischemia. Both studies were performed in all patients within 4 hours of ED presentation and the agreement between ECHO and ARMPI was found to be high, with a concordance of 89%. However, in patients with resolution of symptoms, a negative ECHO does not exclude ACS.

Cost Savings

Adding an imaging study for evaluation of chest pain does not save cost unless it reduces the number of admissions and/or decreases the length of stay. To study the economic impact of additional testing, Heller et al.[43] performed a net cost analysis and estimated the potential cost savings from reduced hospital admissions with the increased diagnostic cost of imaging. Using a model in which patients with normal perfusion

imaging are discharged home, they estimated that hospital admissions would be reduced by 57%. With a mean cost of $487 for nuclear imaging in U.S. hospitals (including technical and professional charges), the mean individual cost savings was $4,258 as shown in Figure 7-13. However, because of other high clinical risk indicators of CAD or recurrent symptoms, not all patients with normal images would be discharged. When the authors analyzed cost savings with a scenario of only 80% of patients being discharged, the cost savings were still substantial.

Radensky et al.[64] showed potential cost-effectiveness of ARMPI in a retrospective observation model, and Stowers et al.[65] in a small study had shown that ARMPI and early exercise stress testing can reduce in-hospital costs and decrease length of stay. These studies demonstrate that despite the added cost of the study itself, if decisions to hospitalize are based on imaging results, significant savings would occur.

CONCLUSIONS

Patients presenting to the ED with chest pain constitute a very heterogeneous population mixed with a small but high-risk group for short-term ad-

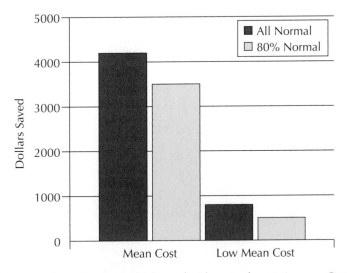

Figure 7-13.   Potential cost savings of patients discharged with normal acute images. Cost savings of patients discharged with normal acute images. Data from Heller et al.[44]

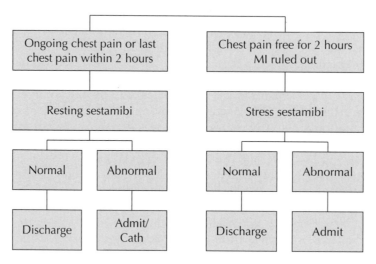

Figure 7-14.   Imaging in suspected acute coronary syndrome and nondiagnostic ECG.

verse cardiac events and litigation potential. Several clinical protocols and diagnostic modalities have been evaluated, among which ARMPI appears to be an accurate and cost-effective tool for identifying the high-risk as well as low-risk groups for appropriate management of this challenging clinical problem. ARMPI can be effectively employed in institutions with appropriate resources.[66] An algorithm for its use is included in Figure 7-14.

REFERENCES

1. *New Imaging Test Helps ER Docs Separate out Faster Patients in Danger of Heart Attack from Other ER Patients.* Press Release, November 10, 1999. Agency for Health Care Policy and Research, Rockville, MD. *www.ahrq.gov/news/press/pr1999/selkr3pr.htm.*
2. Fuster V, Badimon L, Badimon JJ, Chesebro JH. The pathogenesis of coronary artery disease and the acute coronary syndromes (first of two parts). *N Engl J Med* 1992;326:242–250.
3. Fuster V, Badimon L, Badimon JJ, Chesebro JH. The pathogenesis of coronary artery disease and the acute coronary syndromes (second of two parts). *N Engl J Med* 1992;326:310–318.
4. Falk E, Shah PK, Fuster V. Coronary plaque disruption. *Circulation* 1995;92:657–671.
5. Karlson BW, Herlitz J, Wiklund O, et al. Early prediction of acute myocardial infarction from clinical history, examination and electrocardiogram in the emergency room. *Am J Cardiol* 1991;68:171–175.
6. Pope JH, Aufderheide TP, Ruthazer R, et al. Missed diagnoses of acute cardiac ischemia in the emergency department. *N Engl J Med* 2000;342:1163–1170.
7. McCarthy BD, Beshansky JR, D'Agostino RB, Selker HP. Missed diagnosis of acute myocardial infarction in the emergency department: Results from a multicenter study. *Ann Emerg Med* 1993;22:579–582.
8. Lee TH, Rouan GW, Weisberg MC, et al. Clinical characteristics and natural history of patients with acute myocardial infarction sent home from the emergency room. *Am J Cardiol* 1987;60:219–224.
9. Schor S, Behar S, Modan B, et al. Disposition of presumed coronary patients from an emergency room. A follow-up study. *JAMA* 1976;236(8):941–943.
10. Hamm CW, Goldmann BU, Heeschen C, et al. Emergency room triage of patients with acute chest pain by means of rapid testing for cardiac troponin T or troponin I. *N Engl J Med* 1997;337:1648–1653.
11. Antman E, Sacks D, Rifai N, et al. Time to positivity of a rapid bedside assay for cardiac-specific troponin T predicts prognosis in acute coronary syndromes: a Thrombolysis in Myocardial Infarction (TIMI) IIA substudy. *J Am Coll Cardiol* 1998;31:326–330.
12. Gibler WB, Runyon JP, Levy RC, et al. A rapid diagnostic and treatment center for patients with chest pain in the emergency department. *Ann Emerg Med* 1995;25:1–8.
13. Gomez MA, Anderson JL, Karagounis LA, et al. An emergency department–based protocol for rapidly ruling out myocardial ischemia reduces hospital time and expense: results of a randomized study (ROMIO). *J Am Coll Cardiol* 1996;28:25–33.
14. Mikhail MG, Smith FA, Gray M, et al. Cost-

effectiveness of mandatory stress testing in chest pain center patients. *Ann Emerg Med* 1997;29:88–98.

15. Tatum JL, Jesse RL, Kontos MC, et al. Comprehensive strategy for the evaluation and triage of the chest pain patient. *Ann Emerg Med* 1997;29:116–125.

16. Katz DA. Risk stratification in unstable angina: The role of clinical prediction models. *J Am Coll Cardiol* 2000;36:1809–1811.

17. Braunwald E. *Diagnosis and Managing Unstable Angina.* [Rockville, Md]: U.S. Dept. of Health and Human Services, Public Health Service, Agency for Health Care Policy and Research, National Heart, Lung, and Blood Institute, [1996] 01-Jan-1996; vii, 201 p. AHCPR publication; no. 97-N010; Clinical practice guideline. Guideline technical report no. 10; AHCPR pub. no. 97-N010.

18. Braunwald E. Unstable angina: A classification. *Circulation* 1989;80:410–414.

19. Calvin JE, Klein LW, VandenBerg BJ, et al. Risk stratification in unstable angina. Prospective validation of the Braunwald classification. *JAMA* 1995; 273:136–141.

20. Bilodeau L, Theroux P, Gregoire J, et al. Technetium-99m sestamibi tomography in patients with spontaneous chest pain: Correlations with clinical, electrocardiographic and angiographic findings. *J Am Coll Cardiol* 1991;18:1684–1691.

21. Zarling EJ, Sexton H, Milnor P. Failure to diagnose acute myocardial infarction: The clinicopathologic experience at a large community hospital. *JAMA* 1983;250:1177–1181.

22. Antman EM, Tanasijevic MJ, Thompson B, et al. Cardiac-specific troponin I levels to predict the risk of mortality in patients with acute coronary syndromes. *N Engl J Med* 1996;335:1342–1349.

23. Polanczyk C, Johnson P, Cook E, Lee T. A proposed strategy for utilization of creatine kinase-MB and troponin I in the evaluation of acute chest pain. *Am J Cardiol* 1999; 83:1175–1179.

24. Gardner CJ, Brown S, Hagen-Ansert S, et al. Guidelines for cardiac sonographer education: Report of the American Society of Echocardiography Sonographer Education and Training Committee. *J Am Soc Echocardiogr* 1992;5:635–639.

25. Pearlman AS, Gardin JM, Martin RP, et al. Guidelines for optimal physician training in echocardiography. Recommendations of the American Society of Echocardiography Committee for Physician Training in Echocardiography. *Am J Cardiol* 1987;60:158–163.

26. Lewis WR, Amsterdam EA, Turnipseed S, Kirk JD. Utility and safety of immediate exercise testing of low risk patients with coronary artery disease presenting to the emergency department with chest pain. *Circulation* 1997;96:I–270.

27. Nesto RW, Kowalchuk GJ. The ischemic cascade:

Temporal sequence of hemodynamic, electrocardiographic and symptomatic expressions of ischemia. *Am J Cardiol* 1987;59:23C–30C.

28. Boden WE, McKay RG. Optimal treatment of acute coronary syndromes—an evolving strategy. *N Engl J Med* 2001;344:1939–1942.

29. Carr EAJ, Beierwalters WH, Wegst AV, et al. Myocardial scanning with rubidium-86. *J Nucl Med* 1962;3:76–82.

30. Carr EAJ, Gleason G, Shaw J, et al. The direct diagnosis of myocardial infarction by photoscanning after administration of cesium-131. *Am Heart J* 1964;68:627–636.

31. Romhilt DW, Adolph RJ, Sodd VJ, et al. Cesium-129 myocardial scintigraphy to detect myocardial infarction. *Circulation* 1973;48:1242–1251.

32. Wackers FJ, Schoot JB, Sokole EB, et al. Noninvasive visualization of acute myocardial infarction in man with thallium-201. *Br Heart J* 1975;37(7):741–744.

33. Wackers FJ, Sokole EB, Samson G, et al. Value and limitations of thallium-201 scintigraphy in the acute phase of myocardial infarction. *N Engl J Med* 1976;295:1–5.

34. Maseri A, Parodi O, Severi S, Pesola A. Transient transmural reduction of myocardial blood flow demonstrated by thallium-201 scintigraphy, as a cause of variant angina. *Circulation* 1976;54(2):280–288.

35. Wackers FJ, Lie KI, Liem KL, et al. Potential value of thallium-201 scintigraphy as a means of selecting patients for the coronary care unit. *Br Heart J* 1979;41:111–117.

36. Ritchie JL, Zaret BL, Strauss HW, et al. Myocardial imaging with thallium-201: A multicenter study in patients with angina pectoris or acute myocardial infarction. *Am J Cardiol* 1978;42:345–350.

37. Wackers FJ, Lie KI, Liem KL, et al. Thallium-201 scintigraphy in unstable angina pectoris. *Circulation* 1978;57:738–742.

38. Brown KA, Okada RD, Boucher CA, et al. Serial thallium-201 imaging at rest in patients with unstable and stable angina pectoris: relationship of myocardial perfusion at rest to presenting clinical syndrome. *Am Heart J* 1983;106:70–77.

39. Freeman MR, Williams AE, Chisholm RJ, et al. Role of resting thallium-201 perfusion in predicting coronary anatomy, left ventricular wall motion, and hospital outcome in unstable angina pectoris. *Am Heart J* 1989;117:306–314.

40. Varetto T, Cantalupi D, Altieri A, Orlandi C. Emergency room technetium-99m sestamibi imaging to rule out acute myocardial ischemic events in patients with nondiagnostic electrocardiograms. *J Am Coll Cardiol* 1993;22:1804–1808.

41. Hilton TC, Thompson RC, Williams HJ, et al. Technetium-99m sestamibi myocardial perfusion

imaging in the emergency room evaluation of chest pain. *J Am Coll Cardiol* 1994;23:1016–1022.

42. Varetto T, Cantalupi D, Cerruti A. Tc 99m sestamibi and 2D-echo imaging for rule-out of acute ischemia in patients with chest pain and non-diagnostic ECG [abstract]. *Circulation* 1994;90:I-367.

43. Hilton TC, Fulmer H, Abuan T. Ninety-day follow-up of patients in the emergency department with chest pain who undergo initial single-photon emission computed tomographic perfusion scintigraphy with technetium 99m-labeled sestamibi. *J Nucl Cardiol* 1996;3:308–311.

44. Kontos MC, Jesse RL, Schmidt KL, et al. Value of acute rest sestamibi perfusion imaging for evaluation of patients admitted to the emergency department with chest pain. *J Am Coll Cardiol* 1997;30:976–982.

45. Heller GV, Stowers SA, Hendel RC, et al. Clinical value of acute rest technetium-99m tetrofosmin tomographic myocardial perfusion imaging in patients with acute chest pain and nondiagnostic electrocardiograms. *J Am Coll Cardiol* 1998;31:1011–1017.

46. Udelson JE, Beshansky JR, Ballin DS, et al. Myocardial perfusion imaging for evaluation and triage of patients with suspected acute cardiac ischemia. A randomized controlled trial. *JAMA* 2002;288:2693–2700.

47. Miller TD, Christian TF, Hopfenspirger MR, et al. Prognosis in patients with spontaneous chest pain, a nondiagnostic electrocardiogram, normal cardiac enzymes, and no evidence of severe resting ischemia by quantitative technetium 99m sestamibi tomographic imaging. *J Nucl Cardiol* 1998;5:64–72.

48. Smitherman TC, Osborn RC Jr, Narahara KA. Serial myocardial scintigraphy after a single dose of thallium-201 in men after acute myocardial infarction. *Am J Cardiol* 1978;42:177–182.

49. Duncan BH, Heller GV. Acute rest myocardial perfusion imaging in the evaluation of patients with chest pain syndromes. *ACC Curr J Rev* 1999;8:52–56.

50. Rizik DG, Healy S, Margulis A, et al. A new clinical classification for hospital prognosis of unstable angina pectoris. *Am J Cardiol* 1995;75:993–997.

51. Goldman L, Cook EF, Johnson PA, et al. Prediction of the need for intensive care in patients who come to the emergency departments with acute chest pain. *N Engl J Med* 1996;334:1498–1504.

52. Selker HP, Griffith JL, D'Agostino RB. A tool for judging coronary care unit admission appropriateness, valid for both real-time and retrospective use. A time-insensitive predictive instrument (TIPI) for acute cardiac ischemia: A multicenter study. *Med Care* 1991;7:610–627.

53. Lee TH, Goldman L. Evaluation of the patient with acute chest pain. *N Engl J Med* 2000;342:1187–1195.

54. Katz D. Barriers between guidelines and improved patient care: An analysis of AHCPR. *Health Serv Res* 1999;34(Part II):377–389N.

55. Kontos MC, Kurdziel KA, Ornato JP, et al. A nonischemic electrocardiogram does not always predict a small myocardial infarction: Results with acute myocardial perfusion imaging. *Am Heart J* 2001;141:360–366.

56. Kontos MC, Arrowood JA, Paulsen WH, Nixon JV. Early echocardiography can predict cardiac events in emergency department patients with chest pain. *Ann Emerg Med* 1998;31:550–557.

57. Young GP, Green TR. The role of single ECG, creatinine kinase, and CKMB in diagnosing patients with acute chest pain. *Am J Emerg Med* 1993;11:444–449.

58. Lüscher MS, Thygesen K, Ravkilde J, Heickendorff L. Applicability of cardiac troponin T and I for early risk stratification in unstable coronary artery disease. *Circulation* 1997;96:2578–2585.

59. Polanczyk CA, Lee TH, Cook EF, et al. Cardiac troponin I as a predictor of major cardiac events in emergency department patients with acute chest pain. *J Am Coll Cardiol* 1998;32:8–14.

60. Kontos MC, Jesse RL, Anderson FP, et al. Comparison of myocardial perfusion imaging and cardiac troponin I in patients admitted to the emergency department with chest pain. *Circulation* 1999;99:2073–2078.

61. Duca MD, Giri S, Wu AH, et al. Comparison of acute rest myocardial perfusion imaging and serum markers of myocardial injury in patients with chest pain syndromes. *J Nucl Cardiol* 1999;6:570–576.

62. Kim SC, Adams SL, Hendel RC. Role of nuclear cardiology in the evaluation of acute coronary syndromes. *Ann Emerg Med* 1997;30:210–218.

63. Kontos MC, Arrowood JA, Jesse RL, et al. Comparison between 2-dimensional echocardiography and myocardial perfusion imaging in the emergency department in patients with possible myocardial ischemia. *Am Heart J* 1998;136:724–733.

64. Radensky PW, Hilton TC, Fulmer H, et al. Potential cost effectiveness of initial myocardial perfusion imaging for assessment of emergency department patients with chest pain. *Am J Cardiol* 1997;79:595–599.

65. Stowers SA, Eisenstein EL, Wackers FJ, et al. An economic analysis of an aggressive diagnostic strategy with single photon emission computed tomography myocardial perfusion imaging and early exercise stress testing in emergency department patients who present with chest pain but nondiagnostic electrocardiograms: Results from a randomized trial. *Ann Emerg Med* 2000;35:17–25.

66. Hutter AM, Amsterdam EA, Jaffe AS. 31st Bethesda Conference. Emergency Cardiac Care. Task force 2: Acute coronary syndromes: Section 2B—Chest discomfort evaluation in the hospital. *J Am Coll Cardiol* 2000;35:853–862.

CHAPTER 8

Indications for Equilibrium Radionuclide Angiography

Thomas H. Hauser
Peter G. Danias

INTRODUCTION

Equilibrium radionuclide angiography (ERNA) was first introduced in the early 1970s[1] and was quickly established as the most accurate technique for measurement of left ventricular ejection fraction (LVEF). Several early studies demonstrated an excellent correlation of LVEF as measured by ERNA with values obtained by cardiac catheterization contrast ventriculography.[2–4] In one of these, Burow et al.[2] evaluated 17 patients with suspected coronary artery disease (CAD) with both ERNA and contrast ventriculography and reported an excellent correlation of LVEF values ($r = 0.93$). ERNA was shown to have a high degree of reproducibility with low inter- and intra-observer variability that compared favorably to existing cardiac imaging modalities.[5–7] Wackers et al.[5] measured LVEF in 83 randomly selected patients who were referred for ERNA and found an inter-observer variability of 1.6% and an intra-observer variability of 1.4%.

In 70 patients who underwent ERNA on two separate occasions, there was a mean variability of only 3.7% between the first and subsequent values for LVEF. ERNA was thus established as the most reproducible test for the assessment of left ventricular systolic function. ERNA is also referred to as radionuclide ventriculography (RVG), radionuclide cineangiography (RNCA), and multiple gated blood pool imaging (MUGA).

IMAGE ACQUISTION AND ANALYSIS

ERNA is performed by labeling the patient's red blood cell pool with a radioactive tracer and measuring radioactivity over the anterior chest with a suitably positioned gamma camera. The number of counts recorded per unit of time is proportional to the blood volume. Thus, a direct volumetric assessment of the cardiac chambers can be performed throughout the cardiac cycle.

Blood pool labeling is routinely performed with technetium 99m (Tc-99m), which achieves high red cell labeling, has a relatively short half-life (6 hours), and has an emission photo peak (140 keV) close to the maximal sensitivity of the gamma camera crystal. Labeling can be done in vitro by incubating a small autologous blood sample with Tc-99m or, more commonly, in vivo with the direct intravenous injection of Tc-99m pertechnetate.[8] The in vivo labeling technique is more convenient for most patients since it involves one venipuncture instead of two, is less time consuming, and is less costly. Although red blood cell labeling is generally more efficient with the in vitro techniques, more than 80% of the injected radionuclide usually binds to red blood cells with the in vivo approach.

Shortly after the injection, the labeled red blood cells equally distribute throughout the entire blood pool. Image acquisition is performed for 800 to 1,000 heartbeats for each projection (see below), corresponding to a time period of 5 to 10 minutes, depending on the heart rate. Data acquisition is gated to the electrocardiogram (ECG). The RR interval is divided into 16 to 32 equal phases (gating windows), and counts are recorded separately for each phase. At the end of the acquisition, the counts are summed for all cardiac cycles, and images obtained for each phase are then displayed in sequence, creating a cine-loop of the entire cardiac cycle.

ERNA images are obtained in the anterior, left posterior oblique (LPO), and modified left anterior oblique (mLAO) projections to best visualize all cardiac chambers and provide indirect information for all left ventricular walls. The anterior projection best visualizes the right atrium, right ventricle, and anterolateral left ventricle and apex. The LPO projection best visualizes the inferior, apical, and anterolateral left ventricle. The LAO projection best separates the left and right ventricles. An additional cranial orientation (frequently achieved with slant-hole collimators) may be used to separate the left atrium and ventricle (mLAO view). The LAO projection visualizes the septal, anterolateral, and posterolateral

left ventricle. The LAO or mLAO projections are used for measurement of LVEF, because in these views the left ventricle is free of any overlap from other cardiac chambers.

Measurement of Ejection Fraction

The ejection fraction is calculated directly from counts measured in the left ventricle at end-diastole and end-systole. Using the LAO (or mLAO) projection, a region of interest (ROI) is positioned to include the entire left ventricle at end-diastole (first frame of acquisition, corresponding to the R wave of the ECG). A second ROI is positioned around the left ventricle at end-systole. The number of counts in each ROI is the sum of the counts from the labeled blood in the ventricular cavity plus the background activity from Tc-99m that has been absorbed in overlying soft tissues. The number of counts of the labeled blood pool is proportional to the corresponding blood volume. The ejection fraction can then be calculated from the formula:

$$\text{LVEF} = \frac{\left(\begin{array}{c}\text{End-diastolic}\\\text{counts}\end{array}\right) - \left(\begin{array}{c}\text{End-systolic}\\\text{counts}\end{array}\right)}{\left(\begin{array}{c}\text{End-diastolic}\\\text{counts}\end{array}\right) - (\text{Background})}$$

The LVEF can be determined at rest, during exercise, or with pharmacologic inotropic stimulation. For stress ERNA, only the LAO or mLAO projection is used, and multiple shorter acquisitions are performed at graded levels of stress.

Measurement of Ventricular Volumes

The left ventricular volume can be calculated from the ventricular cavity counts if the blood radioactivity per unit of volume is known.[9] For this purpose, a sample of blood is drawn during image acquisition, and the blood radioactivity is measured. A simple mathematical conversion is then used to calculate the left ventricular volume, after correction for attenuation. This correction requires several assumptions regarding chest wall composition and the distance of the heart from the anterior chest wall.[10] The standard error of this method is 10 to 35 mL.[11]

Evaluation of Regional Systolic Function

As previously discussed, ERNA visualizes the left ventricular cavity and not the left ventricular walls. Therefore, only inferences can be made regarding regional systolic function. Regional ejection fraction can be calculated by segmenting the left ventricle and measuring counts independently for each segment at end-systole and end-diastole. More commonly, however, regional wall motion is assessed qualitatively from visual inspection of the cine loop. A circumferential inward motion of the left ventricular cavity contour and decrease of the number of counts suggests normal regional systolic function, while the relative delay of count reduction in a focal area suggests hypokinesis of the adjacent left ventricular wall.

An additional tool for evaluation of regional systolic function is phase analysis. For this, counts for each ventricular segment are measured independently and the corresponding time-count activity curves are constructed. These sinusoidal curves are normally all in phase. If there is regional left ventricular dysfunction, one or more of the regional time-count curves will be out of phase. The phase difference is encoded with different color maps, thereby presenting a visual display of the timing of contraction of each segment. The degree of phase difference is related to the severity of the wall motion abnormality. Hypokinesis is suggested when there is only a slight phase difference. Complete reversal of the contraction pattern suggests regional dyskinesis and is caused by focal left ventricular aneurysm or severe conduction abnormality (e.g., left bundle branch block).

Evaluation of Diastolic Function

ERNA has been proposed as a sensitive method to evaluate left ventricular diastolic function.[11] The left ventricular time–activity curve can be used to quantify volume changes with time. This requires high temporal resolution, which can be achieved with the acquisition of a larger number of phases per cardiac cycle.[12] The peak filling rate is most commonly used to assess diastolic function. However, because it is dependent on preload, afterload, LVEF, and heart rate,[13,14] the peak filling rate may vary considerably in serial measurements for the same patient without an actual change in left ventricular diastolic function. Other parameters, such as time to peak filling rate and filling fraction, have also been described as correlates of diastolic function,[11] but their use is limited.

APPLICATION TO CLINICAL PROBLEMS

The major advantage of ERNA is that it provides a highly accurate and reproducible noninvasive measurement of LVEF. Image acquisition and study quality are not significantly affected by overweight and obesity, conditions that limit the applicability of most other cardiac noninvasive modalities. Furthermore, image acquisition occurs in a relatively short time (usually < 30 minutes) and with minimal risk to the patient. Finally, in addition to the assessment to of both regional and global LVEF, ERNA can also be used for accurate measurement of the RVEF and ventricular volumes.

The values of the LVEF as determined by ERNA, cardiac magnetic resonance imaging (MRI), and echocardiography are not interchangeable. Preliminary data on myocardial infarction (MI) survivors with left ventricular systolic dysfunction, who were evaluated with ERNA, echocardiography, and cardiac MRI, have suggested that ERNA and cardiac MRI compared favorably to echocardiography.[15] Previous studies have also shown that echocardiography has significantly higher variability in measurement of LVEF than does ERNA[16–18] and is not suitable for patients who require precise serial measurements of LVEF.[19] Although cardiac MRI has exquisite accuracy and reproducibility and is currently considered the most accurate technique for determination of LVEF and ventricular volumes,[18] ERNA is more widely available and less costly. In practice, ERNA is often used as the best available clinical test for evaluation of the LVEF.[20–23]

In 1995, the American Heart Association (AHA) and the American College of Cardiology (ACC) convened a task force to evaluate the use of cardiac radionuclide imaging, and recommendations for the appropriate use of ERNA in clinical practice were published.[24] These recommendations are listed in Table 8-1 and discussed in the following sections.

Cardiotoxic Chemotherapy

Several chemotherapy agents, including the anthracycline derivatives (such as doxorubicin [adriamycin], daunorubicin, and idarubicin), cyclophosphamide,[25,26] taxol,[27] interferon[28,29] and interleukins,[30] are effective therapies for a variety of malignancies but also have associated cardiac toxicity. For some of these chemotherapies, the cardiac adverse effects are dose related, and treatment may result in severe systolic dysfunction and congestive heart failure (CHF). Accordingly, careful monitoring of left ventricular function is warranted in patients receiving chemotherapy. Upon detection of systolic dysfunction, the continuation of any chemotherapy needs to be reassessed, and alternative therapies should be considered with the risk of additional cardiotoxicity weighed against the expected chemotherapeutic benefit. Due to its high accuracy and reproducibility, ERNA is indicated to serially monitor LVEF for early detection of cardiac toxicity.[31] Echocardiography has been found to be inadequate for this purpose.[19]

The toxicity of the anthracycline derivatives, particularly doxorubicin, has been studied extensively. Lefrak et al.[32] first reported dose-related doxorubicin cardiac toxicity in 1973. Congestive heart failure occurred in 30% of patients who were treated with a cumulative dose of > 550 mg/m², while of those treated with < 550 mg/m², only one in 366 developed CHF. A later study further clarified the dose–response of doxorubicin cardiac toxicity. The average incidence of cardiac toxicity with doxorubicin is 2.2% but rises to 3.5% at a dose of 400 mg/m², 7% at a dose of 550 mg/m², and 18% at 700 mg/m².[33] The outcome of patients who develop CHF is poor, with a 1-year survival of approximately 50%.[34] The chemotherapeutic effect of doxorubicin is also dose related. Decreasing the dose in an attempt to limit cardiac toxicity may compromise treatment efficacy.[35]

Because myocardial damage can occur prior to any measurable decrement in LVEF,[36,37] several strategies have been attempted to identify those patients treated with doxorubicin who are at increased risk for the development of CHF. Prior cardiomyopathy has been identified as the main risk factor, while other heart diseases do not confer an increased risk.[38] Cardiac catheterization is not useful for assessment of the risk for progressive cardiac dysfunction during therapy.[39] Endomyocardial biopsy is effective for detecting the presence of myocardial fibrosis resulting from doxorubicin toxicity, but it is limited by sampling error and has associated risk.[40,41]

Titrated chemotherapy guided by serial measurements of LVEF with ERNA has been shown to prevent the development of CHF.[42] In patients with a normal LVEF at baseline, an absolute decline in LVEF of more than 15% predicts subsequent decline if therapy with doxorubicin is continued, even in the absence of symptoms.[43] By limiting the decline in LVEF to 10% and using the algorithm shown in Table 8-2, the incidence of heart failure due to doxorubicin cardiac toxicity can be reduced up to fourfold.[44] This strategy allows for a maximal dose of doxorubicin while minimizing the risk of cardiac toxicity. Concomitant use of cyclophosphamide or mediastinal radiation requires reduction in the dose of doxorubicin.[45]

Although exercise ERNA has been proposed as a more sensitive test for anthracycline toxicity,[46] the patient's general condition often limits the ability to exercise.

Table 8-1

Indications for ERNA

	Test
Class I: Usually appropriate and considered useful.	
1. Assessment of initial and serial LVEF in patients receiving chemotherapy with doxorubicin.	
2. Assessment of initial and serial LVEF and RVEF in patients with myocarditis and nonischemic cardiomyopathies.	Rest ERNA
3. Assessment of initial and serial LVEF and RVEF in adults with congenital heart disease.	Rest ERNA
4. Assessment of LVEF prior to cardiac transplantation.	Rest ERNA
5. Assessment of LVEF, RVEF and ventricular volumes in patients with valvular heart disease.	Rest ERNA
6. Assessment of LVEF in patients with chronic ischemic heart disease.	Rest ERNA
7. Assessment of LVEF or RVEF after AMI.	Rest ERNA
8. Assessment of LVEF in patients with unstable angina.	Rest ERNA
Class IIa: Acceptable but usefulness is less well established; the weight of evidence is in favor of usefulness.	
1. Assessment of the effect of drug therapy on LVEF in patients with chronic ischemic heart disease.	Rest ERNA
2. Detection and localization of shunts.	First-pass RNA
3. Quantitation of left to right shunts.	First-pass RNA
4. Diagnosis of right ventricular infarction.	Rest ERNA
5. Diagnosis of chronic ischemic heart disease in symptomatic patients and in selected patients without symptoms.	Stress ERNA
6. Diagnosis of stress-induced ischemia after AMI.	Stress ERNA
7. Planning percutaneous coronary intervention—identifying lesions causing myocardial ischemia.	Stress ERNA
8. Assessment for restenosis after percutaneous coronary intervention.	Stress ERNA
9. Assessment for ischemia after surgical revascularization.	Stress ERNA
Class IIb: Acceptable but usefulness is less well established; can be helpful but not well established by evidence.	
1. Assessment of myocardial viability.	Dobutamine, post-stress or post-NTG ERNA
2. Detection and monitoring of rejection after cardiac transplantation.	Rest ERNA
3. Determination of cardiac involvement in systemic diseases.	Rest ERNA
4. Quantitation of aortic or mitral regurgitation.	Rest ERNA
5. Diagnosis of hypertrophic cardiomyopathy.	Rest ERNA
6. Detection of CAD in the setting of valvular heart disease.	Stress ERNA

Adapted from Ritchie et al. Ref# 24.

Table 8-2

ERNA Protocol During Therapy
with Doxorubicin

1. Baseline study within the first 100 mg/m^2 in all patients.

2. Follow-up studies at approximately 300 mg/m^2 and 450 mg/m^2. The study should be performed at 400 mg/m^2 if there is a history of prior cardiomyopathy or concomitant use of cyclophosphamide or mediastinal radiation.

3. Follow-up studies prior to each dose of doxorubicin after 450 mg/m^2.

4. Discontinuation of doxorubicin if the LVEF declines $\geq$ 10% from the baseline study or if the absolute value of the LVEF is $\leq$ 30%.

Based on the algorithm of Schwartz et al.[44]

Other Cardiotoxic Substances

Mediastinal radiation,[47] alcohol,[48] cocaine,[49] and iron[50] all have direct cardiotoxic effects and may cause dilated cardiomyopathy. ERNA can be useful by providing an accurate measurement of LVEF, both initially to diagnose systolic dysfunction and then serially to monitor the effects of therapy. ERNA is particularly useful for close follow-up of transfusion-dependent patients with beta-thalassemia who frequently develop cardiomyopathy from iron overload.[50-52] The efficacy of iron chelation therapy can be assessed using serial measurements of LVEF using ERNA.

Valvular Heart Disease

The timing of surgery for aortic valve replacement is critically important. It is necessary to separate patients who are likely to have a benign course from those who may develop progressive left ventricular dilation, CHF, or sudden death. In asymptomatic patients with a normal resting LVEF, a combination of left ventricular wall thickness (measured by echocardiography) and LVEF at rest and with exercise (measured by ERNA) can identify those patients at risk for sudden death.[53,54] The first sign of ventricular

dysfunction is an abnormal LVEF response to exercise.[55-62] However, most patients with a normal LVEF at rest and an abnormal LVEF with exercise do not progress over 4 years,[63] and thus immediate valve replacement is not recommended. Instead, close monitoring of resting systolic function with serial measurements of LVEF with ERNA is indicated.[64] Aortic valve replacement can then be pursued if there is a decrement in resting LVEF, even if the patient is asymptomatic. If surgery is delayed until the onset of symptoms of heart failure or until moderate to severe left ventricular dysfunction develops, up to 50% of patients may have a poor outcome.[65]

After aortic valve replacement, LVEF frequently improves if it is abnormal at the time of surgery.[66] Late improvement of LVEF usually occurs in patients who have an improvement of their LVEF within the first 6 months.[67] The resting LVEF remains the major predictor of death or CHF.[68]

With significant mitral regurgitation, the measured LVEF is frequently normal even in patients with underlying systolic dysfunction, because a significant fraction of the stroke volume is ejected into the low-pressure left atrium rather than the aorta. This greatly reduces the left ventricular afterload and creates an apparent high value for the LVEF. A decreased LVEF in the setting of significant mitral regurgitation suggests severe underlying systolic dysfunction and implies a poor prognosis with either medical or surgical therapy.[69,70] The right heart can also be affected if pulmonary hypertension develops. When right ventricular dysfunction ensues, early mortality is high with both medical and surgical therapy.[70]

Although ERNA cannot directly assess the severity of aortic stenosis, it can identify the functional consequences of its presence.[71,72] Left ventricular hypertrophy can be indirectly assessed by the presence of diastolic dysfunction. The LVEF typically is normal early in the disease. As the disease progresses, serial measurements demonstrate a gradual reduction in LVEF, which often improves after surgical or percutaneous intervention.[73] Echocardiography is better for assessment of aortic stenosis, as it provides structural detail of the aortic valve, measurement of LVEF, quantitation of left ventricular hypertrophy by direct visualization of the ventricular walls, and quantitation of the hemodynamic significance of the degree of stenosis.

ERNA is also not particularly useful for the assessment of mitral stenosis. As in aortic stenosis, ERNA can detect the functional consequences of its presence.[74] Mitral stenosis is characterized by a normal LVEF, normal left ventricular cavity size, and variable enlargement of the right ventricle.[75] ERNA can identify patients with a depressed LVEF or RVEF in whom valve replacement may be less effective.[76] Echocardiography is routinely used to assess mitral stenosis, as it provides structural detail of the mitral valve, a hemodynamic assessment of the severity of stenosis, and measurement of the LVEF.

Coronary Artery Disease

CAD is the leading cause of death in the United States and the principal cause of CHF.[77] In patients with CAD, the greatest value of ERNA is for the precise measurement of LVEF. This is particularly important for patients with heart failure and for patients being considered for cardiac transplantation. In the 1970s, ERNA was the only imaging modality that could evaluate regional wall motion abnormalities, short of invasive contrast ventriculography, but the introduction of echocardiography has largely replaced ERNA for routine evaluation of LVEF and particularly regional systolic function.

The LVEF at rest is one of the most important prognostic factors in chronic CAD and is inversely associated with mortality.[78–81] The LVEF with exercise similarly provides strong prognostic information. A drop in LVEF with stress is associated with severe CAD and predicts poor outcome at 2 to 5 years.[82–84]

For patients with CHF, medical therapy with angiotensin-converting enzyme (ACE) inhibitors, diuretics, digoxin, and beta blockers has been shown to improve symptoms and prolong survival.[24,78,81,85,86] With optimal therapy, LVEF can often improve.[86,87] Cardiac transplantation is a treatment option for patients who are not candidates for coronary revascularization and are refractory to maximal medical therapy. The principal objective criterion for transplantation eligibility is a severe reduction of LVEF, usually less than 20%.[88] ERNA is commonly used to provide an accurate assessment of LVEF for patients being considered for cardiac transplantation.

ERNA may rarely be useful in the setting of acute coronary syndromes and can localize the area of involvement of an acute myocardial infarction (AMI).[89] Right ventricular infarction can also be identified using ERNA.[90,91] The LVEF at rest is strongly predictive of the risk of in-hospital death[92] and survival after discharge[93,94] in patients with AMI.

ERNA has been used to evaluate the functional changes after reperfusion therapy and predict the likelihood of future adverse events.[95–99] The LVEF with exercise can improve after percutaneous coronary intervention, providing objective evidence for relief of ischemia.[100] Wallis et al.[101] found that, in patients who have undergone coronary artery bypass surgery, the response of the LVEF to exercise was the best predictor of infarction or death over 9 years of follow-up, better than the knowledge of coronary anatomy or number of bypass grafts.

Exercise ERNA can be used for the diagnosis of chronic, stable CAD. In subjects without CAD, the exercise LVEF increases by at least 5%,[11] while in patients with CAD there is either no change or a decline of the LVEF with exercise. The average reported sensitivity for the diagnosis of CAD is approximately 90% with a specificity of 85%.[102] The exercise LVEF obtained by ERNA provides additional prognostic information compared with myocardial perfusion scintigraphy alone,[103] although with the advent of ECG-gated single photon emission tomography (SPECT), simultaneous assessment of perfusion and post-stress function can now be performed[104–106] (see Chapter 13), and in most laboratories, has replaced exercise ERNA.

Hypertensive Heart Disease

Chronic hypertension results in cardiac pathology that can be identified with ERNA. Left ventricular hypertrophy is often present, and the associated diastolic dysfunction can be detected by a low peak filling rate.[107,108] ERNA is able to identify an increased thickness of the interventricular septum (visualized between the left and right ventricles in the mLAO projection) but not of the other left ventricular walls. The LVEF is usually normal until the late stages of the disease. Patients with left ventricular hypertrophy frequently have an abnormal LVEF response to exercise.[109,110] Although ERNA may be helpful, echocardiography is the preferred imaging modality for patients with hypertensive heart disease.

Hypertrophic Cardiomyopathy

ERNA can reveal several abnormalities in patients with hypertrophic cardiomyopathy. A hyperdynamic LVEF, prominent thickening of the interventricular septum, and impaired diastolic function are typically found.[111,112] Volumetric measurement often reveals a small left ventricular cavity. The finding of a low LVEF in a patient with hypertrophic cardiomyopathy implies a poor prognosis.[113]

Dilated Cardiomyopathy

ERNA reveals the characteristically depressed LVEF and enlarged left ventricular cavity and severe global hypokinesis present in dilated cardiomyopathy.[114,115] Though the absence of focal wall motion abnormalities suggests a nonischemic cardiomyopathy, considerable overlap may exist.[114,115] Therefore, regionality of wall motion abnormalities alone is an unreliable criterion for identification of etiology of cardiomyopathy in individual patients. As with those patients who have CHF due to ischemic cardiomyopathy, ERNA is particularly useful in this population for serial evaluation of LVEF for assessment of treatment efficacy and for evaluation of prognosis.[24,86,87] In patients referred for cardiac transplantation, a precise measurement of the LVEF is of great importance[88] and is usually obtained with ERNA.

After Cardiac Transplantation

Progressive ventricular dysfunction and rejection account for most deaths in patients who receive a cardiac transplant.[116] ERNA has been used to monitor for the occurrence of rejection and to identify patients who may be at increased risk for further decline in LVEF. Because of an altered position of the heart within the chest cavity, the ERNA imaging projection usually needs to be modified to provide an accurate calculation of the LVEF.[117]

Although patients can have severe rejection documented on endomyocardial biopsy without a change in the LVEF,[118] more commonly a decrement in the LVEF is seen. The change in LVEF may be rather small, but is usually detectable with ERNA. Follansbee et al.[119] found that the LVEF declined from 63% to 59% in the progression from "no rejection" to "mild rejection" as demonstrated by endomyocardial biopsy. The LVEF further declined to 57% in patients who progressed to "moderate rejection." However, a decline in the LVEF after heart transplantation does not always signify rejection.[120] In the absence of rejection, the LVEF decline was initially reported to not influence late survival,[118] but a more recent study suggested that patients with an LVEF of < 40% at 1 year were at increased risk for future cardiac events.[121]

Clinical Research

The ability to detect a treatment effect, or generally a difference between two groups, depends not only on the effect size (actual difference to be measured), but also on the measurement error of the test that is used. A highly accurate and reproducible test provides high statistical power for detection of a given difference with even a small sample size.[122–124] From both clinical trial design and implementation perspectives, having a small study sample size is preferable: The likelihood to maintain study population homogeneity increases, recruitment is completed in a timely fashion, and costs are minimized. Accordingly, in clinical trials in which LVEF (or the change thereof) is the outcome measure, the use of highly accurate and reproducible methodology has advantages. ERNA has long been the preferred modality to measure LVEF in clinical trials, has been the reference standard against which other imaging modalities have been compared, and has only recently challenged by cardiac MRI for this role.

Intracardiac Shunts

The presence and severity of a left-to-right shunt can be evaluated with radionuclide angiography (RNA) using the first-pass technique.[125] For this technique images are obtained immediately after injection of the radioactive tracer and without ECG gating. The injection must be rapid, so that the radioactive injectate travels as a discrete bolus. Images are obtained as the bolus makes its first pass through the circulation and are obtained only in the anterior projection. In the presence of a left-to-right shunt, there is early recirculation of radioactivity, best demonstrated by obtaining a pulmonary time–activity curve. An ROI is placed over one of the lungs, usually the right one, and counts are measured over time. The normal pulmonary time–activity curve has a rapid upslope and a gradual downslope. The presence of a second peak on the downslope of the curve indicates early recirculation due to the presence of a left-to-right shunt.

The severity of the left-to-right shunt can be quantified using a gamma variate fit model.[126–128] The fitted curve is subtracted from the pulmonary time–activity curve, producing the time–activity curve for the labeled red blood cells that underwent early recirculation. A second gamma variate function is then fitted to this time–activity curve, and the area under the curve is calculated. Because the area under the curve is

proportional to blood flow, the ratio of pulmonary blood flow (Qp) to systemic blood flow (Qs) can be calculated[129,130]:

$$\frac{Qp}{Qs} = \frac{A1}{(A1 - A2)}$$

where A1 and A2 are the areas under the first and second gamma variate fits, respectively. This method can be reliably used for left-to-right shunts that generate a Qp/Qs ratio of 1.2 to 3.0.

First-pass RNA is useful in the diagnosis of left-to-right shunts caused by atrial septal defects, ventricular septal defects, and patent ductus arteriosus. It can also confirm resolution of shunting after repair of the defect or, if not completely repaired, it can quantify the amount of residual shunting.[131,132]

LIMITATIONS OF ERNA

ERNA is contraindicated in lactating and pregnant women because of the concern of ionizing radiation exposure. However, the uniform whole-body radiation exposure for a single ERNA is quite small (620 mrem), approximately twice the annual amount of natural environmental radiation the average person receives in the United States.

ECG gating becomes unreliable in patients with arrhythmia and significant variability of the RR interval. Modified acquisition and postprocessing methods, such as the list mode acquisition, have been implemented and are clinically used to correct for RR variability.[133–135] With this approach, the frequency distribution of the RR interval is plotted for the duration of the acquisition. The operator can then select a narrow range for acceptance around the mode of distribution to retrospectively minimize variability. However, even with such approaches, ERNA cannot be reliably performed in the presence of marked arrhythmia.

Both obtaining the optimum projection for separation of the ventricles and defining the ventricular contours are operator dependent. Poor technique can introduce measurement error.

SUMMARY

ERNA is a highly accurate and reproducible method for measurement of the LVEF. Patients with clinical conditions that require careful serial measurements of LVEF, such as those who are undergoing chemotherapy with cardiotoxic agents, those with heart failure, and those considered for transplantation, derive the most benefit from evaluation with ERNA. ERNA can also provide additional information about left ventricular cavity size and regional systolic function, although in practice it is infrequently the first-choice test for these evaluations.

REFERENCES

1. Strauss HW, Zaret BL, Hurlye PJ, et al. A scintiphotographic method for measuring left ventricular ejection fraction in man without cardiac catheterization. *Am J Cardiol* 1971;28:575–580.
2. Burow RD, Strauss HW, Singleton R, et al. Analysis of left ventricular function from multiple gated acquisition cardiac blood pool imaging. Comparison to contrast angiography. *Circulation* 1977;56:1024–1028.
3. Folland ED, Hamilton GW, Larson SM, et al. The radionuclide ejection fraction: A comparison of the radionuclide techniques with contrast angiography. *J Nucl Med* 1977;18:1159–1166.
4. Ashburn WL, Schelbert HR, Verba JW. Left ventricular ejection fraction—a review of several radionuclide angiographic approaches using the scintillation camera. *Prog Cardiovasc Dis* 1978;20:267–284.
5. Wackers FJ, Berger HJ, Johnstone DE, et al. Multiple gated cardiac blood pool imaging for left ventricular ejection fraction: Validation of the technique and assessment of variability. *Am J Cardiol* 1979;43:1159–1166.
6. Nichols K, Adatepe MH, Isaacs GH, et al. A new scintigraphic method for determining left ventricular volumes. *Circulation* 1984;70:672–680.
7. Greenberg BH, Drew D, Botvinick EH, et al. Evaluation of left ventricular performance by gated radionuclide angiography. *Clin Nucl Med* 1980;5:245–254.
8. Hegge FN, Hamilton GW, Larson SM, et al. Cardiac chamber imaging: A comparison of red blood cells labeled with Tc-99m in vitro and in vivo. *J Nucl Med* 1978;19:129–134.
9. Massie BM, Kramer BL, Gertz EW, et al. Radionuclide measurement of left ventricular volume: Comparison of geometric and count based methods. *Circulation* 1982;65:725–730.
10. Links JM, Becker LC, Shindledecker JG, et al. Measurement of absolute left ventricular volume from gated blood pool studies. *Circulation* 1982;65:82–90.
11. Arrighi JA, Dilsizian V. Radionuclide angiography in coronary and noncoronary heart disease: Technical background and clinical applications. In Harbert JC, Eckelman WC, Neumann RD. *Nuclear medicine: Diagnosis and therapy.* New York: Thieme Medical Publishers, Inc., 1996.
12. Bacharach SL, Green MV, Borer JS. Left ventricular peak ejection rate, peak filling rate, and ejection fraction: Frame rate requirements at rest and during exercise. *J Nucl Med* 1979;20:189–195.
13. Brutsaert DL, Housmans PR, Goethals MA. Dual control of relaxation: Its role in the ventricular function in the mammalian heart. *Circ Res* 1980;47:637–652.
14. Bianco JA, Filiberti AW, Baker SP, et al. Ejection fraction and heart rate correlate with diastolic peak filling rate at rest and during exercise. *Chest* 1985;88:107–113.
15. Reichek N, Vido D, Axel L, et al. LV ejection fraction following acute MI: Echo, MUGA and MRI—preliminary results from the MARRVEL study. *J Am Coll Cardiol* 2000;35:464A (Abstract).
16. van Royen N, Jaffe CC, Krumholz HM, et al. Comparison and reproducibility of visual echocardiographic and quantitative radionuclide left ventricular ejection fractions. *Am J Cardiol* 1996;7:843–850.
17. Gottsauner-Wolf M, Schedlmayer-Duit J, Porenta G, et al. Assessment of left ventricular function: Comparison between radionuclide angiography and semiquantitative two-dimensional echocardiographic analysis. *Eur J Nucl Med* 1996;3:1613–1618.
18. Bellenger NG, Burgess MI, Ray SG, et al. Comparison of left ventricular ejection fraction and volumes in heart failure by echocardiography, radionuclide ventriculography and cardiovascular magnetic resonance; are they interchangeable? *Eur Heart J* 2000;2:1387–1396.
19. Nousiainen T, Vanninen E, Jantunen E, et al. Comparison of echocardiography and radionuclide ventriculography in the follow-up of left ventricular systolic function in adult lymphoma patients during doxorubicin therapy. *J Intern Med* 2001;49:297–303.
20. Todino V, Rubini G, Cuocolo A. Assessment of left ventricular function by ECG-gated myocardial perfusion scintigraphy with image inversion technique: Comparison with equilibrium radionuclide angiography. *J Nucl Cardiol* 1999;6:605–611.
21. Nosir YF, Salustri A, Kasprzak JD, et al. Left ventricular

ejection fraction in patients with normal and distorted left ventricular shape by three-dimensional echocardiographic methods: A comparison with radionuclide angiography. *J Am Soc Echocardiogr* 1998;11:620–630.

22. Acar P, Maunoury C, Antonietti T, et al. Left ventricular ejection fraction in children measured by three-dimensional echocardiography using a new transthoracic integrated 3D-probe. A comparison with equilibrium radionuclide angiography. *Eur Heart J* 1998;19:1583–1588.

23. Calnon DA, Kastner RJ, Smith WH, et al. Validation of a new counts-based gated single photon emission computed tomography method for quantifying left ventricular systolic function: Comparison with equilibrium radionuclide angiography. *J Nucl Cardiol* 1997;4:464–471.

24. Ritchie JL, Bateman TM, Bonow RO, et al. Guidelines for clinical use of cardiac radionuclide imaging. A report of the American Heart Association/American College of Cardiology Task Force on Assessment of Diagnostic and Therapeutic Cardiovascular Procedures, Committee on Radionuclide Imaging, developed in collaboration with the American Society of Nuclear Cardiology. *Circulation* 1995;91:1278–1303.

25. Strashun A. Drug toxicity. In: Wagner HN, Szabo Z, Buchanan J, eds. *Principles of Nuclear Medicine.* Philadelphia: WB Saunders Company, 1996.

26. Gottdeiner JS, Applebaum FR, Ferrars, BJ, et al. Cardiotoxicity associated with high dose cyclophosphamide therapy. *Arch Intern Med* 1981;141:758–763.

27. Klein JL, Rey PM, Dansey RD, et al. Cardiac sequelae of doxorubicin and paclitaxel as induction chemotherapy prior to high-dose chemotherapy and peripheral blood progenitor cell transplantation in women with high-risk primary or metastatic breast cancer. *Bone Marrow Transplant* 2000;25:1047–1052.

28. Cohen MC, Huberman MS, Nesto RW. Recombinant alpha-2 interferon related cardiomyopathy. *Am J Med* 1988;85:549–551.

29. Deyton LR, Walker RE, Kovacs JA. Reversible cardiac dysfunction associated with interferon alpha therapy in AIDS patients with Kaposi's sarcoma. *N Engl J Med* 1989;321:1246–1249.

30. Du Bois JS, Udelson JE, Atkins MB. Severe reversible global and regional ventricular dysfunction associated with high-dose interleukin-2 immunotherapy. *J Immunother Emphasis Tumor Immunol* 1995;18:119–123.

31. Alexander J, Dainiak N, Berger HJ, et al. Serial assessment of doxorubicin cardiotoxicity with quantitative radionuclide angiocardiography. *N Engl J Med* 1979;300:278–283.

32. Lefrak EA, Pitha J, Rosenheim S, et al. A clinicopathologic analysis of doxorubicin cardiotoxicity. *Cancer* 1973;32:302–314.

33. Van Hoff DD, Layard MM, Basa P, et al. Risk factors for doxorubicin induced congestive heart failure. *Ann Intern Med* 1979;91:710–717.

34. Felker GM, Thompson RE, Hare JM, et al. Underlying causes and long-term survival in patients with initially unexplained cardiomyopathy. *N Engl J Med* 2000;342:1077–1084.

35. O'Bryan RM, Baker LH, Gottlieb JE, et al. Dose response evaluation of doxorubicin in human neoplasia. *Cancer* 1977;39:1940–1948.

36. Bristow MR, Mason JW, Billingham ME, et al. Dose-effect and structure function relationships in doxorubicin cardiomyopathy. *Am Heart J* 1981;88:168–175.

37. Druck MN, Gulenchyn KY, Evans WK, et al. Radionuclide angiography and endomyocardial biopsy in the assessment of doxorubicin cardiotoxicity. *Cancer* 1984;53:1667–1674.

38. Choi BW, Berge JH, Schwartz PG, et al. Serial radionuclide assessment of doxorubicin cardiotoxicity with quantitative radiounuclide angiography. *N Engl J Med* 1979;300:278–293.

39. Bristow MR, Lopez MB, Mason JW, et al. Efficacy and cost of cardiac monitoring in patients receiving doxorubicin. *Cancer* 1982;50:32–41.

40. Bristow MR, Mason JW, Billingham ME, et al. Doxorubicin cardiomyopathy: Evaluation by phonocardiography, endomyocardial biopsy and cardiac catheterization. *Ann Intern Med* 1978;88:168–175.

41. Ganz WI, Sridhar KS, Ganz SS, et al. Review of tests for monitoring doxorubicin-induced cardiomyopathy. *Oncology* 1996;53:461–470.

42. Palmeri ST, Bonow RO, Myers CE, et al. Prospective evaluation of doxorubicin cardiotoxicity by rest and exercise radionuclide angiography. *Am J Cardiol* 1985;58:607–613.

43. Alexander J, Dainik N, Berger HJ, et al. Serial assessment of doxorubicin cardiotoxicity with quantitative radionuclide angiocardiography. *N Engl J Med* 1979;300:278–283.

44. Schwartz RG, McKenzie B, Alexander J, et al. Congestive heart failure and left ventricular dysfunction complicating doxorubicin therapy: Seven-year experience using serial radionuclide angiocardiography. *Am J Med* 1987;82:1109–1118.

45. Torti FM, Bristow MR, Howes AE, et al. Reduced cardiotoxicity of doxorubicin delivered on a weekly schedule assessment by endocardial biopsy. *Ann Intern Med* 1983;99:745–749.

46. Gottdeiner JS, Mathison DJ, Borer JS, et al. Doxorubicin cardiotoxicity: Assessment of left ventricular dysfunction by radionuclide cine-angiography. *Ann Intern Med* 1981;94:430–439.

47. Gottdeiner JS, Katin MJ, Borer JS, et al. Late cardiac effects of mediastinal radiation: Assessment by echocardiography and radionuclide angiography. *N Engl J Med* 1983;308:569–572.

48. Demakis JG, Proskey A, Rahimtoola SH, et al. The natural course of alcoholic cardiomyopathy. *Ann Intern Med* 1974;80:293–297.

49. Weiner RS, Lockhart JT, Schwartz RG. Dilated cardiomyopathy and cocaine abuse. *Am J Med* 1986;81:696–703.

50. Leon MB, Borer JS, Bacharach SL, et al. Detection of early cardiac dysfunction in patients with severe beta-thalassemia and chronic iron overload. *N Engl J Med* 1979;301:1143–1148.

51. Scopinaro F, Banci M, Vania A, et al. Radioisotope assessment of heart damage in hypertransfused thalassaemic patients. *Eur J Nucl Med* 1993;20:603–608.

52. Kucuk NO, Aras G, Sipahi T, et al. Evaluation of cardiac functions in patients with thalassemia major. *Ann Nucl Med* 1999;13:175–179.

53. Borer JS, Hochreiter C, Herrold EM, et al. Prediction of indications for valve replacement among asymptomatic or minimally symptomatic patients with chronic aortic regurgitation and normal left ventricular performance. *Circulation* 1998;97:525–534.

54. Borer JS, Kligfield P. Aortic regurgitation: Making management decisions. *Am Coll Cardiol J Rev* 1995;4:30–32.

55. Bassand JP, Faivre R, Berthout P, et al. Factors influencing the variation of ejection fraction during exercise in chronic aortic regurgitation. *Eur J Nucl Med* 1987;13:419–425.

56. Borer JS, Bacharach SL, Green MV, et al. Exercise-induced left ventricular dysfunction in symptomatic and asymptomatic patients with aortic regurgitation: Assessment with radionuclide cineangiography. *Am J Cardiol* 1978;42:351–357.

57. Dehmer GJ, Firth BG, Hillis LD, et al. Alterations in left ventricular volumes and ejection fraction at rest and during exercise in patients with aortic regurgitation. *Am J Cardiol* 1981;48:17–26.

58. Firth BG. The value of rest and exercise radionuclide ventriculography as compared to echocardiography in the detection of left ventricular dysfunction in patients with chronic aortic regurgitation. *Herz* 1984;9:279–287.

59. Lewis SM, Riba Al, Berger HJ, et al. Radionuclide angiographic exercise left ventricular performance in chronic aortic regurgitation: Relationship to resting echocardiographic dimension and systolic wall stress index. *Am Heart J* 1982;103:498–504.

60. Massie BM, Kramer BL, Loge D, et al. Ejection fraction response to supine exercise in asymptomatic aortic regurgitation: Relation to simultaneous hemodynamic measurements. *J Am Coll Cardiol* 1985;5:847–855.

61. Ormerod OJM, Barber RW, Stone DL, et al. A comparison of radionuclide methods of evaluating aortic regurgitation with observations on the effect of exercise and symptoms. *Eur J Nucl Med* 1986;12:72–76.

62. Steingart RM, Yee C, Weinstein L, et al. Radionuclide ventriculographic study of adaptations to exercise in aortic regurgitation. *Am J Cardiol* 1983;51:483–488.

63. Bonow RO, Rosing DR, McIntosh CL, et al. The natural history of asymptomatic patients with aortic regurgitation and normal left ventricular function. *Circulation* 1983;68:509–517.

64. Bonow RO, Carabello B, de Leon AC Jr, et al. Guidelines for the management of patients with valvular heart disease: Executive summary. A report of the American College of Cardiology/American Heart Association Task Force on Practice Guidelines (Committee on Management of Patients with Valvular Heart Disease). *Circulation* 1998;98(18):1949–1984.

65. Bonow RO, Epstein SE. Is preoperative left ventricular function predictive of survival and functional results after aortic valve replacement for chronic aortic regurgitation? *J Am Coll Cardiol* 1987;10:713–716.

66. Borer JS, Herrold EM, Hochreiter C, et al. Natural history of left ventricular performance at rest and during exercise after aortic valve replacement for aortic regurgitation. *Circulation* 1991;84(5 Suppl): III133–III139.

67. Bonow RO, Dodd JT, Maron BJ, et al. Long-term serial changes in left ventricular function and reversal of ventricular dilatation after valve replacement for chronic aortic regurgitation. *Circulation* 1988;78:1108–1120.

68. Bonow RO. Asymptomatic aortic regurgitation: Indications for operation. *J Card Surg* 1994;9(2 Suppl):I70–I73.

69. Phillips HR, Levine FH, Carter JE, et al. Mitral valve replacement for isolated mitral regurgitation: Analysis of clinical course and late post-operative left ventricular ejection fraction. *Am J Cardiol* 1981;48:647–654.

70. Hochreiter C, Niles N, Devereux RB, et al. Mitral regurgitation: Relationship of non-invasive descriptors of right and left ventricular performance to clinical and hemodynamic findings and to prognosis in medically and surgically treated patients. *Circulation* 1986;73:900–912.

71. Borer JS, Jason M, Devereux RB, et al. Function of the hypertrophied left ventricle at rest and during exercise: Hypertension and aortic stenosis. *Am J Med* 1983;75:34–39.

72. Borer JS, Wencker D, Hochreiter C. Management decisions in valvular heart disease: The role of radionuclide-based assessment of ventricular function and performance. *J Nucl Cardiol* 1996;3:72–81.

73. McKay RG, Safian RD, Lock JE, et al. Assessment of left ventricular and aortic valve function after aortic balloon valvuloplasty in adult patients with critical aortic stenosis. *Circulation* 1987;75:192–203.

74. Morise AP, Goodwin C. Exercise radionuclide angiography in patients with mitral stenosis: Value of right ventricular response. *Am Heart J* 1986;112:509–517.

75. Kriss JP, Enright LP, Hayden WG, et al. Radioisotope angiocardiography: Wide scope of applicability in diagnosis and evaluation of therapy in diseases of the heart and great vessels. *Circulation* 1971;43:792–808.

76. Boucher CA, Okada RD, Pohost GM. Current status of radionuclide imaging in valvular heart disease. *Am J Cardiol* 1980;46:1153–1163.

77. *2001 Heart and Stroke Statistical Update*. Dallas: American Heart Association, 2001.

78. The SOLVD Investigators. Effect of enalapril on survival in patients with reduced left ventricular ejection fractions and congestive heart failure. *N Engl J Med* 1991;325:293–302.

79. Harris PJ, Harrell FE Jr, Lee KL, et al. Survival in medically treated coronary artery disease. *Circulation* 1979;60:1259–1269.

80. Mock MB, Ringqvist I, Fisher LD, et al. Survival of medically treated patients in the coronary artery surgery study (CASS) registry. *Circulation* 1982;66:562–568.

81. Pfeffer M, Braunwald E, Moye L, et al. for the SAVE Investigators. Effect of captopril on mortality and morbidity in patients with left ventricular dysfunction after myocardial infarction: Results of the survival and ventricular enlargement trial. *N Engl J Med* 1992;327:669–677.

82. Jones RH, Floyd RD, Austin EH, et al. The role of radionuclide angiocardiography in the preoperative prediction of pain relief and prolonged survival following coronary artery bypass grafting. *Ann Surg* 1983;197:743–754.

83. Lee KL, Pryor DB, Pieper KS, et al. Prognostic value of radionuclide angiography in medically treated patients with coronary artery disease: A comparison with clinical and catheterization variables. *Circulation* 1990;82:1705–1717.

84. Pryor DB, Harrell FE Jr, Lee KL, et al. Prognostic indicators from radionuclide angiography in medically treated patients with coronary artery disease. *Am J Cardiol* 1984;53:18–22.

85. The Digitalis Investigation Group. The effect of digoxin on mortality and morbidity in patients with heart failure. *N Engl J Med* 1997;336:525–533.

86. Packer M, Bristow MR, Cohn JN, et al. The effect of carvedilol on morbidity and mortality in patients with chronic heart failure. N *Engl J Med* 1996;334:1349–1355.

87. Clements IP, Miller WL. Effect of metoprolol on rest and exercise left ventricular systolic and diastolic function in idiopathic dilated cardiomyopathy. *Am Heart J* 2001;141:259.

88. Steinman TI, Becker BN, Frost AE, et al. Guidelines for the referral and management of patients eligible for solid organ transplantation. *Transplantation* 2001;71:1189–1204.

89. Underwood SR, Walton S, Laming PJ, et al. Differential sensitivity of radionuclide ventriculography for the detection of anterior and inferior infarction. *Br Heart J* 1988;60:411–416.

90. Starling MR, Dell'Italia LJ, Chaudhuri TK, et al. First transit and equilibrium radionuclide angiography in patients with inferior transmural myocardial infarction: Criteria for the diagnosis of associated hemodynamically significant right ventricular infarction. *J Am Coll Cardiol* 1984;4:923–930.

91. Reduto LA, Berger HJ, Cohen LS, et al. Sequential radionuclide assessment of left and right ventricular performance after acute transmural myocardial infarction. *Ann Intern Med* 1978;89:441–447.

92. Griffin BP, Shah PK, Diamond GA, et al. Incremental prognostic accuracy of clinical, radionuclide and hemodynamic data in acute myocardial infarction. *Am J Cardiol* 1991;68:707–712.

93. Risk stratification and survival after myocardial infarction. *N Engl J Med* 1983;309:331–336.

94. Rogers WJ, Papapietro SE, Wackers FJT, et al. Variables predictive of good functional outcome following thrombolytic therapy in the Thrombolysis in Myocardial Infarction phase II (TIMI II) pilot study. *Am J Cardiol* 1989;63:503–512.

95. Simoons ML, Vos J, Tijssen JGP, et al. Long-term benefit of early thrombolytic therapy in patients with acute myocardial infarction: 5 year follow-up of a trial conducted by the Interuniversity Cardiology Institute of the Netherlands. *J Am Coll Cardiol* 1989;14:1609–1615.

96. Christian TF, Behrenbeck T, Pellikka PA, et al. Mismatch of left ventricular function and infarct size demonstrated by technetium-99m isonitrile imaging after reperfusion therapy for acute myocardial infarction: Identification of myocardial stunning and hyperkinesia. *J Am Coll Cardiol* 1990;16:1632–1638.

97. Cerqueira MD, Maynard C, Ritchie JL, et al. Long-term survival in 618 patients from the Western Washington Streptokinase in Myocardial Infarction Trials. *J Am Coll Cardiol* 1992;20:1452–1459.

98. Borges-Neto S, Shaw LJ, Kesler K, et al. Usefulness of serial radionuclide angiography in predicting cardiac death after coronary artery bypass grafting and comparison with clinical and cardiac catheterization data. *Am J Cardiol* 1997;79:851–855.

99. Rocchi G, Poldermans D, Bax JJ, et al. Usefulness of the ejection fraction response to dobutamine infusion in predicting functional recovery after coronary artery bypass grafting in patients with left ventricular dysfunction. *Am J Cardiol* 2000;85:1440–1444.

100. Kent KM, Bonow RO, Rosing DR, et al. Improved myocardial function during exercise after successful percutaneous transluminal coronary angioplasty. *N Engl J Med* 1982;306:441–446.

101. Wallis JB, Supino PG, Borer JS. Prognostic value of left ventricular ejection fraction response to exercise during long-term follow-up after coronary bypass grafting surgery. *Circulation* 1993;88:II99-II109.

102. Borer JS, Supino P, Wencker D, et al. Assessment of coronary artery disease by radionuclide cineangiography: History, current applications, and future directions. *Cardiol Clin* 1994;12:333–357.

103. Iskandrian AS, Heo J, Kong B, et al. Use of technetium-99m isonitrile (RP-30A) in assessing left ventricular perfusion and function at rest and during exercise in coronary artery disease, and comparison with coronary arteriography and exercise thallium-201 SPECT imaging. *Am J Cardiol* 1989;64:270–275.

104. DePuey EG, Nichols K, Dobrinsky C. Left ventricular ejection fraction assessed from gated technetium-99m-sestamibi SPECT. *J Nucl Med* 1993;34:1871–1876.

105. Williams KA, Taillon LA. Left ventricular function in patients with coronary artery disease assessed by gated tomographic myocardial perfusion images. Comparison with assessment by contrast ventriculography and first-pass radionuclide angiography. *J Am Coll Cardiol* 1996;27:173–181.

106. Faber TL, Cooke CD, Folks RD, et al. Left ventricular function and perfusion from gated SPECT perfusion images: An integrated method. *J Nucl Med* 1999;40:650–659.

107. Inouye I, Massie B, Loge D, et al. Abnormal left ventricular filling: An early finding in mild to moderate systemic hypertension. *Am J Cardiol* 1984; 53:120–126.

108. Cuocolo A, Sax FL, Brush JE, et al. Left ventricular hypertrophy and impaired diastolic filling in essential hypertension: Diastolic mechanisms for systolic dysfunction during exercise. *Circulation* 1990;81:978–986.

109. Wasserman AG, Katz RJ, Varghese PJ, et al. Exercise radionuclide ventriculographic responses in hypertensive patients with chest pain. *N Engl J Med* 1984;311:1276–1280.

110. Christian TF, Zinsmeister AR, Miller TD, et al. Left ventricular systolic response to exercise in patients with systemic hypertension without left ventricular hypertrophy. *Am J Cardiol* 1990;65:1204–1208.

111. Pohost GM, Vignola PA, McKusick KE, et al. Hypertrophic cardiomyopathy: Evaluation by gated cardiac blood pool scanning. *Circulation* 1977;55:92–99.

112. Bonow RO, Rosing DR, Bacharach SL, et al. Effects of verapamil and left ventricular systolic function and diastolic filling in patients with hypertrophic cardiomyopathy. *Circulation* 1981;64:787–796.

113. Seiler C, Jenni R, Vassalli G, et al. Left ventricular chamber dilatation in hypertrophic cardiomyopathy: Related variables and prognosis in patients with

medical and surgical therapy. *Br Heart J* 1995;74:508–516.

114. Bulkley BH, Hutchins GM, Bailey I, et al. Thallium-201 imaging and gated blood pool scans in patients with ischemic and idiopathic congestive cardiomyopathy: A clinical and pathologic study. *Circulation* 1977;55:753–760.

115. Greenberg JM, Murphy JH, Okada RD, et al. Value and limitations of radionuclide angiography in determining the cause of reduced left ventricular ejection fraction: Comparison of idiopathic dilated cardiomyopathy and coronary artery disease. *Am J Cardiol* 1985;55:541–544.

116. Kriett JM, Kaye MP. The Registry of the International Society for Heart and Lung Transplantation: Eighth official report—1991. *J Heart Lung Transplant* 1991;10:491–498.

117. Lee KJ, Wallis JW, Miller TR, et al. The clinical utility of radionuclide ventriculography in cardiac transplantation. *J Nucl Med* 1990;31:1933–1939.

118. Verhoeven PP, Lee FA, Ramahi TM, et al. Prognostic value of noninvasive testing one year after orthotopic cardiac transplantation. *J Am Coll Cardiol* 1996;28:183–189.

119. Follansbee WP, Kiernan JN, Curtiss EI, et al. Changes in left ventricular systolic function that accompany rejection of the transplanted heart: A serial radionuclide assessment of fifty-three consecutive cases. *Am Heart J* 1991;121:548–556.

120. Hartmann A, Maul FD, Huth A, et al. Serial evaluation of left ventricular function by radionuclide ventriculography at rest and during exercise after orthotopic heart transplantation. *Eur J Nucl Med* 1993;20:146–150.

121. Hershberger RE, Ni H, Toy W, et al. Distribution and declines in cardiac allograft radionuclide left ventricular ejection fractions in relation to late mortality. *J Heart Lung Transplant* 2001;20:417–424.

122. Leon AC, Marzuk PM, Portera L. More reliable outcome measures can reduce sample size requirements. *Arch Gen Psychiatry* 1995;52:867–871.

123. Obuchowski NA. Sample size tables for receiver operating characteristic studies. *Am J Roentgenol* 2000;175:603–608.

124. Rippin G. Design issues and sample size when exposure measurement is inaccurate. *Method Inf Med* 2001;40:137–140.

125. Nadel HR, Stilwell ME. Cardiopulmonary nuclear medicine in children. In: Freeman LM, ed. *Nuclear Medicine Annual 1998.* New York, Lippincott-Raven, 1998.

126. Starmer CE, Clark DO. Computer computations of cardiac output using the gamma function. *J Appl Physiol* 1970;28:219–220.

127. Maltz DL, Treves S. Quantitative radionuclide

angiocardiography: Determination of Qp:Qs in children. *Circulation* 1973;47:1049–1056.

128. Askenazi J, Ahnberg DS, Korngold E, et al. Quantitative radionuclide angiocardiography: Detection and quantification of left to right shunts. *Am J Cardiol* 1976;37:382–387.

129. Gelfand MJ, Hannon DW. Nuclear studies of the heart and great vessels. In: Miller JH, Gelfand MH, eds. *Pediatric nuclear imaging.* Philadelphia: WB Saunders, 1994.

130. Wernovsky G, Hurwitz RA, Weindling SN, et al. Heart. In: Treves ST, ed. *Pediatric nuclear medicine.* New York: Springer Verlag, 1981.

131. Kalbaek H, Aldershvile J, Svendsen JH, et al. Evaluation of left to right shunts in adults with atrial septal defect using first-pass radionuclide cardiography. *Eur Heart J* 1992;13:491–495.

132. Kress P, Bitter F, Stauch M, et al. Radionuclide ventriculography: A non-invasive method for the detection of left to right shunts in atrial septal defect. *Clin Cardiol* 1982;5:192–200.

133. Lear JL, Pratt JP. Real-time list-mode processing of gated cardiac blood pool examinations with forward-backward framing. *Eur J Nucl Med* 1992;19:177–180.

134. Vaquero JJ, Rahms H, Green MV, et al. Dynamic circular buffering: A technique for equilibrium gated blood pool imaging. *Comput Biol Med* 1996; 26:113–121.

135. Vemmer T, Steinbuchel C, Bertram J, et al. Cardiac phase-synchronized myocardial thallium-201 single-photon emission tomography using list mode data acquisition and iterative tomographic reconstruction. *Eur J Nucl Med* 1997;24:276–280.

CHAPTER 9

Performing the Test: Exercise and Pharmacologic Stress Testing

Aaron Satran

Robert C. Hendel

INTRODUCTION

Using radiopharmaceuticals to visualize the regional distribution of myocardial perfusion during rest and stress is a well-established modality for the evaluation of known or suspected coronary artery disease (CAD). In 1964, the first scintigraphic images of myocardial perfusion were acquired by Carr and colleagues,[1] while Zaret and coworkers were the first to demonstrate exercise-induced myocardial ischemia using thallium-201 (Tl-201) in 1973.[2] Since then, the field of nuclear cardiology has grown dramatically, and numerous studies have validated the utility of both stress and pharmacologic myocardial perfusion imaging (MPI) for risk assessment and the prediction of future cardiac events. With more than 5 million such studies being performed yearly in the United States alone, understanding the logistics of and options available for nuclear stress testing is paramount.

EXERCISE STRESS TESTING

Whenever possible, exercise is the preferred modality for stress testing, because it allows for a physiologic assessment of functional capacity, hemodynamics, and symptoms. In addition, when compared to pharmacologic stress testing, exercise is associated with less extensive hepatic and gastrointestinal tracer uptake, which significantly improves image quality.[3]

MPI in conjunction with exercise stress testing enhances diagnostic sensitivity and specificity, particularly among patients with resting electrocardiographic (ECG) abnormalities that preclude the interpretation of ST-segment deviation. Similarly, MPI can differentiate true-positive from false-positive ST-segment depression, which is helpful, because among patients referred for exercise ECG testing with a low to intermediate pretest probability of CAD, approximately 40% of those who develop ST-segment depression will not have CAD.[4] When compared to ECG interpretation in isolation, MPI not only provides a more accurate assessment of the extent and severity of disease, but it can also localize ischemia to a particular vascular distribution. MPI is also useful when patients fail to achieve their target heart rate during exercise, because myocardial perfusion abnormalities in response to stress occur earlier than ECG changes.[5] Finally, when combined with exercise, MPI not only improves diagnostic capability, but it is also predictive of short- and long-term cardiac events.[6] This important prognostic ability does not apply to ECG interpretation without concurrent use of the Duke treadmill score or the presence of significant ischemic changes, such as ST-segment elevation (see below).

Logistics and Procedures

The indications and contraindications for exercise MPI are listed in Tables 9-1 and 9-2. Among patients who are capable of physical exercise, MPI is usually performed using one of several standardized treadmill protocols. Individuals who are generally healthy should perform treadmill exercise using the Bruce protocol, which calls for 3-minute stages of gradually increasing speed and grade. Older individuals, or those with limited exercise capacity, can be evaluated with a modified Bruce protocol that incorporates two warm-up stages. Other protocols, such as the Naughton or Weber, use 1- or 2-minute stages with incremental 1-MET increases, and are appropriate for patients with significantly limited exercise tolerance. Cycle ergometers, while less expensive than treadmills, are infrequently used in the United States. They are unfamiliar to many patients, and often preclude maximum levels of exercise due to muscle fatigue. Regardless of the particular protocol or equipment, 6 to 12 minutes of continuous and progressive exercise produces maximal myocardial metabolic demand and is optimal for diagnostic and prognostic purposes.[7-11]

From a procedural standpoint, patients should be instructed not to eat, drink, or smoke

Table 9-1

Indications for Exercise Stress Myocardial Perfusion Imaging

Indication	Class
1. Diagnosis of Ischemic Heart Disease	
Symptomatic or asymptomatic myocardial ischemia	I
Identification of lesions causing myocardial ischemia, if not known	I
Risk stratification prior to noncardiac surgery	I
Screening of asymptomatic patients with a low likelihood of disease	III
2. Assessment of Severity, Prognosis, and Risk Stratification	
Identification of extent and severity of ischemia, and localization of ischemia	I
Presence and/or extent of stress-induced myocardial ischemia after AMI	I
3. Assessment of Interventions and Therapy in Ischemic Heart Disease	
Assessment for restenosis after PCI (symptomatic)	I
Assessment for ischemia after CABG (symptomatic)	I
Assessment of asymptomatic patients after PTCA or CABG with resting ECG abnormalities, or a known abnormal ECG response to exercise	I
Identification of extent and severity of disease in patients whose unstable angina is controlled with medical therapy	IIa
Effect of medical therapy on myocardial perfusion	IIb
Routine assessment of asymptomatic patients after PTCA or CABG	III

AMI = acute myocardial infarction, PCI = percutaneous coronary intervention, CABG = coronary artery bypass grafting, ECG = electrocardiogram.
Class I: Usually appropriate and considered helpful
Class II: Acceptable but usefulness less well established
Class IIa: Weight in favor of usefulness
Class IIb: Can be helpful but not well established
Class III: Generally not appropriate
Adapted from ACC/AHA Guidelines, 1995.

Table 9-2

Contraindications to Exercise Stress Testing

Absolute	Relative[a]
Acute MI (< 2 days)	Left main coronary stenosis
Uncontrolled unstable angina	Moderate valvular stenosis
Uncontrolled, symptomatic arrhythmias	Electrolyte abnormalities
Decompensated CHF	Uncontrolled hypertension (BP > 200/110)
Symptomatic severe aortic stenosis	Tachy- or bradyarrhythmias
Acute PE or pulmonary infarction	Hypertrophic cardiomyopathy or outflow tract obstruction
Acute myocarditis or pericarditis	Mental or physical impairment
Acute aortic dissection	High-grade AV block

MI = myocardial infarction, CHF = congestive heart failure, PE = pulmonary embolism, BP = blood pressure.
[a] Relative contraindications can be suspended if the benefits of exercise stress testing outweigh the risks.
Adapted from ACC/AHA Guidelines, 2002.

for 8 hours prior to exercise testing, and to wear comfortable shoes and loose-fitting clothing. Antihypertensive and antianginal medications can limit the development of ischemia and blunt the physiologic heart rate response during exercise, resulting in a lower level of sensitivity for detecting CAD. Thus, whenever clinically feasible, these medications (beta blockers, calcium channel blockers, and long-acting nitrates) should be tapered and discontinued anywhere from 12 to 48 hours prior to exercise testing,[12] especially if the study is being performed for diagnostic purposes.

After explaining the logistics of the test as well as the potential risks and benefits, informed consent is obtained, after which a brief history and physical examination should be conducted in order to elicit any medical issues that may limit or preclude exercise. An intravenous line is then placed for injection of the radiopharmaceutical agent. During exercise, the heart rate, blood pressure, and ECG should be recorded toward the end of each stage, and with symptoms should they occur. When the endpoint of exercise is reached, the radiopharmaceutical is injected rapidly and followed by a saline flush, and the patient is encouraged to continue exercising for at least 1 to 2 more minutes. Continuation of exercise is crucial because it allows for myocardial extraction of radiopharmaceutical during peak blood flow and maximum ischemic stress. If necessary, the speed and grade of the treadmill can be decreased to allow for continuation of exercise. Following completion of the test, monitoring should continue for at least 5 to 10 minutes or until any symptoms resolve. The indications for terminating exercise MPI, aside from patient fatigue, are listed in Table 9-3.

ECG Interpretation

Prior to any form of single photon emission computed tomography (SPECT) MPI, standard 12-lead ECGs should be recorded along with blood pressure and heart rate in both the supine and standing positions, since postural changes can elicit ST-T–wave abnormalities. Hyperventilation, which can also produce nonspecific ST-segment changes, is no longer recommended as a routine prior to stress testing.[13] If false-positive ST-segment changes due to hyperventilation are suspected, a hyperventilation ECG can always be obtained after the test is complete,[14] and then compared with the maximal ST-segment abnormalities observed during exercise.

Multiple ECG changes can occur as part of the normal physiologic response to exercise, including PR, QRS, and QT interval shortening, and J point, or junctional, depression with rapid, upsloping ST-segments. In the presence of underlying ischemia, the ST-segment classically becomes horizontal during exercise, a finding that may be associated with angina or become more pronounced with increasing workload (Figure 9-1). Abnormal ECG findings during exercise include ≥ 1 mm of horizontal or downsloping ST-

Table 9-3

Indications for Termination of Exercise Stress Testing

Absolute	Relative
Drop in SBP of ≥ 10 mm Hg from baseline despite increasing workload, when evidence of ischemia is present	Drop in SBP of ≥ 10 mm Hg from baseline despite increasing workload, without evidence of ischemia
Moderate–severe angina	Profound ST-segment depression
Ataxia, dizziness, or near syncope	Multifocal PVCs, triplets of PVCs, SVT, heart block, or bradyarrhythmias
Poor perfusion (pallor, cyanosis)	
Technical difficulties	Fatigue, shortness of breath, or claudication
Subject wishes to stop	New bundle branch block or IVCD that cannot be distinguished from ventricular tachycardia
Sustained ventricular tachycardia	
ST segment elevation without Q waves (except in leads V_1 and AVR)	Increasing chest pain
	Hypertensive response (BP > 250/115)

SBP = systolic blood pressure, PVC = premature ventricular complex, SVT = supraventricular tachycardia, IVCD = intraventricular conduction delay, BP = blood pressure. Adapted from ACC/AHA Guidelines, 2002.

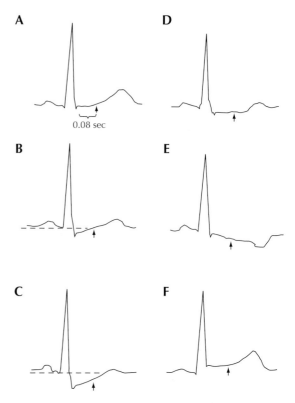

Figure 9-1. Potential ST-segment changes during exercise. **A.** Normal. **B.** Upsloping ST-segment depression that returns to baseline within 0.08 sec (arrow). **C.** Persistent upsloping ST-segment depression. **D.** Horizontal ST-segment depression. **E.** Downsloping ST-segment depression. **F.** ST-segment elevation. Reprinted from Tavel[16] with permission.

segment depression (STD), and 1.5 mm of up-sloping STD, all measured 60 to 80 msec after the J point.[15-17] Of these criteria, downsloping STD is the strongest predictor of underlying CAD. Precordial STD, especially in lead V_5, is more reliable for detecting CAD in patients without prior myocardial infarction (MI) and normal resting ECG's than is STD in the inferior leads, which carries a high false-positive rate.

STD may first appear after exercise is complete or persist during recovery,[18,19] emphasizing the need for continuous monitoring throughout the procedure. STD that begins after the cessa-

tion of exercise is not more significant than STD that occurs during exercise,[20-22] but when ST changes during exercise are equivocal, downsloping STD during recovery indicates a significant ischemic burden, and portends a poor long-term prognosis.[23] In general, true ischemic STD tends to coincide with the termination of exercise, and frequently persists or intensifies for at least 2 to 3 minutes during recovery. If STD does not occur until more than 2 or 3 minutes into recovery, or if it occurs near peak exertion and resolves rapidly in early recovery, a false-positive response is likely.[16,24]

Overall, the diagnostic accuracy of the exercise ECG in isolation is extremely variable, with an overall mean sensitivity and specificity of ~70%, based on meta-analyses of 147 consecutively published reports involving more than 20,000 patients who underwent both coronary angiography and exercise testing.[13] The sensitivity of exercise-induced ECG changes is higher in populations with a greater prevalence of disease, such as the elderly or those with multiple cardiac risk factors. Likewise, specificity is reduced when false-positive results are likely, as when resting ECG abnormalities or confounding clinical conditions are present (see below).

Exercise-induced STD does not reliably predict the location of coronary stenoses.[25] In contrast, the rare finding of exercise-induced ST-segment elevation (STE) without prior MI implies a high-grade coronary lesion,[25,26] and localizes myocardial ischemia quite accurately. Exercise-induced STE in the presence of a previous transmural MI is relatively common and of debatable significance. The mechanism is unclear, but has been ascribed to wall-motion abnormalities or residual viability in the infarcted area.[27–31]

Confounders of Stress ECG Interpretation

The clinical conditions associated with false-positive ST segment responses to exercise are listed in Table 9-4. In addition to postural changes and hyperventilation, several additional factors deserve further comment. *Resting STD* of < 1 mm in the absence of other abnormal findings is nonspecific, but it is also a relatively sensitive marker for significant CAD, and has been shown to be associated with adverse outcomes.[32–36] Thus, exercise-induced ST segment changes can be reasonably well interpreted in this cohort,[13] with the potential exception of patients taking *digoxin* and those with *left ventricular hypertrophy* (LVH). Digoxin produces abnormal ventricular repolarization and STD in response to exercise.[37–39] Similarly, the repolarization abnormalities associated with LVH decrease the specificity

Table 9-4

Confounders of Exercise ECG Interpretation

- Resting ST-segment depression of > 1 mm
- Left bundle branch block
- Right bundle branch block (precludes interpretation of ST-segment changes in leads V_1–V_3)
- Left ventricular hypertrophy
- Digoxin
- Beta blockers or calcium channel blockers (inadequate heart rate response to exercise)
- Other medications (nitrates, antihypertensive agents, antiarrhythmic agents)
- Preexcitation (Wolff–Parkinson–White syndrome)
- Ventricular paced rhythm

Adapted from ACC/AHA Guidelines, 2002.

of any ECG changes during exercise. Thus, current consensus guidelines for stress testing recommend imaging modalities in combination with exercise among patients taking digoxin, or for those with LVH.[13]

Exercise-induced STD usually occurs in the presence of *left bundle branch block* (LBBB), and has no diagnostic significance or association with ischemia.[40] However, during exercise, both increased heart rate and augmented myocardial workload decrease septal blood flow in the setting of LBBB, which often results in falsely abnormal MPI. Therefore, vasodilator pharmacologic stress MPI is the preferred modality when baseline LBBB or a ventricular paced rhythm is present. Exercise in the setting of *right bundle branch block* (RBBB) is associated with nonischemic anterior STD (in leads V_1–V_3) secondary to abnormal repolarization.[41] Nonetheless, ischemic changes can still be interpreted in the presence of RBBB using the left chest leads (V_5 and V_6) and inferior leads (II, III, and aVF) without reduced sensitivity, specificity, or predictive value. The induction of complete right or left bundle branch block during exercise is a nonspecific finding in isolation, but it may suggest myocardial ischemia if noted in conjunction with hemodynamic or clinical symptoms.[16]

Additional Diagnostic Modalities

Aside from exercise-induced STD, other modalities may provide supplementary clinical and prognostic information during and after stress testing. Michaelides et al.[42] evaluated the utility of *right-sided precordial leads* during exercise testing in a group of 245 patients, and found that the sensitivity and specificity of the ECG to detect CAD was enhanced when compared to standard leads, yielding comparable results to those obtained with stress MPI. However, there was a high pretest prevalence of CAD in their patient population, and without confirmatory studies involving larger groups, the routine use of right-sided leads during stress testing is not currently recommended.[13]

The degree of ST-segment displacement relative to the maximum heart rate achieved during exercise, or *ST/HR index,* has also been suggested as a means to enhance the detection of CAD. This measurement can be derived manually or generated by computer, although its use among symptomatic patients has been limited.[43-48] Thus, the ST/HR index has not been validated for routine use during stress testing, but it may be helpful in certain situations, such as when there is equivocal STD associated with a high exercise heart rate.[13] Also of note, *computer processing* of exercise ECG data to calculate STD is part of most standard software programs, but a significant number of false-positive findings can result.[49] Computerized scores or measurements of ST-segment deviation, while useful, should always be preceded by and compared to the raw ECG data, and never used in isolation.

The increase in heart rate during exercise is a function of parasympathetic withdrawal and sympathetic activation, while heart rate recovery immediately after exercise is mediated by reactivation of the parasympathetic nervous system. *Chronotropic incompetence* during exercise in the absence of rate-limiting medications, although variably defined, generally signifies significant cardiac disease, and among patients with known or suspected coronary artery disease is independently associated with higher all-cause mortality.[50] *Heart rate recovery* after exercise can also provide prognostic information. In a study involving 2,428 consecutive patients undergoing exercise MPI, Cole et al.[51] were the first to demonstrate that a delayed decrease in the heart rate during the first minute after exercise was an independent predictor of overall morality regardless of workload, changes in heart rate during exercise, or perfusion defects. Their findings have been independently confirmed in several subsequent studies.[52-55] Adverse outcomes are also more frequent with persistently elevated *systolic blood pressure* after exercise[56] or an inability to adequately augment systolic blood pressure in response to exercise.

Finally, the *Duke treadmill score* is a valuable clinical tool that is used for diagnosis as well as risk assessment and prognosis. It was originally devised by Mark et al.[57] using clinical and ECG data from almost 3,000 inpatients with known or suspected CAD who underwent exercise stress testing prior to coronary angiography. Briefly, the formula incorporates exercise time, ECG changes, and angina to calculate a score from −11 to +5 which has been shown to be a powerful predictor of mortality. It works equally well with men and women, and has subsequently been validated in outpatients, patients at other centers, and in those with resting nonspecific ST-T–wave changes.[57-60]

PHARMACOLOGIC STRESS TESTING

Even when MPI is combined with exercise stress testing, failure to attain an adequate heart rate response during exercise reduces the sensitivity of stress MPI for detecting CAD, diminishes the extent of defects seen on perfusion scintigraphy,[61-65] and can result in a substantial number (up to 25%) of false negative results.[66-68] Many individuals referred for stress testing are elderly, and are unable to perform maximum exercise because of chronic obstructive pulmonary disease (COPD), physical deconditioning, musculoskeletal and peripheral vascular disease, previous stroke, extremity amputation, unfamiliarity with the treadmill, or simply poor motivation. Heart rate responsiveness is also frequently affected by the use of medications, particularly beta blockers. In addition, as noted above, complete LBBB or a ventricular paced rhythm can produce artifactual septal perfusion defects with exercise.

Pharmacologic stress testing is increasingly being utilized for stress perfusion imaging, and currently accounts for nearly 40% of all nuclear stress tests in the United States. Pharmacologic stress MPI has been well validated when compared to exercise MPI in terms of diagnostic sensitivity, specificity, and risk stratification, and can safely be accomplished with vasodilating agents such as adenosine and dipyridamole, or catecholamines such as dobutamine. The indications for pharmacologic stress MPI are listed in Table 9-5.

Vasodilators: Adenosine and Dipyridamole

Adenosine is a small, ubiquitous heterocyclic compound that is produced endogenously in myocardial smooth muscle and vascular endothe-

Table 9-5

Indications for Pharmacologic Vasodilator Stress Imaging

- Inability to perform adequate exercise
- Left bundle branch block
- Ventricular pacemaker
- Concurrent use of medications that may blunt the heart rate response (calcium channel blockers, beta blockers)
- Evaluation of patients very early after acute myocardial infarction (< 3 days) or very early after PCI (< 2 weeks)

PCI = percutaneous coronary intervention
Adapted from the American Society of Nuclear Cardiology Imaging Guidelines, 2001.

lium, or derived via the extracellular dephosphorylation of adenosine triphosphate (ATP) and adenosine diphosphate (ADP). It acts on four known receptor subtypes (A1, A2A, A2B, and A3). When adenosine binds to cardiac-specific A2A receptors, it triggers several reactions, including increased production of adenylate cyclase and intracellular cyclic adenosine monophosphate (cAMP), all of which ultimately lead to coronary vasodilatation. After activating its receptors, adenosine enters endothelial and red blood cells by a facilitated transport mechanism, where it is rapidly inactivated.

Although commonly referred to as such, by definition pharmacologically induced coronary artery vasodilatation is not a "stress test," since it does not significantly increase the rate–pressure product. The vasodilatory effects of adenosine predominate; it produces little, if any, chronotropic or inotropic response.[69] When cardiac A2A adenosine receptors are activated in patients without CAD, resistance vessel blood flow is increased three to five times above baseline levels. In patients with CAD, the resistance vessels distal to a hemodynamically significant stenosis are usually maximally dilated in order to maintain normal resting flow, and are consequently unaffected by adenosine. However, any adjacent myocardium that is supplied by relatively normal coronary arteries will experience a substantial increase in blood flow when exposed to adenosine. This flow disparity translates into relative hypoperfusion of the ischemic myocardium, which can be then be detected by means of MPI (Figure 9-2).

The preprocedure routine for dipyridamole or adenosine stress MPI is similar to that of exercise MPI. In addition to not eating or drinking for 8 hours before testing, patients should not take xanthine derivatives (e.g., aminophylline) or consume caffeine-containing products for 24 hours prior to testing, because xanthines block adenosine receptors, and can cause false-negative results.[70] Neither dipyridamole nor adenosine should be administered if there is a history of asthma or bronchospasm. Other contraindica-

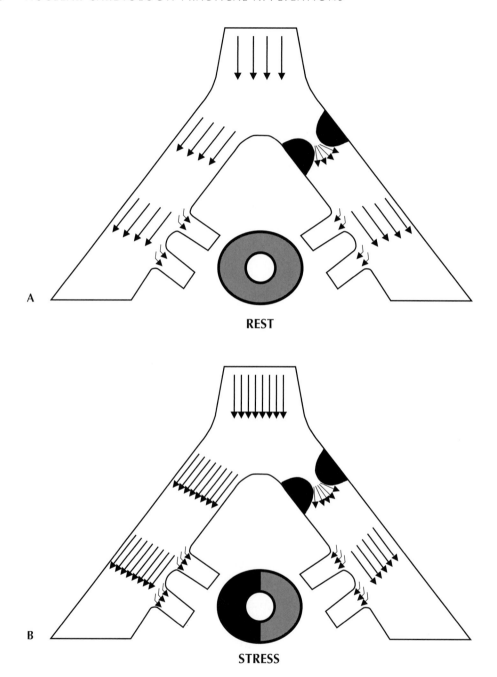

Figure 9-2.   Schematic representation of rest and stress myocardial blood flow. **A.** At rest, the presence of a non–flow-limiting stress does not alter regional perfusion and the representative image appears homogenous. **B.** With vasodilation, coronary blood flow more than doubles. The presence of the stenosis and the limited flow reserve now limits regional perfusion and creates a "defect" on the resultant image.

tions to vasodilatory pharmacologic stress testing include persistent hypotension (systolic blood pressure < 90 mm Hg), unstable angina, or recent acute MI (< 2 days), high-grade AV block without a permanent pacemaker, uncontrolled arrhythmias, and critical aortic stenosis.

Dipyridamole blocks the cellular reuptake of adenosine. It is infused slowly over 4 minutes (0.142 mg/kg/min), at which point maximum vasodilatation is achieved, and the radiopharmaceutical is injected. Frequently, low-level exercise is performed after the infusion is complete in order to minimize side effects, which occur frequently and include headache, flushing, hypotension, nausea, dyspnea, jaw pain, various forms of AV block, and chest discomfort. These effects can often persist for hours because of the lengthy half-life of dipyridamole. Fortunately, major adverse events during dipyridamole stress MPI (death, MI, or stroke) are extremely rare (< 0.001%), as has been demonstrated in more than 73,000 patients.[71] If necessary, the effects of dipyridamole can be reversed with intravenous aminophylline, a competitive adenosine receptor antagonist, although its administration should be delayed for at least 1 minute after the radioisotope injection so as not to compromise the perfusion images.

Adenosine is typically administered at a rate of 140 µg/kg/min over 6 minutes, although protocols using abbreviated 3 or 4 infusions have proven to be equally efficacious.[72–74] Peak vasodilatation after adenosine administration occurs earlier than with dipyridamole, usually within 1 to 2 minutes after the start of the infusion. When using a standard 6-minute protocol, the radiopharmaceutical is injected 3 minutes into the infusion. Exogenous administration of adenosine results in side effects that are similar to those seen with dipyridamole, but they occur more frequently, particularly AV block. Cerqueria et al.[75] prospectively reported the incidence of adenosine-related side effects in a large, multicenter trial. More than 80% of 9,256 patients experienced adverse effects, including flushing (37%), chest pain (35%), dyspnea (35%),

headache (14%), and AV block (8%). However, in contrast to dipyridamole, adenosine has an extremely short half-life (seconds), and thus side effects usually resolve rapidly upon termination of the infusion. Aminophylline may be used, but is rarely necessary. The safety profile of adenosine as a pharmacologic stress MPI agent has been proven through evaluation of more than 15,000 patients.[75,76]

Synthetic Catecholamines: Dobutamine and Arbutamine

Although adenosine and dipyridamole are the preferred agents for pharmacologic stress MPI, they are contraindicated in the presence of asthma or bronchospasm. In such cases, dobutamine can be substituted as a pharmacologic stressor. Dobutamine is a beta-adrenergic receptor agonist with a relatively short biologic half-life (2 minutes) that increases myocardial oxygen demand via positive chronotropic and inotropic effects. It also acts as a vasodilator by increasing blood flow in normal coronary arteries, thereby reducing perfusion pressure distal to significant coronary stenoses.[77–80]

Dobutamine is administered as a continuous infusion, beginning at 5 µg/kg/min for 3 minutes. It is then increased to 10 µg/kg/min for another 3 minutes, and subsequently increased every 3 minutes by 10 µg/kg up to a maximum dose of 40 µg/kg/min. If an adequate heart rate is not achieved, up to 1 mg of atropine can be given to augment the chronotropic response, which safely results in a target heart rate in more than 90% of patients.[81] The radiopharmaceutical is injected one to two minutes after the target heart rate or maximal tolerable dose of dobutamine is reached. The most common side effects of high-dose dobutamine infusion are palpitations, chest pain, and hypertension. Occasionally, patients will experience a hypotensive response to dobutamine because of beta$_2$-adrenergic agonism. Less frequently, ventricular tachycardia (which is rarely sustained) or rapid atrial fibrillation can develop.[82] These adverse effects can be countered with cessation of the dobutamine infusion or by the administration of intravenous beta blockers.

Dobutamine is a safe and effective adjunct to SPECT MPI. The sensitivity, specificity, and diagnostic accuracy of dobutamine stress MPI is comparable to both adenosine and dipyridamole.[83] The prognostic value of dobutamine stress MPI has been questioned, because in the canine model, dobutamine attenuates the myocardial uptake of technetium 99m (Tc-99m) sestamibi, which may result in an underestimation of blood flow heterogeneity seen on perfusion images.[84,85] However, Calnon et al.[86] recently reviewed the clinical outcomes of patients who underwent dobutamine stress MPI at their institution over a 4-year period, and found that this cohort was at high risk for future cardiac events, especially the subgroup of patients with dobutamine-induced STD and abnormal SPECT imaging.

Arbutamine is a synthetic catecholamine with inotropic and chronotropic effects similar to dobutamine, but with fewer peripheral vasodilatory effects and a longer half-life. In a study of 210 patients with CAD, Dennis et al.[87] reported that hemodynamic responses to arbutamine were similar to those seen with exercise, but that arbutamine was more sensitive than exercise for detecting ischemia. Kiat et al.[88] also found that the hemodynamic response and safety profile of arbutamine SPECT MPI were comparable to exercise SPECT, but in their study the sensitivity and diagnostic accuracy of the two modalities were comparable. Overall, although arbutamine may be an effective exercise-simulating agent, it is quite costly, and still has many of the undesirable side effects associated with dobutamine. Arbutamine is still used in animal experiments, but is not clinically available in the United States.

COMBINED EXERCISE AND PHARMACOLOGIC MPI

Combining exercise with pharmacologic stress testing is an attractive option, because it facilitates the assessment of ischemia while still permitting a determination of functional capacity among patients who might not achieve their target heart rate. In addition, concomitant exercise reduces the quantity and severity of adenosine-related side effects, and enhances image quality, possibly resulting in greater detection of ischemia.[89–91]

Exercise has been successfully combined with adenosine[89–94] and dipyridamole,[95–97] using several different protocols. Elliot et al.[89] compared a standard 6-minute adenosine infusion to limited treadmill exercise combined with 4-minute adenosine infusion, and showed a significant reduction in adverse effects as well as improved image quality with the combined protocol (Figure 9-3). Casale et al.[95] studied 100 patients who received an infusion of dipyridamole combined with treadmill exercise to another 100 patients who received dipyridamole alone. They found that their experimental protocol was safe, resulted in fewer side effects, and yielded better-quality perfusion images when compared with standard dipyridamole stress MPI. Stern et al.[96] evaluated dipyridamole infusion combined with different exercise modalities, and concluded that low-level treadmill exercise in combination with

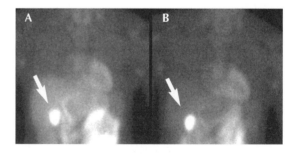

Figure 9-3. Myocardial perfusion imaging: Adenosine versus adenosine + exercise. Panel **A** demonstrates similar intensity in the liver (arrow) as noted in the myocardium following an adenosine infusion. However, when exercise is combined with adenosine (Panel **B**), much less hepatic activity (arrow) is present when compared with the myocardium. Modified from Elliot et al.[89] with permission.

dipyridamole was superior to either handgrip and dipyridamole or dipyridamole alone. Similarly, Igasezewski et al.[97] reported that symptom-limited exercise in combination with dipyridamole was safe and well tolerated, even in elderly patients or those with known significant CAD.

Recently, Holly et al.[98] directly compared standard treadmill exercise to a protocol combining treadmill exercise with a 4-minute adenosine infusion in a group of patients who were thought to be incapable of reaching their target heart rate. The combined adenosine and exercise protocol was well tolerated, with no adverse effects noted as a result of the adenosine infusion. Furthermore, a greater amount of myocardial ischemia was detected using the experimental protocol as compared to exercise alone. In addition, cost savings were significant, because one third less of a dose of adenosine was used with each patient when compared to a standard 6-minute infusion.

In summary, the combination of exercise and pharmacologic MPI is rapidly gaining acceptance as a safe and well-tolerated diagnostic option when choosing a stress test, because it allows for simultaneous assessment of functional capacity and ischemic burden while minimizing or eliminating side effects. These protocols are applicable to a broad range of patients, especially those with marginal exercise tolerance or an inability to temporarily discontinue rate-limiting cardiac medications.

SELECTIVE ADENOSINE A2A RECEPTOR AGONISTS

Adenosine and dipyridamole are well established for use during pharmacologic MPI. However, as noted above, both agents have multiple unpleasant side effects because of their effect on noncardiac adenosine receptors, which can result in patient discomfort and at times cause premature study termination. The intraventricular conduction delays and chest pain that are frequently noted during infusion of adenosine are due to nonselective activation of A1 receptors,[99,100]

while peripheral vasodilatation, bronchoconstriction, and mast cell degranulation that leads to flushing are mediated by A2B receptors.[101,102] Since coronary vasodilatation is mediated by adenosine A2A receptors, selective A2A receptor agonists would seem to offer the advantage of eliminating unwanted side effects while remaining an effective pharmacologic stress agent. In fact, these properties have already been demonstrated in both animal and human trials using various experimental agents. Several different selective A2A receptor agonists are currently in different stages of development and testing, including MRE-0470 (formerly WRC-0470) or binodisine, CGS-21680, ATL-193, ATL-146e, and CVT-3146.[103–106]

CONCLUSIONS

Stress testing in combination with SPECT MPI is a well-established procedure that has been in widespread clinical use for many years. The vast majority of stress testing is performed in order to evaluate either known or suspected CAD. If patients are capable of exercise and have a normal baseline ECG (including complete RBBB and/or < 1 mm of resting STD), they should undergo standard exercise testing without concurrent imaging. If confounding conditions are present, SPECT MPI should be performed along with exercise.

Exercise stress testing with or without SPECT MPI is preferable to any form of pharmacologic stress testing, because it allows for an assessment of functional capacity and provides better quality perfusion images. However, if contraindications to exercise exist, pharmacologic stress with an infusion of adenosine, dipyridamole, or dobutamine can be substituted without diminishing the sensitivity, specificity, or predictive value of SPECT MPI. The side effects of adenosine and dipyridamole, while frequent, are usually inconsequential, and can be easily managed with cessation of the infusion or administration of aminophylline in the case of dipyridamole.

Recent studies combining exercise with adenosine and/or dipyridamole appear to reduce or eliminate these medication-induced side effects while providing an assessment of functional capacity. As such, combined exercise and pharmacologic SPECT MPI may ultimately supplant pharmacologic stress alone among patients who are capable of submaximal exercise. Newer pharmacologic stress agents, which are selective for A2A receptors, appear to be hemodynamically predicable and better tolerated than either adenosine or dipyridamole, while providing comparable imaging data. In the future, they will likely become the pharmacologic stress agents of choice for use during SPECT MPI.

REFERENCES

1. Carr EA, Gleason G, Shaw J, et al. The direct diagnosis of myocardial infarction by photoscanning after administration of cesium-131. *Am Heart J* 1964;68:7627.
2. Zaret BL, Strauss HW, Martin ND, et al. Noninvasive regional myocardial perfusion with radioactive potassium. Study of patients at rest, with exercise and during angina pectoris. *N Engl J Med* 1973;288:809.
3. Jain D, Borges-Neto S, Carrio I, et al. Stress myocardial perfusion imaging protocols. Updated imaging guidelines for nuclear cardiology procedures, part 1. *J Nucl Cardiol* 2001;8:12.
4. Beller GA. Relative merits of cardiovascular diagnostic techniques. In: Braunwald E, Zipes DP, Libby P, eds. *Heart Disease*, 6th ed. Philadelphia: WB Saunders, 2001:426.
5. Esquivel L, Pollock SG, Beller GA, et al. Effect of the degree of effort on the sensitivity of the exercise thallium-201 stress test in symptomatic coronary artery disease. *Am J Cardiol* 1989;63:160.
6. Hachamovitch R, Berman DS, Kiat H, et al. Exercise myocardial perfusion SPECT in patients without known coronary artery disease: Incremental prognostic value and use in risk stratification. *Circulation* 1996;93:905.
7. Chaitman BR. Exercise stress testing. In: Braunwald E, Zipes DP, Libby P, eds. *Heart Disease*, 6th ed. Philadelphia: WB Saunders, 2001:132.
8. Myers J, Froelicher VF. Optimizing the exercise test for pharmacological investigations. *Circulation* 1990; 82:1839–1846.
9. Ellestad MH. *Stress Testing: Principles and Practice*, 4th ed. Philadelphia: FA Davis, 1995.
10. Froelicher VF, Myers J. *Exercise and the Heart*, 3rd ed. Philadelphia: WB Saunders, 1999.
11. Jones NL. *Clinical Exercise Testing*, 4th ed. Philadelphia: WB Saunders, 1997.
12. Ritchie JL, Batemen TM, Bonow RO, et al. Guidelines for clinical use of cardiac radionuclide imaging: A report of the American College of Cardiology/American Heart Association Task Force on assessment of diagnostic and therapeutic cardiovascular procedures (Committee on Radionuclide Imaging), 1995.
13. Gibbons RJ, Balady GJ, Bricker JT, et al. ACC/AHA 2002 guideline update for exercise testing: A report of the American College of Cardiology/American Heart Association Task Force on Practice Guidelines (Committee on Exercise Testing): 2002:12.
14. Chaitman BR. Exercise stress testing. In: Braunwald E, Zipes DP, Libby P, eds. *Heart Disease*, 6th ed. Philadelphia: WB Saunders, 2001:133.
15. Stuart RJ, Ellestad MH: Upsloping ST segments in exercise testing. *Am J Cardiol* 1976;56:13.
16. Tavel ME. Stress testing in cardiac evaluation: Current concepts with emphasis on the ECG. *Chest* 2001;119:907.
17. Eagle KA, Guyton RA, Davidoff R, et al. ACC/AHA guidelines for coronary artery bypass graft surgery: A report of the American College of Cardiology/ American Heart Association Task Force on Practice Guidelines (Committee to Revise the 1991 Guidelines for Coronary Artery Bypass Graft Surgery). American College of Cardiology/American Heart Association. *J Am Coll Cardiol* 1999;34:1262.
18. Froelicher VF. *Exercise and the Heart*, 3rd ed. St. Louis: CV Mosby, 1993.
19. Ellestad MH. *Stress Testing: Principles and Practice*, 3rd ed. Philadelphia: FA Davis, 1986.
20. Rywik TM, Zink NS, Gittings NS, et al. Independent prognostic significance of ischemic ST-segment response limited to recovery from treadmill exercise in asymptomatic subjects. *Circulation* 1998;97:2117.
21. Karnegis JN, Matts J, Tuna N, et al. Comparison of exercise-positive with recovery-positive treadmill graded exercise test. *Am J Cardiol* 1987;60:544.
22. Savage MP, Squires LS, Hopkins JT, et al. Usefulness of ST segment depression as a sign of coronary artery disease when confined to the recovery period. *Am J Cardiol* 1987;60:1405.
23. Rodriguez M, Moussa I, Froning J, et al. Improved exercise test accuracy using discriminant function analysis and "recovery ST slope." *J Electrocardiol* 1993;26:207.
24. Barlow JB. The "false positive" exercise electrocardiogram: Value of time course patterns in assessment of depressed ST segments and inverted T waves. *Am Heart J* 1985;110:1328.
25. Kang X, Berman DS, Lewin HC, et al. Comparative localization of myocardial ischemia by exercise electrocardiography and myocardial perfusion SPECT. *J Nucl Cardiol* 2000;7:140.

26. Galik DM, Mahmarian JJ, Verani MS. Therapeutic significance of exercise-induced ST-segment elevation in patients without previous myocardial infarction. *Am J Cardiol* 1993;72:1.

27. Manvi KN, Ellestad MH. Elevated ST segments with exercise in ventricular aneurysm. *J Electrocardiol* 1972;5:317.

28. Haines DE, Beller GA, Watson DD, et al. Exercise-induced ST segment elevation 2 weeks after uncomplicated myocardial infarction: Contributing factors and prognostic significance. *J Am Coll Cardiol* 1987;9:996.

29. Margonato A, Ballarotto C, Bonetti F, et al. Assessment of residual tissue viability by exercise testing in recent myocardial infarction: Comparison of the electrocardiogram and myocardial perfusion scintigraphy. *J Am Coll Cardiol* 1992;19:948.

30. Margonato A, Chierchia SL, Xuereb RG, et al. Specificity and sensitivity of exercise-induced ST segment elevation for detection of residual viability: Comparison with fluorodeoxyglucose and positron emission tomography. *J Am Coll Cardiol* 1995;25:1032.

31. Lombardo A, Loperfido F, Pennestri F, et al. Significance of transient ST-T segment changes during dobutamine stress testing in Q wave myocardial infarction. *J Am Coll Cardiol* 1996;27:599.

32. Blackburn H. Canadian colloquium on computer-assisted interpretation of electrocardiograms, VI: Importance of the electrocardiogram in populations outside the hospital. *Can Med Assoc J* 1973;108:1262.

33. Cullen K, Stenhouse NS, Wearne KL, et al. Electrocardiograms and 13 year cardiovascular mortality in Busselton study. *Br Heart J* 1982;47:209.

34. Aronow WS. Correlation of ischemic ST-segment depression on the resting electrocardiogram with new cardiac events in 1,106 patients over 62 years of age. *Am J Cardiol* 1989;64:232.

35. Califf RM, Mark DB, Harrel FE Jr, et al. Importance of clinical measures of ischemia in the prognosis of patients with documented coronary artery disease. *J Am Coll Cardiol* 1988;11:20.

36. Harris PJ, Harrell FR Jr, Lee KL, et al. Survival in medically treated coronary artery disease. *Circulation* 1979;60:1259.

37. Sketch MH, Mooss AN, Butler ML, et al. Digoxin-induced positive exercise tests: Their clinical and prognostic significance. *Am J Cardiol* 1981;48:655.

38. LeWinter MM, Crawford MH, O'Rourke RA, et al. The effects of oral propranolol, digoxin, and combination therapy on the resting and exercise electrocardiogram. *Am Heart J* 1977;93:202.

39. Sundqvist K, Atterhög JH, Jogestrand T. Effect of digoxin on the electrocardiogram at rest and during exercise in healthy subjects. *Am J Cardiol* 1986;57:661.

40. Whinnery JE, Froelicher VF Jr, Stuart AJ. The electrocardiographic response to maximal treadmill exercise in asymptomatic men with left bundle block. *Am Heart J* 1977;94:316.

41. Whinnery JE, Froelicher VF Jr, Longo MR Jr, et al. The electrocardiographic response to maximal treadmill exercise in asymptomatic men with right bundle branch block. *Chest* 1977;71:335.

42. Michaelides AP, Psomadaki ZD, Dilaveris PE, et al. Improved detection of coronary artery disease by exercise electrocardiography with use of right precordial leads. *N Engl J Med* 1999;340:340.

43. Okin PM, Kligfield P. Heart rate adjustment of ST segment depression and performance of the exercise electrocardiogram: A critical evaluation. *J Am Coll Cardiol* 1995;25:1726.

44. Fletcher GF, Flipse TR, Kligfield P, et al. Current status of ECG stress testing. *Curr Probl Cardiol* 1998;23:353.

45. Morise AP. Accuracy of heart-rate adjusted ST segments in populations with and without posttest referral bias. *Am Heart J* 1997;134:647.

46. Okin PM, Roman MJ, Schwartz JE, et al. Relation of exercise-induced myocardial ischemia to cardiac and carotid structure. *Hypertension* 1997;30:1382.

47. Viik J, Lehtinen R, Malmivuo J. Detection of coronary artery disease using maximum value of ST/HR hysteresis over different number of leads. *J Electrocardiol* 1999;32(Suppl):70.

48. Froelicher VF, Lehmann KG, Thomas R, et al. The electrocardiographic exercise test in a population with reduced workup bias: Diagnostic performance, computerized interpretation, and multivariable prediction. Veterans Affairs Cooperative Study in Health Services #016 (QUEXTA) Study Group. Quantitative Exercise Testing and Angiography. *Ann Intern Med* 1998;128:965.

49. Milliken JA, Abdollah H, Burggraf GW. False-positive treadmill exercise tests due to computer signal averaging. *Am J Cardiol* 1990;65:946.

50. Lauer MS, Francis GS, Okin PM, et al. Impaired choronotropic response to exercise stress testing as a predictor of mortality. *JAMA* 1999;281:524.

51. Cole CR, Blackstone EH, Pashkow FJ, et al. Heart-rate recovery immediately after exercise as a predictor of mortality. *N Engl J Med* 1999;341:1351.

52. Cole CR, Foody JM, Blackstone EH, et al. Heart rate recovery after submaximal exercise testing as a predictor of mortality in a cardiovascularly healthy cohort. *Ann Int Med* 2000;132:552.

53. Diaz LA, Brunken RC, Blackstone EH, et al. Independent contribution of myocardial perfusion defects to exercise capacity and heart rate recovery for prediction of all-cause mortality in patients with known or suspected coronary heart disease. *J Am Coll Cardiol* 2001;37:1558.

54. Watanabe J, Thamilarasan M, Blackstone EH, et al. Heart rate recovery immediately after treadmill exercise and left ventricular systolic dysfunction as predictors of

mortality: The case of stress echocardiography. *Circulation* 2001;104:1911.

55. Nishime EO, Cole CR, Blackstone EH, et al. Heart rate recovery and treadmill exercise score as predictors of mortality in patients referred for exercise ECG. *JAMA* 2000;284:1392.

56. Shetler K, Marcus R, Froelicher VF, et al. Heart rate recovery: Validation and methodologic issues. *J Am Coll Cardiol* 1999;34:754.

57. Mark DB, Hlatky MA, Harrel FE Jr, et al. Exercise treadmill score for predicting prognosis in coronary artery disease. *Ann Intern Med* 1987;106:793.

58. Kwok JM, Miller TD, Christian TF, et al. Prognostic value of a treadmill exercise score in symptomatic patients with nonspecific ST-T abnormalities on resting ECG. *JAMA* 1999;282:1047.

59. Mark DB, Shaw L, Harrell FE Jr, et al. Prognostic value of a treadmill exercise score in outpatients with suspected coronary artery disease. *N Engl J Med* 1991;325:849.

60. Bruce RA, DeRouen TA, Hossack KF. Pilot study examining the motivational effects of maximal exercise testing to modify risk factors and health habits. *Cardiology* 1980;66:111.

61. Iskandrian AS, Heo J, Askenase A, et al. Dipyridamole cardiac imaging. *Am Heart J* 1988;15:432.

62. Brown KA: Prognostic value of thallium-201 myocardial perfusion imaging: A diagnostic tool comes of age. *Circulation* 1991;83:363.

63. Brown KA, Rowen MA. Impact of antianginal medications, peak heart rate, and stress level on the prognostic value of a normal exercise myocardial perfusion imaging study. *J Nucl Med* 1993;34:1467.

64. Iskandrian AS, Heo J, Kong B, et al. Effect of exercise level on the ability of thallium-201 tomographic imaging in detecting coronary artery disease: Analysis of 461 patients. *J Am Coll Cardiol* 1989;14:1477.

65. Heller GV, Ahmed I, Tilkemeier PL, et al. Influence of exercise intensity on the presence, distribution, and size of thallium-201 defects. *Am Heart J* 1992;123:909.

66. Casale PN, Buiney TE, Strauss HW, et al. Simultaneous low-level treadmill exercise and intravenous dipyridamole stress thallium imaging. *Am J Cardiol* 1988;62:799.

67. Stern S, Greenberg ID, Come RA. Qualification of walking exercise required for improvement of dipyridamole thallium-201 image quality. *J Nucl Med* 1992;33:2061.

68. Igasezewski AP, McCormick LX, Heslip PG, et al. Safety and clinical utility of combined intravenous dipyridamole symptom-related exercise stress test with thallium-201 imaging in patients with known or suspected coronary artery disease. *J Nucl Med* 1993;34:2053.

69. Verani MS. Stress approaches: Techniques. In: Pohost GM, Berman DS, O'Rourke RA, Shah PM, eds. *Imaging in Cardiovascular Medicine.* Philadelphia: Lippincott Williams and Wilkins, 2000:155.

70. Bottcher M, Czernin J, Sun KT, et al. Effect of caffeine on myocardial blood flow at rest and during pharmacological vasodilation. *J Nucl Med* 1995; 36:2016.

71. Lette J, Tatum JL, Fraser S, et al. Safety of dipyridamole testing in 73,806 patients: The Multicenter Dipyridamole Safety Study. *J Nucl Cardiol* 1995;2:3.

72. Treuth MG, Reyes GA, He ZX, et al. Tolerance and diagnostic accuracy of an abbreviated adenosine infusion for myocardial scintigraphy: A randomized, prospective study. *J Nucl Cardiol* 2001;8:548.

73. O'Keefe JH Jr, Bateman TM, Handlin LR, et al. Four versus 6-minute infusion protocol for adenosine thallium-201 single photon emission computed tomography imaging. *Am Heart J* 1995;129:482.

74. Villegas BJ, Hendel RC, Dahlberg ST, et al. Comparison of 3 versus 6-minute infusions of adenosine in thallium-201 myocardial perfusion imaging. *Am Heart J* 1993;126:103.

75. Cerqueria MD, Verani MS, Schwaiger M, et al. Safety profile of adenosine stress perfusion imaging: Results from the Adenoscan Multicenter Trial Registry. *J Am Coll Cardiol* 1994;23:384.

76. Abreu A, Mahmarian JJ, Nishimura S, et al. Tolerance and safety of pharmacologic coronary vasodilatation with adenosine in association with thallium-201 scintigraphy in patients with suspected coronary artery disease. *J Am Coll Cardiol* 1991;18:730.

77. Coma-Canella I. Dobutamine stress test to diagnose the presence and severity of coronary artery lesions in angina. *Eur Heart J* 1991;12:1198.

78. Mazeika PK, Nadazin A, Oakley CM. Dobutamine stress echocardiography for detection and assessment of coronary artery disease. *J Am Coll Cardiol* 1992; 19:1203.

79. Previtali M, Lanzarini L, Ferrario M, et al. Dobutamine versus dipyridamole echocardiography in coronary artery disease. *Circulation* 1991;83(Suppl 3):27.

80. Martin TW, Seaworth JF, John JP, et al. Comparison of adenosine, dipyridamole, and dobutamine in stress echocardiography. *Ann Intern Med* 1992;116:190.

81. Elhendy A, Valkema R, van Domburg RT, et al. Safety of dobutamine–atropine stress myocardial perfusion scintigraphy. *J Nucl Med* 1998;39:1662.

82. Hays JT, Mahmarian JJ, Cochran AJ, et al. Dobutamine thallium-201 tomography for evaluating patients with suspected coronary artery disease unable to undergo exercise or pharmacologic stress testing. *J Am Coll Cardiol* 1993;21:1583.

83. Geleijnse ML, Elhendy A, Fioretti PM, et al. Dobutamine stress myocardial perfusion imaging. *J Am Coll Cardiol* 2000;36:2017.

84. Calnon DA, Glover DK, Beller GA, et al. Effects of dobutamine stress on myocardial blood flow, [99mTc-]

sestamibi, and systolic wall thickening in the presence of coronary artery stenoses: Implications for dobutamine stress testing. *Circulation* 1997;96:2353.

85. Wu JC, Yun JJ, Heller EN, et al. Limitations of dobutamine for enhancing flow heterogeneity in the presence of single coronary stenosis: Implications for technetium-99m-sestamibi imaging. *J Nucl Med* 1998;39:417.

86. Calnon DA, McGrath PD, Doss AL, et al. Prognostic value of dobutamine stress technetium-99m-sestamibi single-photon emission computed tomography myocardial perfusion imaging: Stratification of a high-risk population. *J Am Coll Cardiol* 2001;38:1511.

87. Dennis CA, Pool PE, Perrins EJ, et al. Stress testing with closed-loop arbutamine as an alternative to exercise. *J Am Coll Cardiol* 1995;26:1151.

88. Kiat HS, Iskandrian AS, Villegas BJ, et al. Arbutamine stress thallium-201 single-photon emission computed tomography using a computerized closed-loop delivery system. Multicenter trial for evaluation of safety and diagnostic accuracy. *J Am Coll Cardiol* 1995;26:1159.

89. Elliot MD, Holly TA, Leonard SM, et al. Impact of an abbreviated adenosine protocol incorporating adjunctive treadmill exercise on adverse effects and image quality in patients undergoing stress myocardial perfusion imaging. *J Nucl Cardiol* 2000;7:584.

90. Thomas GS, Prill NV, Majmundar H, et al. Treadmill exercise during adenosine infusion is safe, results in fewer adverse reactions, and improves myocardial perfusion image quality. *J Nucl Cardiol* 2000;7:439.

91. Muller-Suur R, Eriksson SV, Standberg LE, et al. Comparison of adenosine and exercise stress test for quantitative perfusion imaging in patients on beta blocker therapy. *Cardiology* 2001;95:112.

92. Pennell DJ, Mavrogeni SI, Forbat SM, et al. Adenosine combined with dynamic exercise for myocardial perfusion imaging. *J Am Coll Cardiol* 1995;25:1300.

93. Jamil G, Ahlberg AW, Ellliot MD, et al. Impact of limited treadmill exercise on adenosine Tc-99m sestamibi SPECT myocardial perfusion imaging in patients with coronary disease. *Am J Cardiol* 1999;84:400.

94. Samady H, Wackers FJTh, Joska TM, et al. Pharmacologic stress perfusion imaging with adenosine: Role of simultaneous low-level treadmill exercise. *J Nucl Cardiol* 2002;9:188.

95. Casale PN, Buiney TE, Strauss HW, et al. Simultaneous low-level treadmill exercise and intravenous dipyridamole stress thallium imaging. *Am J Cardiol* 1988;62:799.

96. Stern S, Greenberg ID, Come RA. Qualification of walking exercise required for improvement of dipyridamole thallium-201 image quality. *J Nucl Med* 1992;33:2061.

97. Igasezewski AP, McCormick LX, Heslip PG, et al. Safety and clinical utility of combined intravenous dipyridamole symptom-related exercise stress test with thallium-201 imaging in patients with known or suspected coronary artery disease. *J Nucl Med* 1993;34:2053.

98. Holly TA, Satran A, Bromet DS, et al. The impact of adjunctive adenosine infusion during exercise myocardial perfusion imaging: Results of the Both Exercise and Adenosine Stress Test (BEAST) trial. *J Nucl Cardiol*: 2003;10:291.

99. Bertolet BD, Belardinelli L, Franco EA, et al. Selective attenuation by N-0681 (N6-endonorboran-2-yl-9-methyladenie) of cardiac A1 adenosine receptor-mediated effects in humans. *Circulation* 1996;93:1871.

100. Gaspardone A, Crea F, Versaci F. Muscular and cardiac adenosine-induced pain is mediated by A1 receptors. *J Am Coll Cardiol* 1995;25:251.

101. Linden J, Thai T, Figler H, et al. Characterization of human A(2B) adenosine receptors: Radioligand binding, western blotting, and coupling to G(q) in human embryonic kidney 293 cells and HMC-1 mast cells. *Mol Pharmacol* 1999;56:705.

102. Auchampach JA, Jin X, Wan TC, et al. Canine mast cell adenosine receptors: Cloning and expression of the A3 receptor and evidence that degranulation is mediated by the A2B receptor. *Mol Pharmacol* 1997;52:846.

103. Glover DK, Ruiz M, Yang JY, et al. Pharmacological stress thallium scintigraphy with 2-cyclohexyl-methylidenehydrazinoadenosine (WRC-0470): A novel, short-acting adenosine A2A receptor agonist. *Circulation* 1996;94:1726.

104. He ZX, Cwajg E, Hwang W, et al. Myocardial blood flow and myocardial uptake of (201)Tl and (99m)Tc-sestamibi during coronary vasodilation induced by CGS-21680, a selective adenosine A2A receptor agonist. *Circulation* 2000;102:438.

105. Glover DK, Ruiz M, Takehana K, et al. Pharmacological stress myocardial perfusion imaging with the potent and selective A2A adenosine receptor agonists ATL193 and ATL146e administered by either intravenous infusion of bolus injection. *Circulation* 2001;104:1181.

106. Trochu JN, Zhao G, Post H, et al. Selective A2A adenosine receptor agonist as a coronary vasodilator in conscious dogs: potential for use in myocardial perfusion imaging. *J Cardiovasc Pharmacol* 2003;41:132.

CHAPTER 10

Radionuclide Myocardial Perfusion Imaging Protocols

Raymond Taillefer

INTRODUCTION

Introduction of technetium 99m (Tc-99m)-labeled myocardial perfusion imaging (MPI) radiopharmaceuticals with different biological characteristics and more data on the effective use of thallium 201 (Tl-201) especially for myocardial viability assessment, has resulted in several and very different imaging protocols. This multitude of protocols has created some confusion, mainly to the referring physician, who is not always familiar with all the new imaging developments. Various factors must be taken into consideration when designing a new protocol such as physical characteristics of the radionuclide, the dosimetry related to the radiotracer, its physical and biological half-lives, myocardial redistribution, biodistribution in adjacent organs to the heart, degree of contamination from a previous study, improvement of laboratory logistics, the clinical question to be addressed, patient convenience, and cost-effectiveness. However, optimiza-

tion of the imaging results and the best diagnostic accuracy for a given specific clinical indication remain the major goals of any new imaging protocol. The purpose of this chapter is to briefly review the most important imaging protocols currently used in nuclear cardiology laboratories and to compare their relative advantages and disadvantages.

THALLIUM 201 IMAGING PROTOCOLS

Although Tl-201 has been the major radiopharmaceutical used for MPI for more than 15 years, its use in a single radiotracer protocol without concomitant Tc-99m-labeled myocardial perfusion agents (known as dual radionuclide study) is very limited in 2003. Except for myocardial viability assessment, the standard stress-redistribution protocol, as described more than 25 years ago,[1] is rarely used in clinical practice since several nuclear cardiology laboratories have opted for either the dual-radionuclide approach or the Tc-99m-labeled perfusion agents for both rest and stress studies. Many modifications to the so-called standard stress-redistribution injection protocol were mostly designed to improve the value of Tl-201 imaging for myocardial viability assessment.

The following major characteristics of Tl-201 must be considered when imaging protocols are designed: (1) the dosimetry of Tl-201 limits its injected dose to a total of 4.0 to 4.5 mCi; (2) the myocardial half-life of Tl-201 is approximately 2 to 3 hours; (3) there is a significant myocardial redistribution of Tl-201 following its intravenous injection; (4) active transport mechanisms (Na–K–ATPase pump) are involved in the myocyte uptake of Tl-201, an important characteristic for its use in viability assessment; (5) the physical half-life of Tl-201 is 73 hours.

Figure 10-1 summarizes seven major protocols involving Tl-201 as a single radiopharmaceutical. According to the standard or traditional imaging protocol (number 1), a dose of 2 to 3.5 mCi of Tl-201 is injected intravenously at peak stress (treadmill, bicycle, or pharmalogic intervention) and the patient continues the exercise for one or two more minutes to allow for a better myocardial uptake and better heart-to-background ratio. Single photon emission computed tomography (SPECT) imaging starts within 5 to 10 minutes (stress imaging) after the injection. Approximately 3 to 4 hours later, a second imaging session (called delayed or redistribution imaging) is performed. This part of the study is also referred as the rest study, although this does not correspond to a real injection at rest. Various studies have shown that this protocol has a high accuracy in the diagnosis and prognosis of coronary artery disease (CAD); however, it often underestimates myocardial viability.[2–3] Effectively, up to 60% of patients with fixed perfusion defects on the traditional stress-redistribution protocol may have viable myocardium in the area with the nonreversible defect. In these cases, it is likely that the delay of 4 hours between the stress and

redistribution phases is too short to allow for a complete myocardial redistribution of Tl-201. Several modifications to this traditional protocol have been proposed, especially to improve the accuracy of Tl-201 imaging for myocardial viability assessment.

Protocols number 2 through 7 in Figure 10-1 illustrate some of these most important modifications of Tl-201 imaging specifically designed to assess myocardial viability. With the stress-immediate reinjection protocol (number 2), a smaller dose of Tl-201 (1.0 mCi) is reinjected at rest immediately after the stress imaging session. Although this protocol might improve the viability assessment, it suffers from two significant disadvantages: (1) many patients may not need a second dose of Tl-201 since the conventional approach may have provided all the necessary diagnostic information without the increasing cost of the second Tl-201 dose, and (2) the total allowable dose has to be divided for the stress and for the reinjection, decreasing the counting statistics of the stress study, sometimes resulting in a suboptimal quality study. Another similar approach (number 3, delay-reinjection protocol) is to reinject a second dose of Tl-201 (1.0 mCi) at rest, immediately after the delayed or redistribution study has been completed. Delayed-reinjection study is then performed 45 minutes later. This protocol has an advantage over the previous one: It does not use an unnecessary dose of Tl-201 before the second study (redistribution). If the study shows a reversible perfusion defect, there is no need for a second injection. The split Tl-201 dose still remains with its disadvantages and the protocol is lengthy for the patient.

Late-redistribution imaging (number 4) is another alternative to the previous ones. In this protocol, a late redistribution imaging session is performed 24 hours after the Tl-201 injection if fixed perfusion defects are detected and if viability assessment is clinically relevant. This modification does not require an additional injection of Tl-201. However, the count statistics are low at 24 hours and the quality of the images is often suboptimal. Protocols number 5 and 6 offer a

1. TRADITIONAL PROTOCOL

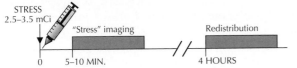

2. STRESS—IMMEDIATE REINJECTION PROTOCOL

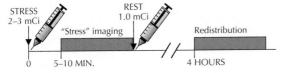

3. DELAY—REINJECTION PROTOCOL

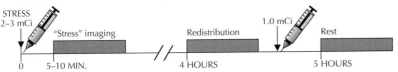

4. LATE REDISTRIBUTION PROTOCOL

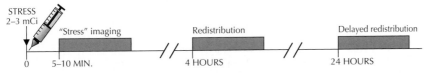

5. LATE REST REINJECTION PROTOCOL (IMMEDIATE REST)

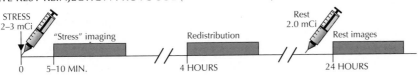

6. SEPARATE STRESS–REST REDISTRIBUTION PROTOCOL

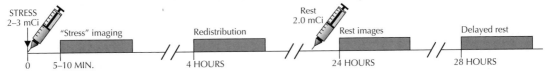

7. STRESS/DELAY–NITRATE PROTOCOL

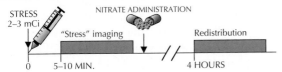

Figure 10-1.   Thallium-201 imaging protocols.

better approach for viability assessment. They both include in a second injection of Tl-201 at rest at least 24 hours after the injection at stress, followed by images. Protocol number 6 also add a fourth imaging session 4 hours after the second injection at rest. This probably represents one of the best approach for both diagnostic and viability assessment. If there is a fixed perfusion defect on the conventional protocol and if viability assessment is clinically relevant, the patient is asked to come back the day after for a second injection of Tl-201 at rest followed by two imaging sessions, one performed 30 minutes later and the second one 4 hours later. This is the most complete protocol in which a second dose of Tl-201 is used only when necessary and the quality of the images is not jeopardized.

Finally, another alternative (which is good for both Tl-201 and Tc-99m-labeled perfusion agents) is to administer isosorbide dinitrate (20 mg) orally (or nitrospray, 0.6 mg) after imaging at stress in order to accelerate redistribution (protocol number 7).[4]

The choice of Tl-201 imaging protocol will depend on the clinical question to be answered and on the results of the conventional protocol. Furthermore, laboratory logistics and ability of the patients to come back for the second study are to be taken into consideration.

TC-99M-LABELED PERFUSION AGENT IMAGING PROTOCOLS (TC-99M-SESTAMIBI AND TC-99M-TETROFOSMIN)

Unlike Tl-201, Tc-99m-sestamibi and Tc-99m-tetrofosmin do not significantly redistribute in the myocardium after their injection. This characteristic offers interesting advantages in clinical practice:

1. Imaging after the stress injection is much more flexible than with Tl-201.
2. Image acquisition can be repeated if there is a significant patient motion or instrument malfunction.

3. It is likely that the image will not be "degraded" by increased respiratory movements, "upward creep" movement of the heart, or rapid myocardial redistribution, as seen when imaging is performed rapidly after an injection of Tl-201.

Because of the absence of significant myocardial redistribution, two separate injections of these two agents, one with the patient at rest and one during stress, are required to differentiate ischemia from scar. Given the 6-hour physical half-life of Tc-99m, a 24-hour separation between the two injections is optimal to minimize background radioactivity for the second set of images. In clinical practice, however, having patients undergo imaging on two separate days may sometimes be inconvenient or impractical. Having all the information from both studies available on a single day is highly desirable in many cases. For these reasons, both 2-day and 1-day protocols for rest and stress imaging have been developed.

For 2-day studies, the Tc-99m-labeled agent is injected at stress, followed 24 or 48 hours later by a second injection at rest (Figure 10-2). Alternatively, the order of the injections can be reversed, with the rest study being performed first. If the stress study is performed first, 20 to 30 mCi (according to the body weight, 0.30 mCi/kg) is injected at peak stress, and imaging is begun 15 to 60 minutes later. The next day the patient is injected with 20 to 30 mCi at rest, and image acquisition is begun 60 to 90 minutes later with Tc-99m-sestamibi and 15 to 45 minutes with Tc-99m-tetrofosmin. If the rest study is done first, 20 to 30 mCi is injected at rest, and imaging is begun 60 to 90 minutes later for Tc-99m-sestamibi and earlier with Tc-99m-tetrofosmin. The next day, the patient is injected with 20 to 30 mCi at peak stress, and imaging is started 15 to 60 minutes later.

The advantages of the 2-day protocol are the following: The 2-day stress–rest protocol has been suggested to be best for novice users of these agents. It is the ideal one based on the

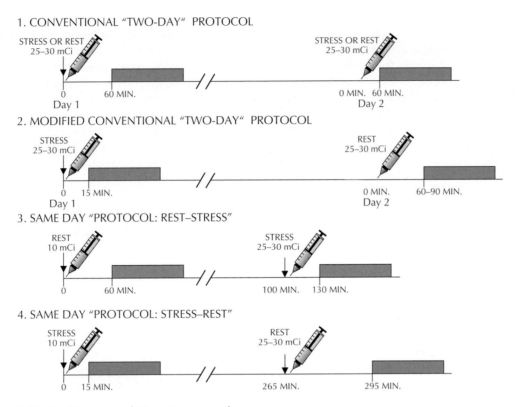

Figure 10-2.   Tc-99m-sestamibi imaging protocols.

physical half-life of Tc-99m. The 2-day protocol also provides scheduling flexibility in that a patient need only be scheduled for a single study on a given day. The 2-day stress–rest protocol offers also the possibility of eliminating the rest study in cases when the stress study is strictly normal. However, as with Tl-201, the ability to judge a single Tc-99m-labeled agent image as strictly normal requires a good deal of experience.

Initial studies with Tc-99m-sestamibi showed that 1 hour after stress injection appeared to be a favorable time for image acquisition because the liver activity has significantly decreased.[5–7] Using the higher-contrast imaging afforded with SPECT, some investigators have further shortened the injection-to-imaging time to 15 minutes for exercise studies.[8] Thus, after a stress injection of Tc-99m-sestamibi, the liver clearance is rapid enough to permit image acquisition as early

as 15 minutes. However, after a rest injection or injection after pharmacologic intervention such as dipyridamole or adenosine, the best compromise is achieved between 60 and 90 minutes after Tc-99m-sestamibi injection. However, earlier imaging can be performed with Tc-99m-tetrofosmin and Tc-99m-furifosmin. Imaging beyond 2 hours after injection is not recommended unless previous images showed a persistent significantly increased subdiaphragmatic activity from small bowel or stomach activity secondary to an enterogastric reflux.[9–10] Although initial reports have suggested to use either a glass of milk or a small fatty meal in order to stimulate gallbladder emptying and decrease liver uptake, feeding decreased the activity in the gallbladder but had no effect on liver parenchyma activity.

In some clinical circumstances, making a rapid diagnosis may be useful or essential. In such cases, the 1-day protocols are a good alternative.[11] A 1-day protocol may be necessary for practical reasons as well. For example, it may be difficult or even impossible for a patient to come to the nuclear medicine or cardiology laboratory on two separate days. The 1-day protocols offer convenience for patients and rapid availability of results. There are two different 1-day protocols according to the injection sequence of the rest and the stress studies.

A dose of Tc-99m-labeled agent is injected at stress or at rest followed the same day by a second, higher dose at rest or at stress (Figure 10-2, protocols 3 and 4). The initial 1-day protocol has been suggested by Taillefer et al.[12] who have used a rest–stress sequence. The Tc-99m-sestamibi doses of 8 to 10 mCi at rest and 25 to 30 mCi at stress were empirically chosen based on preliminary data obtained in their laboratory. The rest–stress dose ratio of approximately 1:3 was also empirically determined, taking into consideration the time interval of 2 hours and the rest–stress injection sequence. A lower ratio can be used, but doing so necessitates increasing the time interval between the two injections. Rest–stress and stress–rest injection sequences for 1-day Tc-99m-sestamibi studies have been compared. Taillefer et al.[12] concluded that a rest–stress sequence is preferable when using a 1-day protocol with a short time interval (< 2 hours) between the two Tc-99m-sestamibi injections, because the rest image performed initially represents a "true" rest study. This is not necessarily the case with the stress–rest sequence due to cross-talk from the stress study present in the rest images. In the rest–stress protocol, there is no "contamination" on the rest study from previous Tc-99m-sestamibi injection. If the stress–rest sequence is used with a longer time interval or with a higher dose at rest, it is likely that results will improve.[13]

Heo et al.[14] compared a rest–stress and a stress–rest protocol for Tc-99m-sestamibi SPECT imaging in 32 patients. They also showed that the rest–stress protocol provided better image contrast and an increased ability to detect reversibility

of perfusion defects. However, the investigators reported that the images obtained using either of the two 1-day protocols were of high quality, and diagnostic results were equivalent. The 1-day stress–rest protocol offers advantages that must be taken into consideration: It allows for elimination of the rest study if the stress study is found to be normal. Furthermore, this sequence offers scheduling similar to that of Tl-201 imaging, which may be more convenient for the nuclear medicine or cardiology staff.

DUAL-RADIONUCLIDE IMAGING PROTOCOLS

Although both 2-day and 1-day Tc-99m-sestamibi imaging protocols have their respective advantages, they also present some disadvantages. In order to avoid these limitations (mainly the relatively long time necessary to complete both rest and stress studies) and also to allow for optimal assessment of perfusion and myocardial viability in a single study, Berman et al.[15] have introduced a dual-radionuclide imaging protocol (Figure 10-3). This protocol consists of an injection of 3.0 to 3.5 mCi of Tl-201 at rest and injection of 25 to 30 mCi of Tc-99m-sestamibi at stress. SPECT imaging starts 10 to 15 minutes after the initial injection of Tl-201 at rest. Immediately following Tl-201 imaging, the patient performs an exercise. At near maximal exercise, a dose of 25 to 30 mCi of Tc-99m-sestamibi is injected. SPECT imaging starts 15 to 30 minutes later. The separate-acquisition dual-radionuclide imaging procedure can be completed in approximately 2 hours. Due to the small contribution of Tl-201 photons into the Tc-99m energy window, this separate-acquisition approach does not require any specific physical correction, contrary to the initial procedure that has been suggested, in which a single imaging period with multiple energy windows to simultaneously detect both Tl-201 (corresponding to rest study) and Tc-99m (corresponding to the stress study) was used (Figure 10-3, protocol 1). This approach of a single acquisition is very attractive in clinical practice because it requires only one image acquisition,[16] it may significantly improve patient throughput, and there is a perfect alignment of both rest and stress images since they are simultaneously acquired. However, a simple and validated method to correct for the spillover of both radionuclides does not exist at the present time.

The dual-radionuclide Tl-201/Tc-99m-sestamibi imaging approach (with two separate acquisitions) has been popularized and extensively validated by the investigators at Cedars-Sinai Medical Center[17–19] and other groups.[20–21] Their results demonstrated a high diagnostic accuracy with good correlation with coronary angiography and "standard" Tc-99m-sestamibi imaging. The dual-radionuclide study also has been compared to rest–stress Tc-99m-sestamibi imaging to evaluate the degree of defect reversibility. In segments with no prior myocardial infarction (MI), the segmental agreement between rest Tl-201 and rest Tc-99m-sestamibi was 97% (kappa: 0.79, $p < 0.001$), whereas in segments with MI the segmental agreement was 98% (kappa: 0.93, $p < 0.001$). The agreement for defect reversibility pattern (normal, transient, or fixed) was 95% (kappa: 0.89, $p < 0.001$).

The dual-radionuclide imaging protocol is relatively shorter than a 1-day Tc-99m-sestamibi protocol and thus can be used to increase patient throughput. It also has the advantage of combining the use of the optimal radionuclide for exercise imaging (Tc-99m-sestamibi) and the optimal radiotracer for myocardial viability assessment (Tl-201). However, this protocol presents some disadvantages. The physical characteristics of the two radionuclides involved are quite different, resulting in a different count density (related to the difference in the injected doses and in the characteristics of emitted photons). This may affect the evaluation of the degree of defect reversibility, especially in patients with prior MI and an abnormal Tl-201 rest study.[22–23] Furthermore, the quality of the rest Tl-201 studies is sometimes suboptimal. Financial impact must also be taken into consideration since two different radionuclides are involved. Depending on the availability and the cost of the radiotracers, the dual-radionuclide protocol may be more expensive. Nevertheless, this protocol has been shown to be as accurate as rest–stress Tc-99m-sestamibi imaging protocol.

The dual-radionuclide imaging protocol can also be modified (Figure 10-3, protocol 3), according to the clinical indication. It has been shown that a 15-minute delay between the injection of Tl-201 at rest and the imaging may sometimes be not sufficient to accurately assess myocardial viability in patients with resting hypoperfusion.[24] This modification consists of an injection of 3.0 to 3.5 mCi of Tl-201 at rest the day (usually the evening) before the stress study. The next day, an 18-to-24-hour Tl-201 redistribution image is performed. As for the "standard" protocol, Tc-99m-sestamibi is injected at stress immediately after Tl-201 rest imaging. This delay of 18 to 24 hours following the Tl-201 injection at rest permits a more complete redistribution in viable myocardium. The main disadvantages are that this protocol is lengthy (at least 24 hours), it requires modifications of laboratory logistics (injection of Tl-201 in the evening before the stress test), and the quality of the 18 to 24-hour Tl-201 images is frequently suboptimal. However, it is an attractive approach for both detection of CAD and assessment of myocardial viability. Finally, it offers another approach to cardiac investigation with radionuclide techniques.

TCN-99M-NOET IMAGING PROTOCOLS

TcN-99m-NOET is a new radiopharmaceutical under clinical investigation and not approved yet for clinical use. At the present time, the number of reported clinical imaging protocols is very limited. Since TcN-99m-NOET demonstrates some degree of myocardial redistribution, similar to Tl-201, Fagret et al.[25] have used a stress-redistribution imaging protocol with TcN-99m-NOET. They showed a similar diagnostic accuracy between the two agents with such imaging proto-

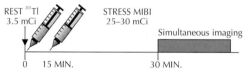

1. INITIAL PROTOCOL WITH SIMULTANEOUS ACQUISITION

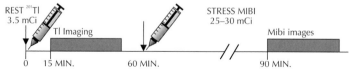

2. STANDARD DUAL RADIONUCLIDE PROTOCOL

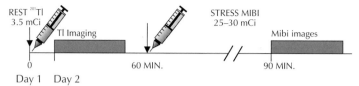

3. TWO-DAY INJECTION PROTOCOL

Figure 10-3. Dual-radioisotope imaging protocols.

col. More comparative data will be needed, but it is likely that if these results are confirmed by other studies, imaging protocols similar to those used for Tl-201 could be applicable to TcN-99m-NOET MPI.

CONCLUSION

Many radionuclide MPI agents are now commercially available with their specific characteristics. Although many of these differ, all these radiotracers share the same utilization, that is the diagnostic and evaluation of patients with CAD. All various imaging protocols have their relative advantages and disadvantages. Even though the variety of protocols may seem confusing, they are all necessary in order to fulfill their ultimate goal: providing the best quality and best diagnostic procedures.

REFERENCES

1. Pohost GM, Zir LM, Moore RH, et al. Differentiation of transiently ischemic from infarcted myocardium by serial imaging after a single dose of thallium-201. *Circulation* 1977;55:294–302.

2. Cloninger KG, DePuey EG, Garcia EV, et al. Incomplete redistribution in delayed thallium-201 single photon emission computed tomographic (SPECT) images: An overestimation of myocardial scarring. *J Am Coll Cardiol* 1988;12:955–963.

3. Kiat H, Berman DS, Maddahi J, et al. Late reversibility of tomographic myocardial thallium-201 defects: An accurate marker of myocardial viability. *J Am Coll Cardiol* 1988;12:1456–1463.

4. He ZX, Darcourt J, Guignier A, et al. Nitrates improve detection of ischemic viable myocardium by thallium-201 reinjection SPECT. *J Nucl Med* 1993; 34:1472–1477.

5. Worsley DF, Fung AY, Coupland DB, et al. Comparison of stress-only vs. stress-rest technetium-99m methoxyisobutylisonitrile myocardial perfusion imaging. *Eur J Nucl Med* 1992;19:441–444.

6. Taillefer R, Dupras G, Sporn V, et al. Myocardial perfusion imaging with a new radiotracer, technetium-99m-hexamibi (methoxy isobutyl isonitrile): Comparison with thallium-201 imaging. *Clin Nucl Med* 1989;14;89–96.

7. Taillefer R, Lambert R, Dupras G, et al. Clinical comparison between thallium-201 and Tc-99m-methoxy isobutyl isonitrile (hexamibi) myocardial perfusion imaging for detection of coronary artery disease. *Eur J Nucl Med* 1989;15:280–286.

8. Taillefer R, Lambert R, Bisson G, et al. Myocardial technetium-99m-labeled sestamibi single-photon

emission computed tomographic imaging in the detection of coronary artery disease: Comparison between early (15 minutes) and delayed (60 minutes) imaging. *J Nucl Cardiol* 1994;1:441–448.

9. Hassan IM, Mohammad MMJ, Constantinides C, et al. Problems of duodenogastric reflux in Tc-99m hexa MIBI planar, tomographic and bull's eye display. *Clin Nucl Med* 1989;14:286–289.

10. Middleton GW, Williams JH. Significant gastric reflux of technetium-99m MIBI in SPECT myocardial imaging. *J Nucl Med* 1994;35:619–620.

11. Taillefer R. Technetium-99m sestamibi myocardial imaging: Same-day rest–stress studies and dipyridamole. *Am J Cardiol* 1990;66:80–84E.

12. Taillefer R, Gagnon A, Laflamme L, et al. Same day injections of Tc-99m methoxy isobutyl isonitrile (hexamibi) for myocardial tomographic imaging: Comparison between rest–stress and stress–rest injection sequences. *Eur J Nucl Med* 1989;15:113–117.

13. Picard M, Franceschi M, Sia BST, et al. Tc-99m-methoxyisobutyl isonitrile (MIBI): Comparing a one- and two-day protocol for the assessment of transient ichemia. *J Nucl Med* 1988;29:851 (abstract).

14. Heo J, Kegel J, Iskandrian AS, et al. Comparison of same-day protocols using technetium-99m-sestamibi myocardial imaging. *J Nucl Med* 1992;33:186–191.

15. Berman DS, Kiat H, Friedman JD, et al. Separate acquisition rest thallium-201/stress technetium-99m sestamibi dual-isotope myocardial perfusion single-photon emission computed tomography: A clinical validation study. *J Am Coll Cardiol* 1993; 22:1455–1464.

16. Yang DC, Ragasa E, Gould L, et al. Radionuclide simultaneous dual-isotope stress myocardial perfusion study using the "three window technique". *Clin Nucl Med* 1993;18:852–857.

17. Berman D, Friedman J, Kiat J, et al. Separate acquisition dual isotope myocardial perfusion SPECT: Results of a large clinical trial. *J Am Coll Cardiol* 1992;19:202A (abstract).

18. Kiat H, Germano G, Friedman J, et al. Comparative feasibility of separate or simultaneous rest thallium-201/stress technetium-99m-sestamibi dual-isotope perfusion SPECT. *J Nucl Med* 1994;35:542–548.

19. Kiat H, Germano G, VanTrain K, et al. Quantitative assessment of photon spillover in simultaneous rest Tl-201/stress Tc-sestamibi dual isotope perfusion SPECT. *J Nucl Med* 1992;33:854–855.

20. Heo J, Wolmer I, Kegel J, et al. Sequential dual-isotope SPECT imaging with thallium-201 and technetium-99m-sestamibi. *J Nucl Med* 1994;35:549–553.

21. Weinmann P, Foult JM, LeGuludec M, et al. Dual-isotope myocardial imaging: Feasibility, advantages and limitations. Preliminary report on 231 consecutive patients. *Eur J Nucl Med* 1994;21:212–215.

22. Wackers FJT. The maze of myocardial perfusion imaging protocols in 1994. *J Nucl Cardiol* 1994;1:180–188.

23. Siebelink HMJ, Natale D, Sinusas AJ, et al. Quantitative comparison of single-isotope and dual-isotope stress–rest single-photon emission computed tomographic imaging for reversibility of defects. *J Nucl Cardiol* 1996;3:483–493.

24. Dilsizian V, Rocco TP, Freedman NMT, et al. Enhanced detection of ischemic but viable myocardium by the reinjection of thallium after stress-redistribution imaging. *N Engl J Med* 1990;323:141–146.

25. Fagret D, Marie PY, Brunotte F, et al. Myocardial perfusion imaging with technetium-99m-Tc NOET: Comparison with thallium-201 and coronary angiography. *J Nucl Med* 1995;36:936–943.

CHAPTER 11

Quality Control for Myocardial Perfusion Imaging

April Mann

INTRODUCTION

Quality control in nuclear cardiology is a multiple-step process that begins before the patient enters the laboratory, occurs during the acquisition, and continues after the patient leaves the laboratory. It requires attention from the technologist as well as the physician. Requirements for imaging system quality control are based on Nuclear Regulatory Commission (NRC) and agreement state requirements.[1-4] The requirements and frequency may vary from state to state and institution to institution. However, the basic premise of why it is necessary is the same in all situations: to ensure adequate camera performance, identify any potential sources of error or artifact within an acquisition, and ultimately to provide the patient and referring physician with the best-quality information possible. If quality control procedures are not followed, it may lead to an equivocal or falsely interpreted study, which may result in increased downstream costs as well as poor outcomes.

QUALITY CONTROL BEFORE THE ACQUISITION

There are several required and recommended equipment quality control procedures that should be performed on each imaging system.[2,5] The recommended frequency of the procedures may vary among equipment manufacturers; however, all are important to ensure proper system performance (Table 11-1). These tasks consist of daily, weekly, and quarterly system testing.

Daily

Energy Peaking Energy peaking (photopeak analysis) should be performed daily to verify that the camera is counting photons using the correct energy.[2,3] Each imaging system should be checked before use to ensure that the camera peaking electronics are functioning properly, that the energy window has not drifted and that the energy spectrum is the appropriate shape.

Table 11-1

Recommended Frequency for Gamma
Camera Quality Control Procedures

Test	Frequency
Energy peaking	Daily
Uniformity	Daily
Sensitivity	Daily or weekly
Resolution and linearity	Weekly
Center of rotation	Weekly
SPECT phantom evaluation	Quarterly

During the procedure, the pulse height analyzer's energy window should be manually or automatically placed over the correct photopeak energy. It is recommended that no greater than a 2% energy window be used in order to obtain the most accurate peak energy.[2,6] If the test is performed intrinsically, a point source should be placed at least 1.5 meters away from the surface of the camera detector. If performed extrinsically, a sheet source should be used. In either case, the source should be enough to flood the entire field of view (FOV).

Verifying the photopeak daily will help prevent artifacts that may occur due to inappropriate photons entering the acquisition and degrading image quality. An off-centered photopeak may also result in poor count statistics, which will result in a poor-quality image.[2-4] If dual-isotope procedures are being performed, on some older imaging systems it may be necessary to perform this procedure between each acquisition of thallium 201 (Tl-201) and technetium 99m (Tc-99m) isotopes.

Daily Uniformity Flood A daily uniformity flood should be performed to analyze system performance and to ensure the sensitivity response of the system is uniform across the detector surface.[2-7] This is performed by exposure of the detector surface to a radioactive source. The recommended method is to perform this procedure intrinsically using a Tc-99m point source of approximately 100 to 500 µCi in ≤ 0.5 mL of volume. The point source should be placed in the center and at a distance of approximately five useful fields of view (UFOV) away from the detector surface. An acquisition should be performed for approximately 2 to 5 million counts using a 20% energy window.[2,5] This may also be performed extrinsically using a 57-Cobalt sheet source. This method is performed frequently on dual-head camera systems because the acquisition can be performed on both detectors at the same time. It is important to remember, however, that during the uniformity analysis of extrinsic floods, the outer 10 to 20% of the FOV should not be considered due to possible edge packing.[2,5]

After the acquisition of the flood field uniformity, the image should be evaluated visually, and a computerized analysis should be performed to measure the performance of the system. Central FOV and UFOV parameters should be < 5%. This analysis should be performed following manufacturers' protocols and will be specific to each imaging system. If nonuniformities are detected, the system should not be used until service is performed. Severe artifacts, such as malfunctioning photomultiplier tubes, will be easily detected (Figure 11-1). Smaller abnormalities may be more difficult to detect, however. These

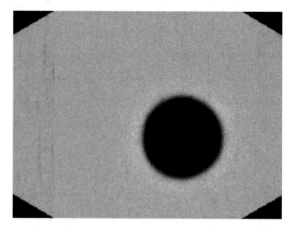

Figure 11-1. Illustration of a uniformity flood that had a cluster of photo multiplier tubes not functioning.

small, undetected nonuniformities may produce artifacts within patient acquisitions and result in a misinterpretation of the study.[5–8]

Weekly

Center of Rotation   A center of rotation (COR) should be performed weekly in order to ensure and maintain the detector's electronic matrix alignment.[2,5–8] This is the x-axis position of the actual axis of rotation as seen by the image matrix.[5] If a COR error occurs, it may produce what has been characterized as a "doughnut"-shaped or "tuning fork" artifact (Figure 11-2).[2] This artifact may appear similar to an artifact caused by patient motion on the perfusion images. This error becomes more pronounced if the deviation widens, particularly > 2 pixels in a 64 × 64 matrix. Smaller deviations may not produce an artifact but could result in decreased spatial resolution and image contrast.[2,5]

Several manufacturers have recommended camera-specific protocols to follow when performing COR procedures. Most recommend using a 500 to 750 μCi point source placed off center in the field of view at approximately 4 to 8 inches away from the detector surface.[2,5] The acquisition is then performed using similar parameters as a standard SPECT. An analysis of this acquisition should be performed, and for any misalignment of > 0.5 pixels of the x-axis, the COR should be recalibrated (Figure 11-3).

System Resolution and Linearity Test   System spatial resolution and linearity evaluation should be performed weekly. This procedure is performed to document spatial resolution over

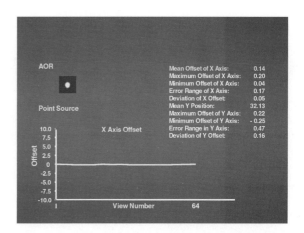

Figure 11-3.   Example of a COR analysis. Mean x offset should be less than 0.5, and evaluation of the graph should be performed for any deviation as well.

time, as well as evaluate the detector's ability to produce straight lines.[2,5] This procedure should be performed intrinsically using a radioactive point source and a test phantom. This evaluation should not be performed extrinsically because the patterns of the lead bars in the phantom and the lead septa of the collimator may interfere with one another causing artifacts.

There are several bar phantoms available commercially that may be used for this test. The most common used are the parallel-line-equal-spaced (PLES), orthogonal hole, and four-quadrant phantoms.[2,5] The four-quadrant phantom has four sections of differing thickness lead bars that are equally spaced. If this type of phantom is used routinely, it should be placed over the detector surface so that each differing size lead bar is in a different position from the previously performed test (rotated 90 degrees from the previously placed position). This will allow the most tightly spaced bars of the phantom to appear over the entire surface of the detector every fifth acquisition. This will provide the most thorough evaluation of the entire detector surface over time.[2,5]

Acquisition parameters for the resolution and linearity test should be similar to those used to perform a daily uniformity flood. Upon completion,

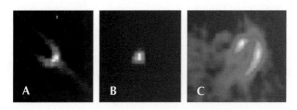

Figure 11-2.   **A.** Tuning fork artifact. **B.** Normal COR image. **C.** Apical artifact a result of COR deviation.

the image should be evaluated visually to assess the straightness of the lines produced by the bar phantom and for how well each different-size lead bar is visualized (Figure 11-4). The test should be stored in an electronic format for comparison of system resolution over time. As a decrease in resolution appears (loss of visualization of individual bars) maintenance should be performed. Manufacturers may supply software to evaluate linearity and resolution that should be used when available.

Quarterly

SPECT Phantom   The National Electrical Manufacturers' Association (NEMA) recommends that SPECT phantoms be performed quarterly.[3-4] This allows for the evaluation of an imaging system's performance and limitations by providing a comparative means to judge previous performance with the most recent phantom acquisition.[2,5] Commercially available multipurpose Plexiglas and water-filled SPECT phantoms have attenuation and scattering properties similar to that of tissue, thus simulating clinical conditions in a three-dimensional view. This allows for a realistic comparison of system performance similar to that in the clinical setting. Therefore, acquisition parameters used should be similar to that of standard SPECT.

QUALITY CONTROL DURING THE ACQUISITION

The previous section focused on quality control procedures related to the imaging system and should be performed prior to the image acquisition. There are also several quality control techniques that should be performed during the acquisition to help achieve an optimal and interpretable study.[5,9]

In order to optimize image quality, it is necessary to ensure patient comfort, utilize appropriate imaging protocols, perform appropriate camera setup and acquisition parameters, and recognize potential sources of internal and external attenuation and artifacts. Artifacts and errors that occur during an acquisition may be the result of inappropriate camera setup or may be patient related (Table 11-2). Understanding potential sources of artifact and using proper imaging techniques may reduce potential errors due to artifact and increase overall test specificity.[5]

Protocols and Acquisition Setup

There are four commonly used imaging protocols for stress myocardial perfusion imaging (MPI).[2] These include 1- and 2-day Tc-99m–labeled isotope protocols, dual-isotope (Tl-201

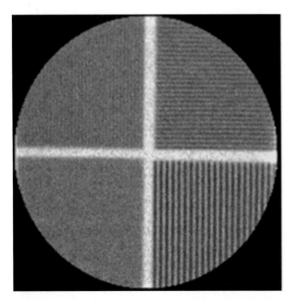

Figure 11-4.   Example of four-quadrant bar phantom.

Table 11-2
Potential Sources of Artifacts Associated with Image Acquisition

Acquisition Setup	Patient-Related Artifacts
Collimation	Soft tissue attenuation
Radius	Extracardiac activity
Positioning	Motion
Number of Projections	Irregular R-R interval with gated SPECT

rest/Tc-99m–labeled stress) protocol and Tl-201 stress/delay protocol (see Chapter 10). The protocol of choice for each laboratory should be based on the patient population being studied (inpatient vs. outpatient), the logistical considerations of the laboratory, and the availability of personnel, including physician, nurse, and technologist. It is important to then maintain consistency with a chosen protocol. This will allow better recognition of abnormalities/artifacts based on deviation from standards.

There are several aspects that should be considered when performing acquisition setup. These include collimation, scan radius, number of projections, counts per projection, matrix size, and patient positioning.[2,5,10–17] When positioning the patient, it is necessary to center the heart in the field of view and reproduce this position for both the rest and stress. The scan radius should be as close to the patient as possible. If it is too large, excessive blurring may occur, resulting in contrast loss, resolution loss, and spatial distortion.[7,10–13]

The number of projections and time per projection are also very important.[7,10–13] In order to acquire a high-quality image set, the study must contain the appropriate count density. Perfusion defects may be created simply due to poor count statistics. To ensure each is optimal, it is necessary to customize the acquisition parameters to the protocol being performed and the imaging system being used. Manufacturers' system recommendations and various published imaging guidelines may be used as a reliable reference.[2]

Potential Sources of Error During the Acquisition

An important reason to continue quality control techniques during the acquisition is to help reduce artifacts and errors that may occur.[2,5,9,18–19] These artifacts can be camera related, as discussed in a previous section; however, they are more commonly related to the patient. The most common cause of artifacts includes soft tissue attenuation, extracardiac activity, patient motion, and an irregular heart rate (R-R interval) with gated SPECT.

Soft Tissue Attenuation Soft tissue attenuation is a common source of artifact on myocardial perfusion studies.[2,5,9] The most common types appear as a result of breast tissue or the diaphragm (Figure 11-5). These generally appear as an apparent localized decrease in count density on an acquired image. The location, size, and severity of the artifact produced are dependent on the attenuation in relation to the myocardium.[19] The severity is also dependent on the energy of the photon being acquired. For example, attenuation artifact occurs more frequently with the use of Tl-201 due to the lower (80 keV) energy in comparison to Tc-99m (140 keV).[18] Generally, attenuation artifacts are fixed; however, if there is a variation in the location between stress and rest it may appear reversible (Figure 11-6).[18] If not recognized as such, these artifacts may result in a false-positive interpretation.

To assist in the prevention of these artifacts it is necessary to use an appropriate imaging protocol and maintain consistency. It is also helpful to image women with the bra off, as this helps position the breast tissue most uniformly between the detector and the myocardium.[5,19] In order to help avoid artifacts resulting from the dia-

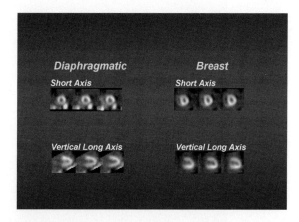

Figure 11-5. Example of diaphragm and breast attenuation. Diaphragm results in a area of decreased activity in the inferior wall and breast attenuation has an area of decreased activity in the anterior wall.

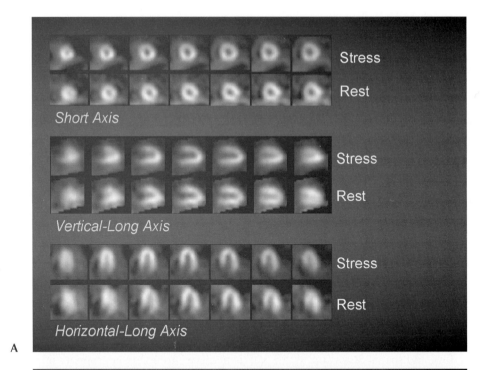

Figure 11-6. **A.** Stress images demonstrate a decrease in photon activity in the anterior wall that complete reverses at rest. **B.** Planar images demonstrate breast shadowing on stress not visualized at rest. This is most likely the cause of the reversible defect.

phragm, stress imaging with Tc-99m–labeled agents should be performed after the patient's heart rate has returned to baseline (15–20 minutes post stress injection).

Other attenuation artifacts may be caused by external sources on the patient. Most common are pendants or necklaces, breast prostheses, or electrocardiogram (ECG) leads left on the patient. To prevent these artifacts, the patient should be asked to remove any metals or other attenuating sources if possible, and the chest area should be visually inspected for these sources before beginning the acquisition.

Extracardiac Activity   Extracardiac activity may also affect myocardial perfusion imaging (MPI).[9,18–19] Such sources may be due to increased liver or bowel activity (Figure 11-7). These artifacts are more common with the Tc-99m–labeled imaging agents. Extracardiac activity may result in inferior wall defects, as it may create the appearance of more counts on the anterior wall.[18] Artifacts may occur during back filter projection and polar plot generation. This can appear as fixed or reversible, depending on activity at both stress and rest.

To assist in prevention of these artifacts, it is necessary to allow for adequate liver clearance when using Tc-99m–labeled imaging agents after injection at rest and/or pharmacologic stress. Whenever possible, it is helpful to encourage some type of exercise with pharmacologic stress to help stimulate liver clearance (Figure 11-8).

Patient Motion   Patient motion is another common cause of artifacts on myocardial perfusion studies.[2,5,18–24] Motion artifact can be related to the camera, but more frequently is a result of patient movement. Motion may occur in the horizontal or vertical axis or occasionally both. When this occurs, misalignment of data during back filter projection produces defects that generally occur in the anterior and posterior wall (Figure 11-9).[5,18–24]

In order to reduce motion artifact, it is important to always explain the procedure thoroughly and make the patient as comfortable as possible. The use of pillows, blankets, and knee supports can be helpful. The inability of a patient to place the arms above the head comfortably may cause patient motion. In this group of patients, it may be helpful to image the patient with the arms at the side.[25]

The raw cine projection data should always be reviewed before the patient is excused from

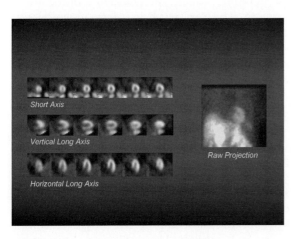

Figure 11-7.   Increased liver activity creates a decrease of activity in the inferior wall.

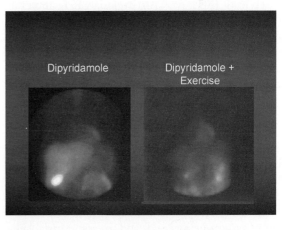

Figure 11-8.   Example of patient pharmacologic stress image with and without supplemental exercise. Both images performed at 30 minutes. Image with supplemental exercise has less liver activity.

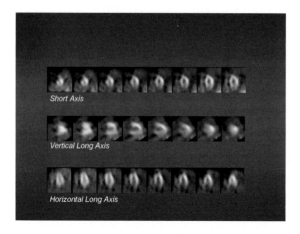

Short Axis

Vertical Long Axis

Horizontal Long Axis

Figure 11-9. Motion artifact appears in the anterior and inferior wall of the myocardium.

the laboratory. If subtle motion is detected, it may be appropriate to apply motion correction software in order to correct the artifact.[5] In some instances, however, the motion may be too severe. The acquisition should then be repeated.

Irregular R-R Interval with Gated SPECT

When performing gated SPECT MPI, the acquisition is triggered from the R-R interval of the three-lead ECG.[26–28] An irregular R-R interval (heart rate) may be a potential source of artifact on these acquisitions. If a patient has an arrhythmia, such as atrial fibrillation or atrial or ventricular premature beats, this may produce a lack of counts in each frame per cardiac cycle. Artifact may occur due to a misrepresentation of end-diastole (ED) and end-systole (ES) in the cardiac cycle. This in turn may cause perfusion artifacts as well as an underestimation of the left ventricular ejection fraction (LVEF).[26–28] While some systems have the capability to prevent this problem during the acquisition, others do not. It is important to understand the limitations of the imaging system being used, and, in some instances, gated SPECT imaging should not be performed on patients with an irregular heart rate in order to preserve image quality.

QUALITY CONTROL AFTER THE ACQUISITION

Quality control should continue even after the patient has been discharged from the laboratory. There are steps that should be taken during processing, display, and interpretation of myocardial perfusion studies to ensure optimal image results and outcomes.

Processing

Processing of a myocardial perfusion study consists of three distinct steps.[2,5] Attention should be given to each step in order to prevent artifacts or errors that may result in a misinterpreted study. Before processing is started, patient raw cine projection data should be evaluated. If any potential problems are visualized, repeating the acquisition should be considered.

The first step in processing is reconstruction. This involves selecting the upper and lower limits of the projection data that will be used to generate the perfusion slices. When selecting the upper and lower limits, care must be taken to ensure the limits are symmetrical, truncation of the myocardium is not occurring, and the limits are reproducible between the stress and rest images. If reconstruction limits are improperly selected, this may produce partial volume effects, difficulties in display scaling, and truncation of the myocardium. This may result in a loss of clinical accuracy.[2,7]

Choosing and applying the appropriate filtering parameters is the next step in processing. Filtering of the data optimizes the signal-to-noise ratio in the tomographic reconstructions, removes inherent reconstruction artifacts, and provides image enhancement.[7,29–32] Considerable care and attention should be given to this step of processing because overfiltering may mask a lesion or defect and underfiltering may create a lesion or defect. Filtering parameters should be chosen for each specific imaging system that allows for the most appropriate image enhancement and quality. These filtering parameters should then be consistent for each image set. For those patients who have low count statistics (i.e., obese patients, infiltrated dose), the acquisition should be performed for a longer time per projection or injected with a higher dose, rather than processed with different filters to increase image quality. Inappropriate filtering of the data may alter the interpretation and reduce clinical sensitivity.[7,29–32]

Reorientation is the last step in processing. This step determines the final creation of the slices, which includes the short, horizontal, and vertical long axis. The reorientation must reflect the accurate long axis of the left ventricle and should be consistent between the stress and rest images. Inappropriate reorientation may create or mask defects, cause geometric distortion of the myocardium, and prevent accurate slice matching during display.[5,7,33–34]

Display and Interpretation

The last two components in the process of MPI are display and interpretation. Quality control techniques should be applied to these aspects of imaging as well in order to complete the process of providing the best-quality information possible.

When displaying myocardial perfusion images, the software used should consist of all short horizontal and vertical long axis slices to include at least eight slices per row.[2,34] The software should also allow one to review the raw cine projection data as well as gated images. This will provide improved efficiency for the interpreter by not having to change between applications to perform a thorough evaluation of the data. The images should be displayed in a linear or monochrome scale (gray or thermal) because some color scales are incremental and may cause a false-positive interpretation. There are several commercially available software programs that incorporate all of these aspects for display.

Interpretation is one of the most important components of a myocardial perfusion study, as it is what allows the referring physician to make clinical decisions on the basis of the results. Referring physicians are looking for a result they can use, in particular a normal or abnormal finding. Equivocal results are not generally helpful.

MPI is best interpreted in a clinical context. Therefore, the interpreter should use all data available, including perfusion images, gated SPECT for wall motion and ejection fraction, stress test findings, and clinical history in order to make a more informed decision.[9] However, it is important that the interpretation as normal or abnormal is the based on the images, not the clinical or stress data.

The sequence of interpretation should be review of the raw cine projection first.[9] This allows visualization of any potential sources that may cause artifacts, on the processed data. It is very important that the interpreting physician is aware and can recognize these artifacts, as they may result in a misinterpretation of the data as discussed earlier in the chapter. Next, the perfusion data should be reviewed for any defects, fixed or reversible. If quantitation is available, it should then be reviewed for comparison. For practices in which there is only one interpreter, quantitation may be a good second reader. Finally, the gated SPECT data should be reviewed to assess wall motion and LVEF. The review of the gated SPECT data may also help resolve questions of true scar due to myocardial infarction (MI) versus artifact with fixed perfusion abnormalities.[26,35]

CONCLUSION

Quality control is a very important component of MPI. It is a process that is continual and requires attention from both the technologist and the physician. It begins before the patients enter the laboratory and continues after they are discharged. In order to achieve optimal image quality, it is important to have a thorough quality control program in place within the laboratory. The explanations and procedures provided are just a few of several components that make up such a program. For a more thorough understanding, it may be helpful to refer to the references provided, as well as several others that are currently available. This process and understanding will result in better referring physician, as well as patient satisfaction, and ultimately result in better patient outcomes.

REFERENCES

1. National Committee on Radiation Protection. *Safe Handling of Radioactive Materials.* Recommendation of NCRP, Report 30. National Bureau of Standards Handbook 92, 1964.
2. DePuey EG, Garcia EV, eds. Instrumentation quality control and performance, In: Updated imaging guidelines for nuclear cardiology procedures, Part 1. *J Nucl Cardiol* 2001;8(1):G5–G10.
3. National Electrical Manufacturer's Association. *Performance Measurements of Scintillation Cameras.* Standards publication no. NU1-1994. Washington, DC: National Electrical Manufacturer's Association, 1994.
4. National Electrical Manufacturer's Association. National Electrical Manufacturer's Association recommendations for implementing SPECT instrumentation quality control. *J Nucl Med Technol* 1999;27:67–72.
5. Nichols KJ, Galt, JR. Quality control for SPECT imaging. In: DePuey EG, Garcia EV, Berman DA, eds. *Cardiac SPECT Imaging*, 2nd ed. Philadelphia: Lippincott Williams and Wilkins, 2001.
6. Early PJ, Sodee DB. Quality assurance. In: *Principles and Practice of Nuclear Medicine*. St. Louis: CV Mosby, 1985.
7. Cullom SJ. Principles of cardiac SPECT imaging. In: DePuey EG, Garcia EV, Berman DA, eds. *Cardiac SPECT Imaging*, 2nd ed. Philadelphia: Lippincott Williams and Wilkins, 2001.
8. Baron JM, Choraguai P. Myocardial single-photon emission computed topography quality assurance. *J Nucl Cardiol* 1996;3:157–166.
9. Port SC, ed. SPECT myocardial perfusion imaging. In: Updated imaging guidelines for nuclear cardiology procedures, Part 2. *J Nucl Cardiol* 1999; 6(2):G67–G77.
10. Breszk JA, Hawman EG. Evaluation of SPECT angular sampling effects: Continuous vs. step and shoot. *J Nucl Med* 1987;28:1308–1314.
11. Galt JR, Garcia EV. Advances in instrumentation for cardiac SPECT. In: DePuey, EG, Garcia EV, and Berman DA, eds. *Cardiac SPECT Imaging*, 2nd ed. Philadelphia: Lippincott Williams and Wilkins, 2001.
12. Maniawski PJ, Morgan HT, Whackers FJ. Orbit-related variation in spatial resolution as a source of artifactual defects in thallium-201 SPECT. *J Nucl Med* 1991;32(5):871–875.
13. Garcia EV, Cooke CD, Van Train KF, et al. Technical aspects of myocardial SPECT imaging with technetium-99m sestamibi. *Am J Cardiol* 1990;66(13):23E.
14. Go RT, MacIntyre WJ, Houser TS, et al. Clinical evaluation of 360° and 180° data sampling techniques for transaxial SPECT thallium-201 myocardial perfusion imaging. *J Nucl Med* 1985;26:695–706.
15. Hoffman EJ. 180° compared with 360° sampling in SPECT. *J Nucl Med* 1982;23:745–746.
16. Maublant JC, Peycelon P, Kwiatkowski F, et al. Comparison between 180° and 360° data collection in technetium-99m MIBI SPECT of the myocardium. *J Nucl Med* 1989;30:295–300.
17. Eisner RL, Nowak DJ, Pettigrew R, et al. Fundamentals of 180° reconstruction in SPECT imaging. *J Nucl Med* 1986;27:1717–1728.
18. DePuey EG. How to detect and avoid myocardial perfusion SPECT artifacts. *J Nucl Med* 1994; 35:699–702.
19. DePuey EG, Garcia EV. Optimal specificity of thallium-201 SPECT through recognition of imaging artifacts. *J Nucl Med* 1989;30:441–449.
20. Friedman J, Berman DS, Van Train K, et al. Patient motion in thallium-201 myocardial SPECT imaging: an easily identified source frequent source of artifactual defect. *Clin Nucl Med* 1988;13:321–324.
21. Cooper JA, Neumann PH, McCandless BK. Effect of patient motion on tomographic myocardial perfusion imaging. *J Nucl Med* 1992;33:1566–1571.
22. Eisner RL. Sensitivity of SPECT thallium-201 myocardial perfusion imaging to patient motion. *J Nucl Med* 1992;33:1571–1573.
23. Geckle WJ, Frank TL, Links JM, et al. Correction for patient motion and organ movement in SPECT: Application to exercise thallium-201 cardiac imaging. *J Nucl Med* 1988;28:441–450.
24. Cooper JA, Neumann PH. Visual detection of patient motion during tomographic myocardial perfusion imaging. *Radiology* 1992;185:283.
25. Toma DM, White MP, Mann A, et al. Influence of arm positioning upon rest/stress Tc-99m sestamibi tomographic imaging. *J Nucl Cardiol* 1999;6:163–168.
26. White MP, Mann A, Saari, MA. Gated SPECT imaging 101. *J Nucl Cardiol* 1998;5:523–526.
27. Cullom SJ, Case JA, Bateman TM. Electrocardiographically gated myocardial perfusion SPECT: Technical principles and quality control considerations. *J Nucl Cardiol* 1998;5:418–425.
28. Nichols K, Dorbala S, DePuey EG, et al. Influence of arrhythmias on gated SPECT myocardial perfusion and function quantification. *J Nucl Med* 1999;40:924–934.
29. Galt JR, Hise LH, Garcia EV, et al. Filtering in frequency space. *J Nucl Med Technol* 1986;14:152–162.
30. Zubal GW, Wisniewski G. Understanding Fourier space and filter selection. *J Nucl Cardiol* 1997;4(3):234–243.
31. King MA, Schwiger RB, Doherty PW et al. Two-dimensional filtering of SPECT images using Metz and Wiener filters. *J Nucl Med* 1984;25:1234–1240.

32. Boulfelfel D, Rangayyan RM, Hahn LJ, et al. Prereconstruction restoration of myocardial single photon emission computed tomography images. *IEEE Trans Med Imaging* 1992;11(3):336–341.

33. Borello JA, Clinthorne NH, Rogers WE, et al. Oblique-angle tomography. A restructuring algorithm for transaxial tomographic data. *J Nucl Med* 1981; 22:471–473.

34. The Cardiovascular Imaging Committee, Standardization of cardiac tomographic imaging. *J Am Coll Cardiol* 1992;20:255–256.

35. DePuey EG, Rozanski A. Using gated technetium-99m-sestamibi SPECT to characterize fixed myocardial defects as infarct or artifact. *J Nucl Med* 1995; 36:952–955.

CHAPTER 12

Interpretation of Myocardial Perfusion Imaging

Robert C. Hendel

INTRODUCTION

The review and interpretation of myocardial perfusion images is obviously the most important duty of a nuclear cardiologist. It is critical that image interpretation be performed in a systematic fashion so as to maximize the clinical value of the study and to ensure the highest-quality result of the entire procedure. As discussed extensively in Chapter 11, the quality of the study must be reviewed and technical abnormalities be recognized. Additionally, a comprehensive evaluation of all available imaging data must be performed so as not to exclude potentially vital information.

A number of guidelines and tools have been recommended for the interpretation of myocardial perfusion studies.[1–3] These policies and guidelines have been developed by experts in the field and should be used as a guide to the successful interpretation of myocardial perfusion imaging (MPI) interpretation.

IMAGE DISPLAY

It is highly recommended that myocardial perfusion images be reviewed on a computer monitor as opposed to x-ray film or paper. While other media may provide useful information, the resolution of a computer monitor screen and the flexibility in adjusting a variety of parameters, including contrast, thresholds, and colors, makes this the medium that is greatly preferred. The practice of interpreting only "hard copy" images is discouraged, especially in view of the dynamic data, which is available by use of a workstation.

A linear color table is recommended for the interpretation of perfusion images. While linear gray scale is preferred and is recommended by many imaging guidelines, other continuous, linear color tables such as hot body/hot iron revised may also be used effectively (Figure 12-1). A great variety of other color tables are available. It is critical that the interpreter understand the workings of these various color tables. It is usu-

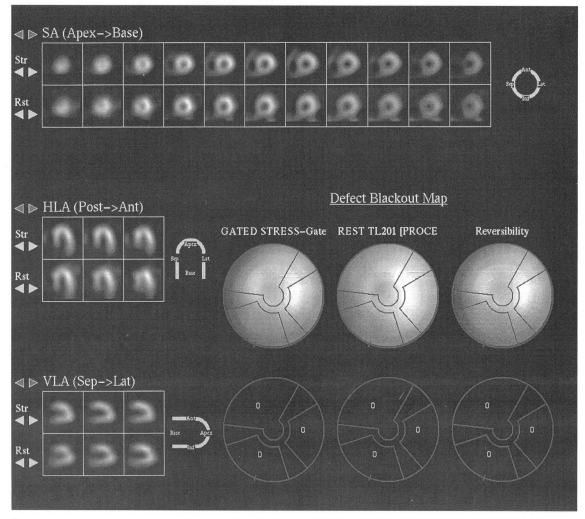

A

Figure 12-1. Exercise/rest dual-isotope myocardial perfusion images (thallium 201 for rest, technetium 99m sestamibi for stress) in a 69-year-old man who presented with atypical chest pain. The myocardial perfusion images were felt to be normal except for the presence of soft tissue attenuation in the inferior and infraseptal regions. These images demonstrate the impact of varying tables. **A.** Gray scale (exponential). (***See also Color Insert***).

ally recommended to avoid color tables with an abrupt transition between each color. Furthermore, it is critical that when a specific color table is used, the scaling should be linear, not exponential, as this will further enhance the appearance of artifacts potentially leading to false-positive results. Irrespective of the color table selected, the most important aspect of the use of these

displays is that the operator be very familiar with the one selected. A bar delineating the color table should also be displayed on screen.

Care should be taken in the review of images to ensure that the particular tomographic slices are aligned. By convention, the stress study is placed in the top row with the resting study below. It is now well accepted that the display of

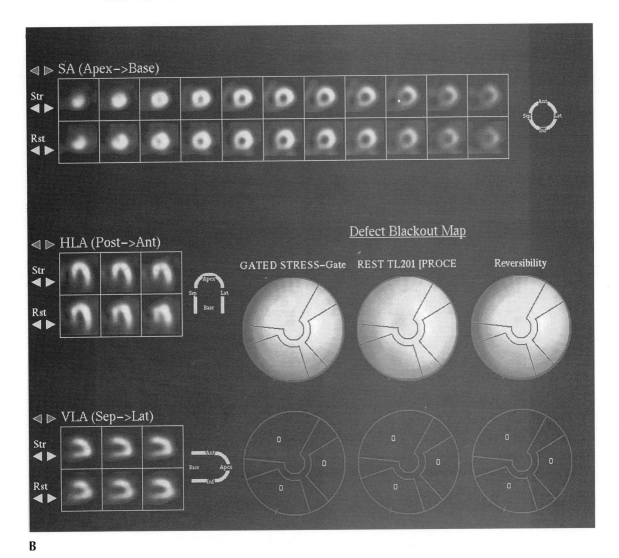

B

Figure 12-1 (continued). B. Hot body (or thermal) (exponential). (*See also Color Insert*).

images should be in a particular format (references), as more than 10 years ago the Joint Guidelines from the American Heart Association, the American College of Cardiology, and the Society of Nuclear Medicine stated the manner in which single photon emission computed tomography (SPECT) images should be displayed.[4]

The top row should present the short-access views, which are obtained by slicing perpendicular to the long axis of the lower left ventricle. By convention, the septum is on the left, with the lateral wall on the right. The slices should be displayed from apex to base (left to right). The long axis should also be presented, demonstrating the data by slicing in a vertical plane (vertical long axis) and a horizontal plane (horizontal long axis). The vertical long-axis views should be displayed with the septal slices positioned on the left and progressing to the lateral wall on the right. The horizontal long axis should be displayed with the inferior slices on the left and moving to the anterior location on the right. All

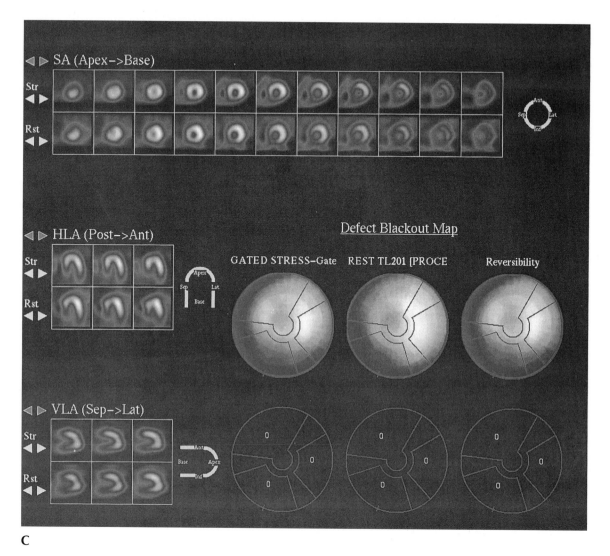

C

Figure 12-1 (continued). C. Warm metal (or CEqual) (linear). (*See also Color Insert*).

images on the SPECT study should be normalized usually to the brightest pixel in the entire study. Flexibility in display software should permit such scaling.

ROTATING (CINE) PLANAR IMAGES

A critical aspect of the interpretation of tomographic data is the review of the raw (un-

processed) projection data.[3] All modern camera systems permit such a review often on the same screen as the SPECT slices. While a sinogram has frequently been used to demonstrate motion and is composed of a sum of the planar data, this method for quality assessment is not ideal and is not recommended. The preferred approach is a review of a cine loop of both the stress and rest planar images usually simultaneously with the tomographic slices.

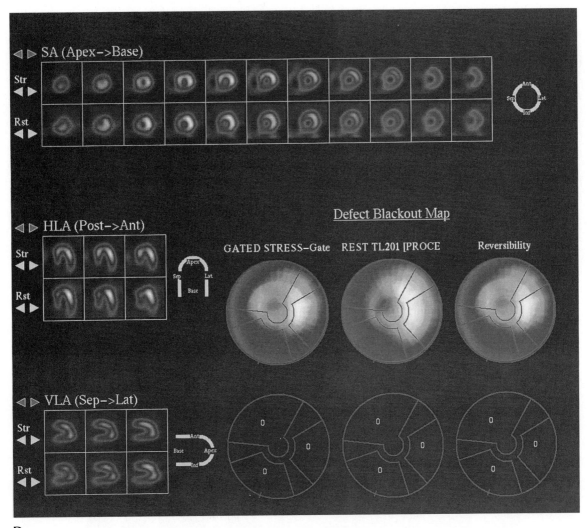

D

Figure 12-1 (continued). **D.** Warm metal (exponential). As can be noted, certain tables must be used with a linear scale, not an exponential relationship (**C, D**). (*See also Color Insert*).

Patient Motion

A review of the rotating images provides clear evidence when there is patient motion, either in a superior–inferior manner or laterally. If substantial motion is present (≥ 2 pixels) repeating the image acquisition is recommended. Motion correction algorithms may also be applied, especially when the patient motion is superior–inferior.

The presence of patient motion may produce artifacts and therefore reduce diagnostic accuracy.[5] Not only do these artifacts resemble ischemic heart disease, but patient motion may create the appearance of multivessel disease. "Upward creep" may also be detected by review of the rotating images. This phenomenon occurs when imaging is performed soon after strenuous exercise and results from the repositioning of the cardiac structures as the respiratory excursion decreases following exercise. Prominent patient motion may result in characteristic defects such as the "hurricane" sign and "flame" occurring at the apex.[6]

Cardiac/Lung Activity

The projection data also provide an assessment of cardiac size and whether prominent lung activity is noted, which frequently is present in the setting of severe left ventricular dysfunction. Perfusion abnormalities may also be noted and confirmed by what is noted on the SPECT slices.

Extracardiac Activity

The rotating planar images should be reviewed for the presence of abnormal activity beyond the boundaries of the myocardial structures. Skin or clothing contamination may mask or mimic a true perfusion abnormality but should be identifiable on the rotating images. The presence of intense subdiaphragmatic activity, either emanating from the liver or from the gastrointestinal (GI) tract, may confound image interpretation. Once such activity is present, it may cause a negative lobe artifact. Intense adjacent activity may cause this reconstruction artifact, for which there is no reliable correction. This type of abnormality may create an artifactual perfusion abnormality or may mask the presence of a true abnormality (Figure 12-2). Ideally, when substantial activity is noted especially in the liver or adjacent bowel loop, image acquisition should be repeated to eliminate this type of artifact.

A variety of neoplastic lesions may also be detected with commonly used radiopharmaceuti-

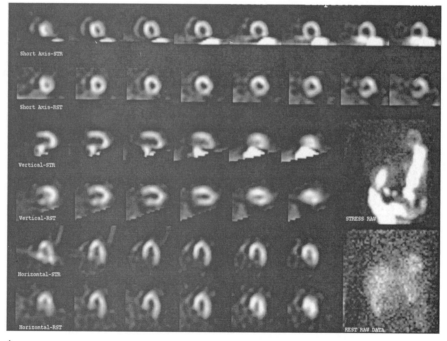

Figure 12-2. Dual-isotope myocardial perfusion images of a patient felt to be at low risk for coronary artery disease. **A.** Prominent activity is noted in a bowel loop immediately adjacent to the infralateral wall on the resting images. This is clearly visible on the resting planar image. These images also demonstrate an apparent reversible inferior wall perfusion defect.

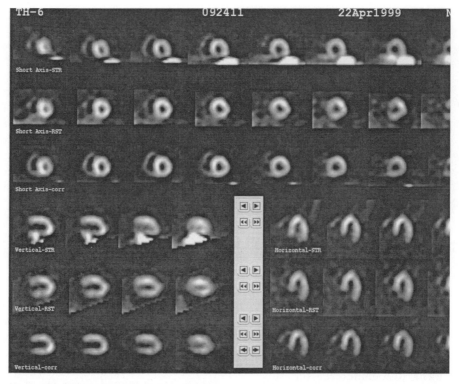

B

Figure 12-2 (continued).   B. The stress and rest images are again shown on the first two rows in the short axis, vertical long axis, and horizontal long axis images. The third row represents repeat image acquisition of the post-stress images following food consumption, defecation, and waiting approximately 2 additional hours. With the subdiaphragmatic/bowel loop activity now removed, there is no perfusion abnormality noted in the inferior wall. (Courtesy of Thomas Holly, MD).

cals.[3] These may reflect either primary or metastatic tumors and include the following types of neoplastic growths: lung, breast, sarcoma, lymphoma, thymoma, parathyroid tumor, thyroid abnormality, and kidney and hepatic tumors.

Finally, the rotating images may reveal contamination by the radiopharmaceutical, occurring either on the skin or clothing, which once again may confound the SPECT image interpretation. Additionally, it is usually possible to distinguish between a neoplastic growth and contamination by review of the rotating images.

Attenuation

Perhaps the greatest value of the rotating images is the ability to demarcate soft tissues, which potentially confound image interpretation. Such soft tissue attenuation may reduce the specificity for coronary artery disease (CAD) detection and is present in up to 40% of all studies.

Photopenic areas may be noted from overlapping breast tissue even when the size of the breast is relatively small. It is often possible to appreciate where the reduction of photons may occur on the SPECT slices by reviewing the cine images (Figure 12-3). Additionally, soft tissue at-

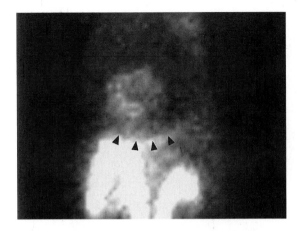

Figure 12-3. An individual frame of the rotating planar images demonstrating prominent soft tissue attenuation from the breast as depicted by the photopenic area (arrowheads). (Reproduced from Hendel et al.[3] with permission.)

tenuation from the diaphragm may obscure the inferior wall, causing a false impression of an inferior wall abnormality. This occurs most commonly in men. Recognition of the superior-placed diaphragm is helpful in the interpretation of images and the enhanced recognition of a potential artifact. When such an abnormality is present, prone imaging may be helpful. Obviously, gated SPECT and attenuation correction methodologies may also be of substantial use in the correction of soft tissue abnormalities.

ANALYSIS OF TOMOGRAPHIC SLICES

A. Image Quality

The first task is to determine whether or not adequate count statistics are present. A number of quality assurance tools are available from most manufacturers that assist in this process. The study should be graded based on overall image quality (poor, fair, good, excellent).

Cavity Size

Left ventricular cavity size may be assessed first by review of the rotating planar images. How-

ever, the overall cavity-to-wall-thickness ratio may be qualitatively determined by looking at the SPECT slices. Additionally, it should be noted if the poststress images reveal a larger left ventricular cavity than noted on the resting study (Figure 12-4). This would be consistent with transient ischemic dilation (TID) of the left ventricular cavity. Usually, about a 20% increase is required when using the dual-isotope protocol[7]; lesser amounts of cavity enlargement is felt to be abnormal when using a single-isotope study. The presence of TID is a marker of multivessel disease and a worsened prognosis. In addition to the visual assessment, quantitative analysis of the TID ratio is available on most software packages.

Perfusion Defect

Defect severity is often described in a qualitative fashion (mild, moderate, severe). A mild abnormality is one in which the clinical significance of the defect is unknown. Such an abnormality may reflect an equivocal finding. This often represents only a 10% reduction of peak tracer activity for a particular study. Moderate and severe defects carry more important diagnostic and prognostic value. Additionally, the extent of the perfusion abnormality may also be qualitatively described as small, medium, or large (Figures 12-5 and 12-6). Although these descriptions are relative, they may be based on objective information from quantitative programs.

In an attempt to describe the severity and extent as a combined value, a variety of scoring systems have been designed, the most popular being the summed stress and summed rest scores. These scores are derived by adding the point value using the range of "0" for normal perfusion to "4" for absent activity for each of either 17- or 20-segment models. As the 17-segment model is now preferred, the summed stress scores should likely use such a semiquantitative system. The difference between the summed stress score and the summed rest score is called the summed difference score and is a measure of reversibility. Usually, individual segments with a $\geq$ 2-grade improvement on the resting study is felt to represent substantial ischemia.

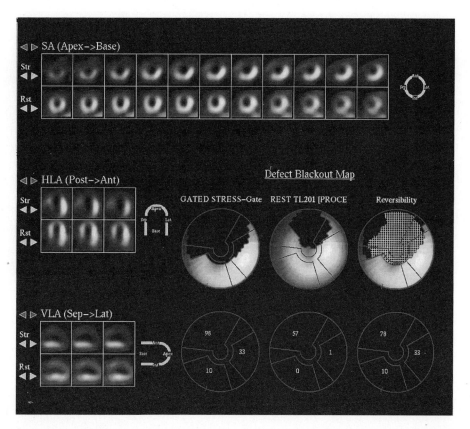

Figure 12-4. Perfusion images from a 31-year-old man with new onset of chest pain, who had limited exercise capacity and developed marked ST segment changes during the stress test. The stress images reveal an extensive, severe defect in the anterior, septal, and apical regions, with substantial reversibility noted on the resting images. Additionally, there is transient enlargement of the left ventricular cavity on the poststress images, relative to the resting study. The transient cavity dilation is most notable on the vertical and horizontal long-axis images; the TID ratio was 1.4. (**See also Color Insert**).

The type of perfusion abnormality should also be described. A fixed perfusion defect (i.e., one that is the same on both the poststress and rest images) is often equated to a myocardial scar, especially when the abnormality is of severe intensity. However, a fixed perfusion abnormality may also reflect severe myocardial ischemia and the presence of myocardial viability. A reversible abnormality is a perfusion abnormality noted on the poststress images, but largely normalizes on the resting images. In many cases some interpreters may use the term *partially reversible*. It is critical to determine whether it is a predominantly re-

versible defect or only a minimally reversible abnormality. Quantitatively, *reversibility* has a variety of definitions, but is often associated with a 20 to 30% improvement in regional activity.

The perfusion abnormalities should also be identified by their location. Standard terminology has now been accepted.[1] The 17-segment model should be used for reference with regard to the nomenclature of such abnormalities (Figure 12-7). However, in general terms, perfusion abnormalities should be described as being present in the apical, anterior, inferior, or lateral walls/regions. The perfusion abnormality may

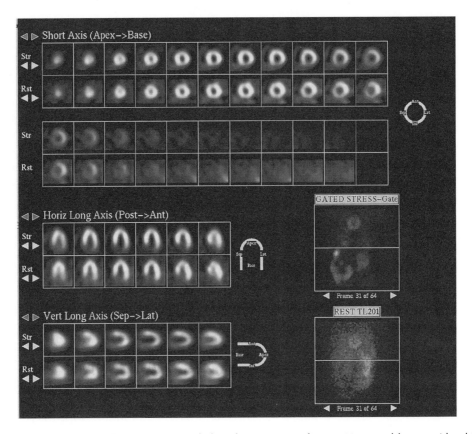

Figure 12-5. Exercise/rest dual-isotope myocardial perfusion images from a 69-year-old man with a history of hypertension, hyperlipidemia, and diabetes who presents with exertional chest pain. There is a small-sized defect of moderate severity involving the basal portion of the inferior wall. This perfusion abnormality appears completely reversible and is consistent with the significant stenosis in the right coronary artery. Subsequent coronary angiography confirms the presence of a 95% right coronary artery stenosis. (**See also Color Insert**).

also be described as occurring within a specific vascular distribution. Obviously, the distribution of an individual coronary artery is highly variable. However, by convention, the 17 segments have been assigned specific vascular distributions so as to standardize interpretation and reporting. As a general rule, the lateral wall is assigned to the circumflex distribution, the anterior and anteroseptal regions to the left anterior descending coronary artery, the inferoseptal and inferior walls to the right coronary artery, and the apex is usually assigned to the left anterior descending distribution, although this is highly variable.

Quantitative Analysis

A variety of software tools are presently available, including the following products that are commercially available. These quantitative programs usually reference an individual patient's data to a normal reference profile. The comparison of individual studies to such a reference is often displayed as a polar map. The "blacked out" segments usually reflect an area of activity that is below the threshold deemed as normal (Figure 12-8). In many cases, it may represent a value such as 2.5 standard deviations below the mean value for a normal patient population; individual programs have specific thresholds. These thresh-

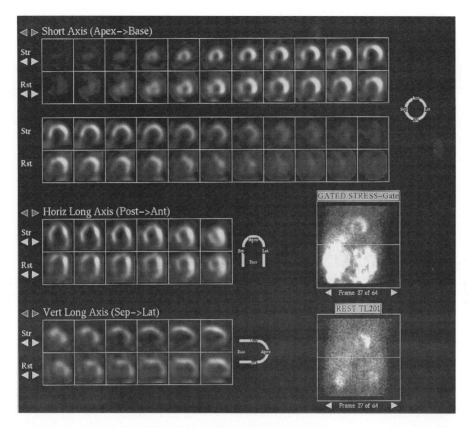

Figure 12-6.   Adenosine/rest dual-isotope myocardial perfusion imaging in a 75-year-old man with a history of known coronary artery disease and status post myocardial infarction. He is currently asymptomatic. The perfusion images demonstrate a large area of severely reduced activity in the inferior and inferoseptal walls, with a moderately severe abnormality noted in the septum and apical regions. No reversibility (ischemia) is noted. (**See also Color Insert**).

olds and normal reference files are often different depending on the radiopharmaceutical. Furthermore, additional techniques, such as attenuation correction, may also alter the profiles. Most important, however, is that the normal reference files are gender specific unless attenuation correction methodology is employed. In addition to the polar map or bull's-eye projection, circumferential profiles may also be created again demonstrating where the count density falls below a specific threshold and is, therefore, deemed abnormal.

Quantitative analysis for most of the software programs has been validated in multiple studies and usually published in pure review journals.

However, it is advised that the quantitative analysis be used as a tool and guide, serving as a "second observer." These quantitative computer-assisted tools should not be used for primary analysis. Following the visual inspection of the tomographic slices, quantitative interpretation may be examined. Any discrepancies or previously unrecognized abnormalities may then be reviewed. However, the individual interpreter must "overread" the computer-assisted interpretations, as many technical problems may develop and lead to false results. Therefore, quantitative analysis is not a substitute for an expert interpretation but should be used as an adjunct to assist the interpreter.

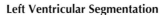

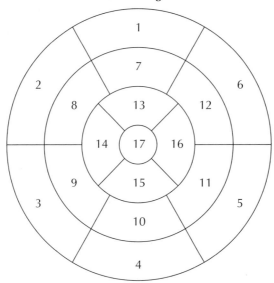

1. Basal anterior
2. Basal anteroseptal
3. Basal inferoseptal
4. Basal inferior
5. Basal inferolateral
6. Basal anterolateral

7. Mid anterior
8. Mid anteroseptal
9. Mid inferoseptal
10. Mid inferior
11. Mid inferolateral
12. Mid anterolateral

13. Apical anterior
14. Apical septal
15. Apical inferior
16. Apical lateral
17. Apex

A

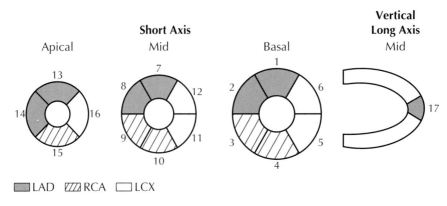

B

Figure 12-7. **A.** A polar-plot depiction of left ventricular segmentation according to the 17-segment model. The recommended nomenclature is noted for each segment below. **B.** The 17-segment model, obtained by three individual short-axis slices as well as one midcavity vertical long-axis slice. A depiction of the coronary artery distribution is also noted. (Reproduced from Cerqueira et al.[1] with permission).

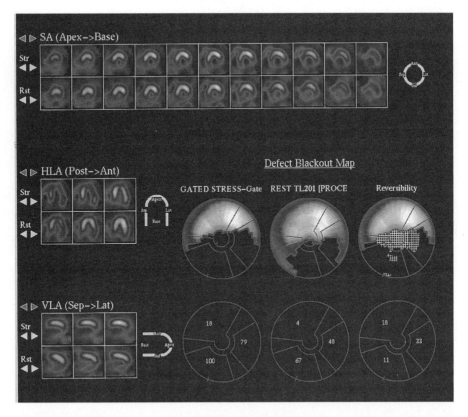

Figure 12-8. Stress/rest perfusion imaging demonstrates a large inferior, interoseptal, and interolateral defect, which has a small area of reversibility (ischemic) in the apex. The polar plots demonstrates the large extent of the defect, with the hatched region indicating reversibility. (*See also Color Insert*).

GATED SPECT

As it is now recommended that gated SPECT be employed for essentially all myocardial perfusion SPECT imaging studies,[8] a standardized approach for the interpretation of gated SPECT data should be employed. This critical component of contemporary perfusion imaging is discussed in detail in Chapter 13. The gated SPECT data are often displayed in different fashions, depending on the software. Irrespective of the display, the most critical information is often demonstrated in the mid ventricular slices from each of the orthogonal axes. Gated SPECT should be displayed as a cine loop, and the interpreter should observe the images for overall global function, examining the endocardial surfaces and their excursion. In addition to the motion of the endocardial walls, myocardial thickening may be determined by the increase in brightness noted on gated SPECT display resulting from the partial volume effect. It is possible that the thickening (brightening) may be normal, although the excursion is abnormal. This is often seen in settings such as following previous cardiac surgery. If there is difficulty localizing the endocardial surfaces, most software will provide "contours" where the computer will provide a line for what it believes the endocardial surface (Figure 12-9). This may be used to assist the interpreter in evaluation of endocardial motion. Regional abnormalities may also be determined

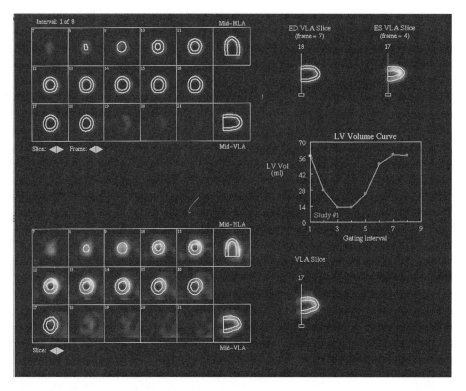

Figure 12-9. Computer-assisted detection of the endocardial surfaces on gated SPECT with the "contours" demonstrating the boundaries of the endocardial and epicardial surfaces (4 D-M SPECT™). (**See also Color Insert**).

especially by examining multiple axes. Similar geographic schema to that noted for perfusion imaging should be employed when describing regional wall motion abnormalities.

A great variety exists with regard to the use of displays for gated SPECT information. While black and white or "hot body/thermal" may demonstrate brightening very effectively, a number of different color tables have also been used to assist in evaluating myocardial brightening or increases in count intensity. Overall, however, the monochromatic color tables are usually recommended.

Gated SPECT Quality

It is critical to have sufficient count density to examine for the accurate interpretation of gated SPECT data. A number of software programs

analyze each of the frames to determine if the count density is adequate. The overall image quality should help the interpreter determine whether or not the study is interpretable. Another concern is that of poor gating, which is manifest as a flashing on the rotating planar images. This is due to variation in the beat–beat interval. For the most part, however, the overall global function data, including the ejection fraction, is still well preserved. If anything, cardiac arrhythmias more often affect the myocardial perfusion data than they do the gated SPECT information and its impact on functional information.

Semiquantitative Description

Global and regional wall motion abnormalities should be defined as normal, hypokinetic, akinetic, or diskinetic. It is possible to further sub-divide the hypokinesis, although it may be very difficult to differentiate between mild and moderate hypokinesis. A five-point scoring system for thickening and wall motion has been described ranging from normal function to mild or moderate hypokinesis, to akinesis and dyskinesis.

Quantitative Analysis

Global left ventricular function may be accurately quantified and described specifically using an ejection fraction determination. Each software program has been well validated and reveals good correlation with other methodologies. When the ejection fraction is > 60%, such as occurring in patients with small left ventricular cavities, it is suggested to describe this as either "normal" or "≥ 60%," as it is somewhat nonsensical to describe an ejection fraction of 92%. More qualitative descriptions may also be used such as "normal function" or those studies possessing mild, moderate, or severely reduced left ventricular systolic function. However, given the overall validation of cardiac software packages, it is recommended to quantitatively describe the ejection fraction. Left ventricular volumes, both end systolic and end diastolic, may also be noted.

Regional wall motion abnormalities and regional myocardial thickening has also been accurately determined using several cardiac software packages. This information is often graphically depicted as a three-dimensional plot. This may be used to assist the interpreter in determinations of abnormal function. However, most of these methods have been less well validated than the global ejection fraction determination. Therefore, the tools for regional determinations should be used as an adjunctive technique to assist the interpreter.

Attenuation Correction

Over the past five years, substantial technological advances have occurred in the field of attenuation-corrected myocardial SPECT perfusion imaging. A number of manufacturers now possess well-validated methods for correcting soft tissue attenuation.[9] Although different techniques have been employed by most vendors, the literature now supports the conclusion that diagnostic specificity is improved. Additionally, it appears that attenuation correction may assist in the improved detection of multivessel disease and left main stenosis. It is also likely that attenuation correction will assist in prognostic applications. It is however, critical to understand the workings of each system, as they are widely different. The interpreter of myocardial perfusion SPECT imaging should note each system's benefits and potential limitations. All attenuation correction methods may cause artifacts, especially when used incorrectly. Therefore, the interpreter should know the specifics of such attenuation correction derived artifacts as well as how effective it is in correcting soft tissue attenuation.

It is critical that the quality of the transmission map used for correcting the admission data be of high quality (Figure 12-10). The counts should be adequate, as determined by the manufacturer, and truncation should be absent or minimal. If the quality of the transmission scan is suboptimal, the attenuation-corrected images should not be used.

It is presently advised that the attenuation corrected images be viewed in conjunction with the review of the uncorrected images. It is critical to understand how the correction occurred and its impact on the images. With the understandings of the benefits and limitations of each system, as well as comparing the uncorrected and corrected information, the interpreter can then gain the true value of attenuation corrected perfusion imaging. Caution is often advised when there is prominent activity from overlying structures such as the bowel or liver. This can directly impact on the interpretation of an inferior wall abnormality. Specifically, if substantial hepatic or subdiaphragmatic activity is present, a true inferior wall perfusion abnormality may be masked by attenuation correction. Importantly, the apex is also far more prominent on attenuation-corrected SPECT images. It is therefore, critical

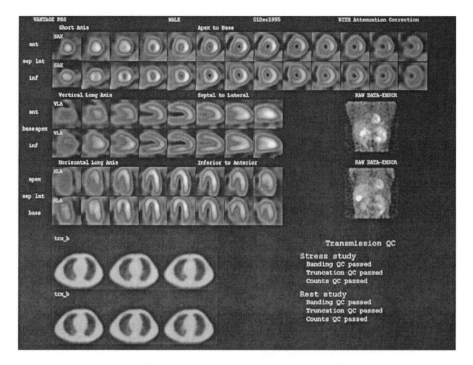

Figure 12-10. Stress images obtained in a 49-year-old man with a low likelihood for coronary artery disease. The top rows demonstrates an inferior and interoseptal wall perfusion abnormality. Following attenuation correction (Vantage Pro™, Philips), a more uniform appearance is present (bottom rows). The bottom portion of the figure depicts the transmission map, which clearly demonstrates the lungs and mediastinal structures. (Courtesy of Gary Heller, MD, PhD).

to understand the "normal" appearance of an attenuation-corrected image. Likewise, the right ventricle is far more prominent on attenuation-corrected SPECT imaging. This does not reflect right ventricular enlargement or hypertrophy, but instead improve visualization of the structure. Obviously, a "learning curve" is required to understand the impact of attenuation correction on the left ventricular apex and right ventricle.

Despite the cautions raised, a system with well-validated attenuation correction techniques should result in uniform tracer distribution on MPI. Such attenuation-corrected scans should also produce gender-independent distribution of myocardial counts. Attenuation-corrected quantitative software is now becoming available and will be further used as an adjunct for MPI. Fi-

nally, the use of attenuation correction permits gated SPECT imaging, although the gated SPECT slices need not be corrected for attenuation, only the summed images.

CONCLUSION

A systematic process of interpretation of myocardial perfusion SPECT images is critical for the highest level of accuracy and clinical utility. Attention must be paid to the quality of MPI data. In recent years, a variety of guidelines and position papers have focused on optimal techniques for image interpretation. A common vocabulary and format also ensures that high-quality interpretation and reporting is achieved. Advanced imaging technology, including quantitative analysis, gated SPECT, and attenuation correction, has improved the value of SPECT imaging, but the "reader" of such images must be cognizant of the advantages and pitfalls for these methods and understand the potential impact of these techniques on the final interpretation.

REFERENCES

1. Cerqueira MD, Weissman NJ, Dilsizian V, et al. Standardized myocardial segmentation and nomenclature for tomographic imaging of the heart: A statement for healthcare professionals from the Cardiac Imaging Committee of the Council on Clinical Cardiology of the American Heart Association. *Circulation* 2002;105:539–542.
2. Port SC, ed. Imaging guidelines for nuclear cardiology procedures, Part II. American Society of Nuclear Cardiology. *J Nucl Cardiol* 1999;6:G47–84.
3. Hendel RC, Gibbons RJ, Bateman TM. Use of rotating (cine) planar projection images and the interpretation of a tomographic myocardial perfusion study. *J Nucl Cardiol* 1999;6:234–240.
4. Standardization of cardiac tomographic imaging. The Cardiovascular Imaging Committee, American College of Cardiology; The Committee on Advanced Cardiac Imaging and Technology, Council on Clinical Cardiology, American Heart Association; and Board of Directors, Cardiovascular Council, Society of Nuclear Medicine. *J Am Coll Cardiol* 1992;20:255–256.
5. Fitzgerald J, Danias PG. Effect of motion on cardiac SPECT imaging: Recognition and motion correction. *J Nucl Cardiol* 2001;8:701–706.
6. Sorrell V, Figueroa B, Hansen CL. The "hurricane sign": Evidence of patient motion artifact on cardiac single-photon emission computed tomographic imaging. *J Nucl Cardiol* 1996;3:86–88.
7. Mazzanti M, Germano G, Kiat H, et al. Identification of severe and extensive coronary artery disease by automatic measurement of transient ischemic dilation of the left ventricular in dual-isotope myocardial perfusion SPECT. *J Am Coll Cardiol* 1996;27:1612–1620.
8. Bateman TM, Berman DS, Heller GV, et al. American Society of Nuclear Cardiology position statement on electrocardiographic gating of myocardial perfusion SPECT scintigrams. *J Nucl Cardiol* 1999;6:470–471.
9. Hendel RC, Corbett JR, Cullom SJ, et al. The value and practice of attenuation correction for myocardial perfusion SPECT imaging: A joint position statement from the American Society of Nuclear Cardiology and the Society or Nuclear Medicine. *J Nucl Cardiol* 2002;9:135–143.

CHAPTER 13

Interpretation of Ventricular Function Using ECG-Gated SPECT Imaging

Gary V. Heller
Sachin Navare

INTRODUCTION

The ability to assess radionuclide myocardial perfusion and function with electrocardiogram (ECG)-gated single photon emission computed tomography (SPECT) imaging has revolutionized the field of nuclear cardiology. Since its advent of 1991, physicians have found the evaluation of myocardial perfusion and function to be beneficial for diagnosis, risk stratification, and clinical decision making in their patients. ECG-gated SPECT imaging has now become routine part of SPECT equipment produced for myocardial perfusion imaging (MPI). For gated SPECT imaging, image data are acquired in synchrony with the ECG signal using a specific number of intervals between consecutive R waves. Counts accumulated during each of these intervals generate individual images. Each individual image is subsequently reconstructed into a tomographic set. At present, using commercially available software, it is standard to acquire 8 frames per cardiac cycle. Since the distribution of the radiopharmaceutical remains stable in the myocardium, the spatial and temporal changes in the tracer activity reflect regional myocardial wall motion and thickening, when the individual frame images are displayed in a cinematic format. Quantitative methods enable measurement of global ventricular function [left ventricular ejection fraction (LVEF) and LV volumes] as well as regional ventricular function (myocardial wall motion and thickening). Currently, over 95% of the laboratories in the United States are now collecting and interpreting ventricular function in addition to perfusion data. The procedure also has its own billing code(s). The procedure itself is fully explained in Chapter 22. This section will discuss the correct interpretation sequence for ECG-gated SPECT imaging as well as the clinical utility and circumstances in which functional information is beneficial.

INTERPRETATION OF ECG-GATED SPECT IMAGING

To maximize the value of functional ECG-gated SPECT data, a systematic approach to interpretation is essential. It should be recognized that ventricular function should be interpreted only in the context of the perfusion data, as the latter has potential to influence the results and the two sets of information are complementary. The sequence of interpretation is listed in Table 13-1. This includes assessment of the raw data, myocardial perfusion, and ventricular function, in that order, and then integrating the clinical information for the final conclusion. Following this algorithm (reading SPECT images before clinical data) allows for "blinded" interpretation of the SPECT images and avoids bias. Interpretation of myocardial perfusion was described in detail in Chapter 12; only relevant information will be repeated.

Evaluation of Unprocessed (Raw) Data

The interpretation of gated SPECT begins with evaluation of the unprocessed data for overall image quality and any information that might impact function. This includes potential attenuation artifacts such as liver, breast, diaphragm, or gut activity. In addition, any patient motion that occurred during the study should be noted. If motion is greater than one pixel in deviation, the study should be "motion corrected" prior to interpretation. Body habitus should also be noted for its potential to produce attenuation, particularly diaphragmatic artifacts.

Inspection of raw data provides clue toward the technical quality of gated SPECT acquisition. In general, images with poor counts should be interpreted with caution as they could be associated with artifacts. Periodic flashing of the display results from gating errors, occurring as a result of wide variation in the cardiac cycle during the acquisition leading to variation in counts between images. Presence of gating errors can be further confirmed by a graph displaying accepted counts as a function of the projection number.

Evaluation of Myocardial Perfusion Data

Tomographic slices of the myocardium should be displayed according to the standardized model recommended by the Cardiac Imaging Committee of the Council on Clinical Cardiology of the American Heart Association.[1] The myocardial slices are defined along three planes perpendicular to the long axis of the left ventricle. The three planes are named short axis, horizontal long axis, and vertical long axis. The myocardium is divided into 17 segments based on three short-axis slices (the apical, midventricular, and basal) and a midventricular vertical long-axis slice.

The stress and the rest slices are aligned and displayed side by side. Interpreters should observe the extent and degree of photon reduction as well as the location of the abnormality. The degree of reversibility (differences between stress and rest) should also be noted. If being used, quantitative confirmation of the visual observations of the perfusion data should be made. The final determination of the presence or absence of perfusion abnormalities should be made using the best judgment of the visual and quantitative data.

Evaluation of Ventricular Function

Ventricular function assessment should be made for both the left and the right ventricle. Care should be taken to interpret both global and regional wall motion, particularly in the left ventri-

Table 13-1

Sequence of Interpretation ECG-gated SPECT Function

1. Observation of unprocessed (raw) data
2. Evaluation of individual perfusion slices
3. Application of quantitative perfusion software
4. Evaluation of individual slices for ventricular function
5. Quantitation of left ventricular ejection fraction
6. Evaluation of three-dimensional images

cle. This is critically important in the presence of a perfusion abnormality. It is generally recommended that at least three short-axis slices and one horizontal and vertical long-axis slice be available. The computer system should allow flexibility to move the interpreting slices into the area of the perfusion abnormality. Once the proper slice orientation is made, both global and regional LV wall motion assessment should be made.

Assessment of Regional Ventricular Function Parameters of regional ventricular function assessed by gated SPECT include segmental myocardial wall motion and myocardial thickening. Segmental wall motion analysis consists of observing both epicardial and endocardial surfaces. Wall motion in one region should be compared to adjacent regions (i.e., inferior compared with anterior). Generally speaking, wall motion is best observed using monochrome display scales (thermal, gray, etc.), while wall thickening is best observed using color scale. Both wall motion and wall thickening contribute to overall evaluation of ventricular function.

A visual semiquantitative assessment of regional wall motion and thickening can be performed using the same 17-segment model used for perfusion assessment. For assessing wall motion, a six-point (0 = normal, 1 = mild hypokinesis, 2 = moderate hypokinesis, 3 = severe hypokinesis, 4 = akinesis and 5 = dyskinesis) scoring system is used.

Assessment of Global Ventricular Function This includes estimation and quantification of LVEF and quantification of LV volumes. Completely automated algorithms, both count based and geometry based, are available for quantifying LVEF and volumes.

The interpreter should first estimate the global LVEF and then confirm with the quantitative software. It is important for the reader to know lower limit of normal for a given software quantitation package, as they differ with other modalities such as cardiac catheterization and echocardiography.

Finally, right ventricular size and wall motion should also be noted to assist in differentiation between ischemic versus nonischemic cardiomyopathies or ideology of symptoms. Reports should reflect the best estimation of ventricular ejection fraction as well as right ventricular function.

Three-Dimensional Display

Several software packages provide a three-dimensional display of LV function. This display is the result of the computerized determination of the epicardial and endocardial surface extending from end-diastole to end-systole. LV wall motion can be evaluated using this display. The information gained from the three-dimensional display can be used to complement the visual impression from individual slices. It should be noted, however, that these data are only as good as the ability of the computer program to accurately reflect ventricular function. Thus, if the data from the ECG-gated study is count poor, the information may be misleading. Therefore, this display should be used only after evaluation of individual slices and determining whether the contours (epicardial and endocardial surfaces) are an accurate reflection of ventricular function.

CLINICAL USE OF ECG-GATED SPECT VENTRICULAR FUNCTION

The clinical utility of ECG-gated SPECT imaging comes in many forms—from the identification of attenuation artifact to assisting in risk stratification (Table 13-2). The approaches all have one common theme: The combined assessment of myocardial perfusion and function together is better than the parts. This section will describe the value of ventricular function in various clinical conditions.

Gated SPECT Imaging to Determine the Etiology of Fixed Perfusion Abnormalities: Attenuation Artifact

Gated SPECT imaging has been proposed as a means of determining attenuation artifact from

Table 13-2

Clinical Use of Ventricular Function Using ECG-gated SPECT Imaging

1. Definition of attenuation artifact
2. Differentiation of ischemic from nonischemic etiologies of dilated cardiomyopathy
3. Evaluation of myocardial viability
4. Evaluation of right ventricular function
5. Evaluation of stunned myocardium
6. Prognosis

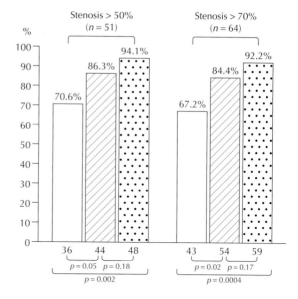

Figure 13-1. Specificity of Tl-201 (open bars), Tc-99m sestamibi perfusion (striped bars) and Tc-99m sestamibi perfusion and gated SPECT (speckled bars) studies for both patients without CAD and the group of normal volunteers. Adapted from Taillefer et al.[3]

coronary artery disease (CAD) in patients with fixed perfusion abnormalities. These abnormalities primarily occur in the inferior and anterior regions. A fixed anterior perfusion abnormality is generally (but not exclusively) seen in female patients due to attenuation artifact from breast while the inferior perfusion abnormality represents diaphragmatic attenuation. The basic assumption using ECG-gated SPECT imaging for this purpose is that a fixed perfusion abnormality associated with CAD should represent either prior myocardial infarction (MI) or stunned myocardium, both of which are associated with wall motion abnormalities. In contrast, if wall motion in the same area as the fixed perfusion abnormality is normal, this should represent attenuation artifact. Thus, a fixed perfusion abnormality with normal wall motion should be considered normal. This interpretation would therefore reduce the number of "false-positive" studies and improve specificity of the procedure. Several studies have been published[2,3] demonstrating improved specificity using this assumption (Figure 13-1).

Correct identification of attenuation artifact also improves reader confidence. In a study by Smanio et al.,[4] interpretation of perfusion and function reduces the number of studies considered "borderline normal or abnormal" and significantly increases the number of studies of normal or abnormal (Figure 13-2). There was no loss in diagnostic accuracy. Such interpretations will allow the referring physician to make better

clinical judgments, possibly reducing unnecessary cardiac catheterizations. Thus, the interpreting physician can feel confident that a fixed perfusion abnormality with normal ventricular function is normal and therefore provide the referring physician with a more definitive answer (normal vs. probably normal or equivocal).

Limitations of Gated SPECT in Interpretation of Distinguishing Attenuation Artifact from CAD

Gated SPECT imaging is limited in distinguishing attenuation artifact in those patients with reversible perfusion abnormalities or those with either stress-only imaging or acute rest myocardial perfusion in the emergency department (ED). In any of these circumstances, if wall motion is normal, one cannot exclude the presence of ischemia as an etiology of the perfusion abnormality. Since ventricular function is assessed 30 to 60 minutes later, any wall motion abnormality created by ischemia would, for the most part, have resolved

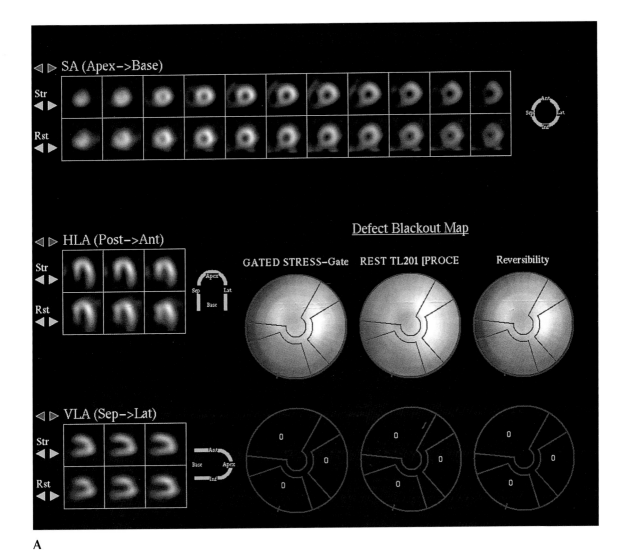

A

Figure 12-1. Exercise/rest dual-isotope myocardial perfusion images (thallium 201 for rest, technetium 99m sestamibi for stress) in a 69-year-old man who presented with atypical chest pain. The myocardial perfusion images were felt to be normal except for the presence of soft tissue attenuation in the inferior and infraseptal regions. These images demonstrate the impact of varying color tables. **A.** Gray scale (exponential).

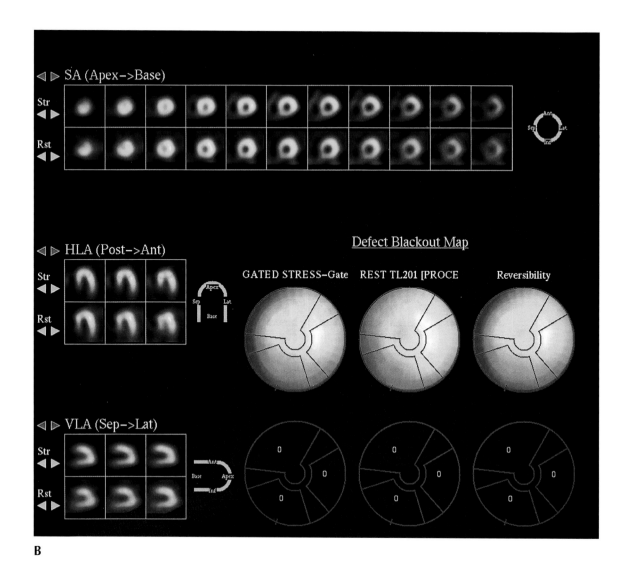

B

Figure 12-1 (continued). **B.** Hot body (or thermal) (exponential).

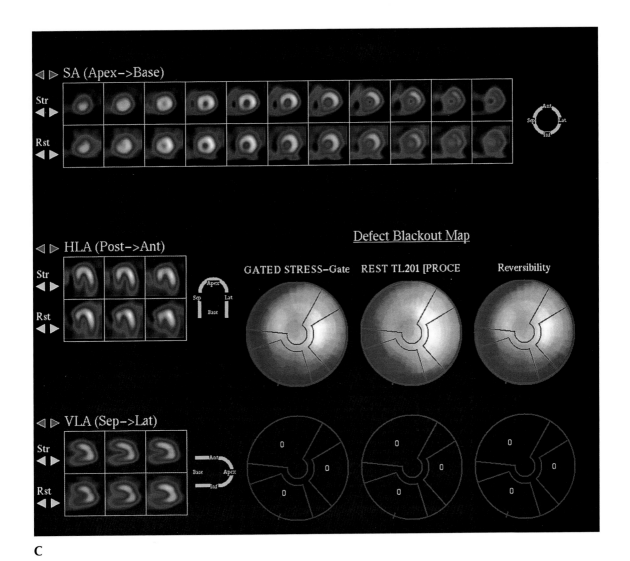

Figure 12-1 (continued). C. Warm metal (or CEqual) (linear).

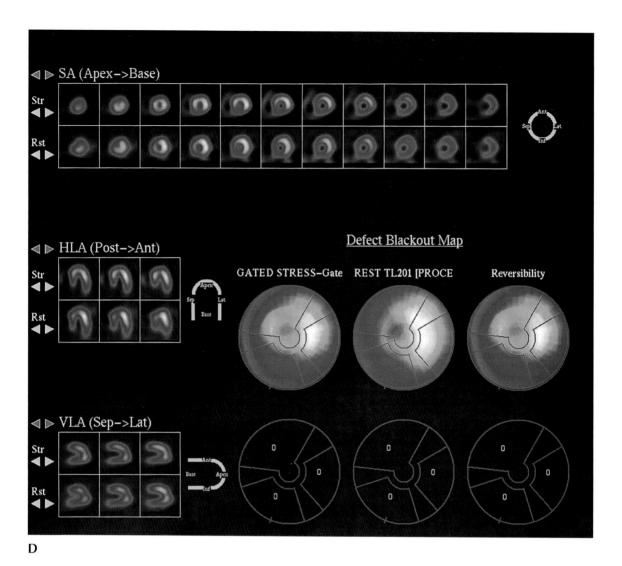

D

Figure 12-1 (continued). **D.** Warm metal (exponential). As can be noted, certain color tables must be used with a linear scale, not an exponential relationship (**C, D**).

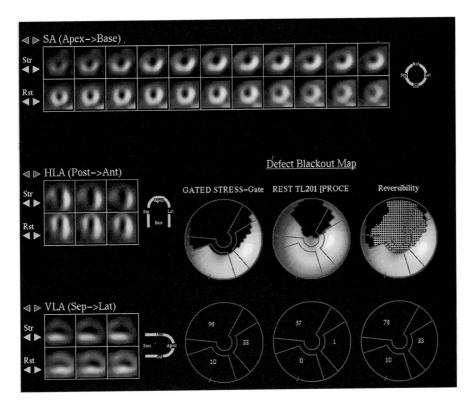

Figure 12-4. Perfusion images from a 31-year-old man with new onset of chest pain, who had limited exercise capacity and developed marked ST segment changes during the stress test. The stress images reveal an extensive, severe defect in the anterior, septal, and apical regions, with substantial reversibility noted on the resting images. Additionally, there is transient enlargement of the left ventricular cavity on the poststress images, relative to the resting study. The transient cavity dilation is most notable on the vertical and horizontal long-axis images; the TID ratio was 1.4.

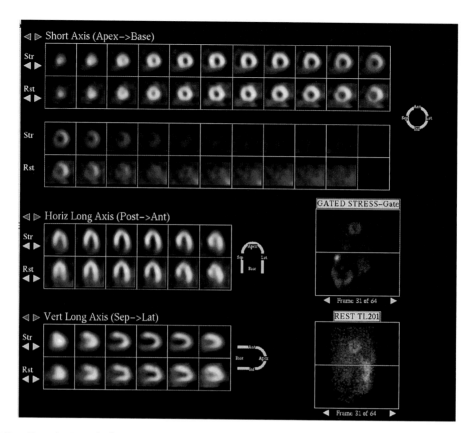

Figure 12-5. Exercise/rest dual-isotope myocardial perfusion images from a 69-year-old man with a history of hypertension, hyperlipidemia, and diabetes who presents with exertional chest pain. There is a small-sized defect of moderate severity involving the basal portion of the inferior wall. This perfusion abnormality appears completely reversible and is consistent with the significant stenosis in the right coronary artery. Subsequent coronary angiography confirms the presence of a 95% right coronary artery stenosis.

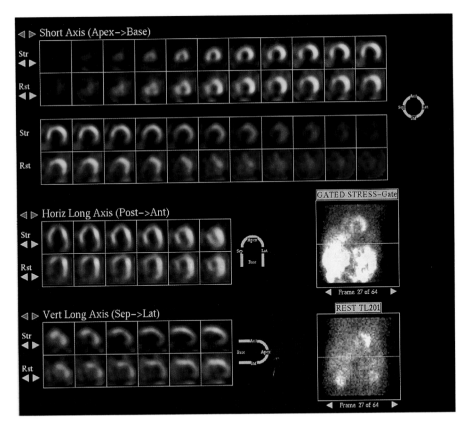

Figure 12-6. Adenosine/rest dual-isotope myocardial perfusion imaging in a 75-year-old man with a history of known coronary artery disease and status post myocardial infarction. He is currently asymptomatic. The perfusion images demonstrate a large area of severely reduced activity in the inferior and inferoseptal walls, with a moderately severe abnormality noted in the septum and apical regions. No reversibility (ischemia) is noted.

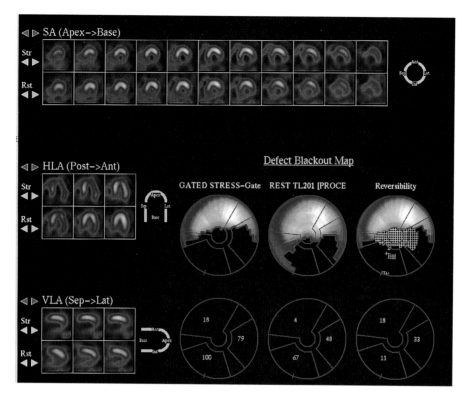

Figure 12-8. Stress/rest perfusion imaging demonstrates a large inferior, interoseptal, and interolateral defect, which has a small area of reversibility (ischemic) in the apex. The polar plots demonstrates the large extent of the defect, with the hatched region indicating reversibility.

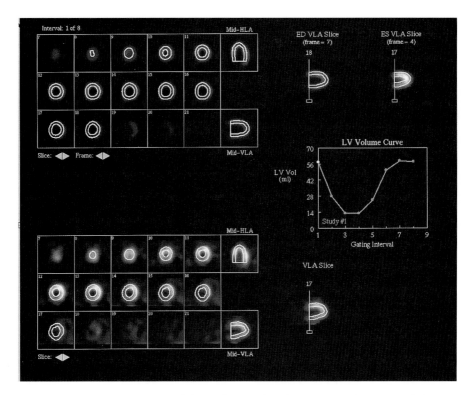

Figure 12-9. Computer-assisted detection of the endocardial surfaces on gated SPECT with the "contours" demonstrating the boundaries of the endocardial and epicardial surfaces (4 D-M SPECT™).

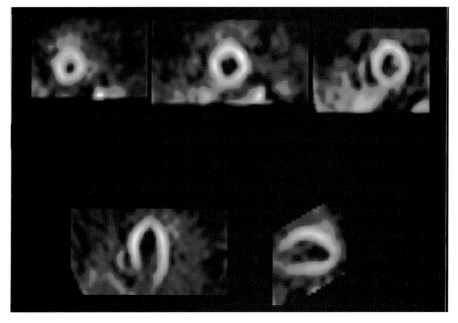

Figure 13-5. Gated-SPECT in 35-year-old female with diabetic cardiomyopathy. Both left and right ventricular cavities were markedly dilated. ECG-gated SPECT imaging demonstrated severe global hypokinesis of both ventricles.

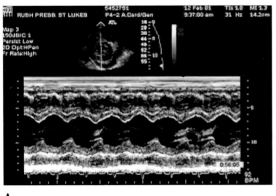

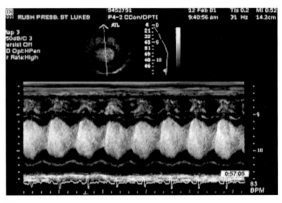

A   **B**

Figure 16-1. M-mode evaluation of LV wall thicknesses and dimensions. **A.** Second harmonics imaging without contrast. IV septum is seen above and pLV posterior wall below with lumen between. **B.** Use of contrast highlights the endocardial–lumen interface. X axis = time; Y axis = distance (1 cm markings).

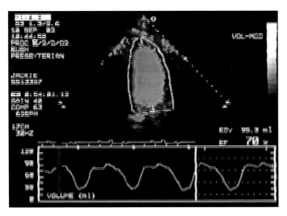

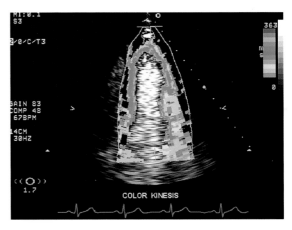

Figure 16-3. Acoustic quantification and online delineation of LV ejection fraction. Note the LVEF of 70% derived from the change in identified endocardium-lumen interface. (Courtesy of Philips Ultrasound.)

Figure 16-4. Color kinesis of the left ventricle. This technique is useful for assessment of relative regional endocardial motion using analysis of the color-coded segments. (Courtesy of Philips Ultrasound.)

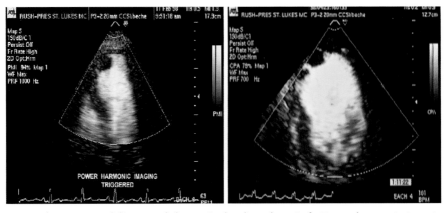

Figure 16-7. Use of contrast to delineate a left ventricular thrombus. **Left:** Power harmonic imaging triggered to the ECG allows delineation of thrombus and myocardial perfusion. **Right:** Harmonic contrast imaging without power allows delineation of thrombus without evaluation of myocardial perfusion.

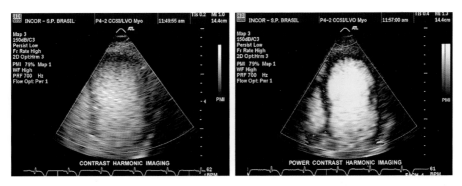

Figure 16-8. Contrast harmonic imaging (**left**) and power contrast harmonic imaging (**right**). The latter allows evaluation of perfusion in the myocardium, and also enhances quantification of LV ejection fraction when used in conjunction with ECG gating and border detection algorithms.

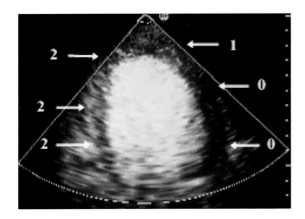

Figure 16-9. Power contrast harmonic imaging perfusion grading scale from 0 (no perfusion) to 2 (normal perfusion).

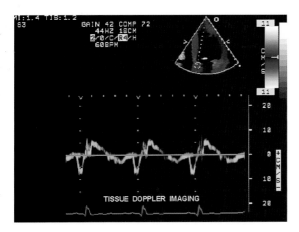

Figure 16-10. Tissue Doppler imaging. The 2D image color coding of general myocardial motion during on time frame (**top**) and pulsed Doppler assessment of regional myocardial motion throughout the cardiac cycle (**bottom**). (Courtesy of Philips Ultrasound.)

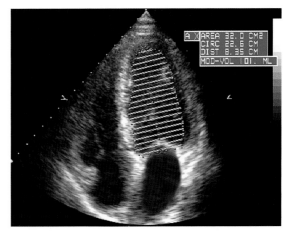

Figure 16-11. Use of internal computer in commercial echocardiography equipment to calculate LV ejection fraction. End diastolic and end systolic frames are chosen for measurements in two planes. This illustrates Simpson's method (biplane method of disks) in one of the tomographic views.

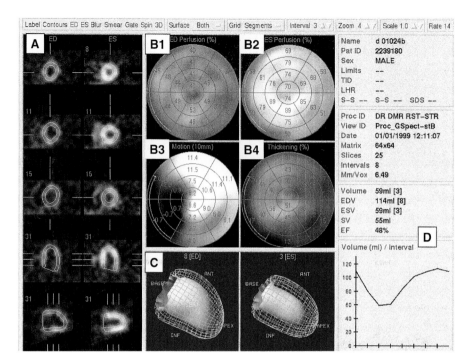

Figure 22-2. Quantification of ejection fraction, regional myocardial wall motion, and thickening from gated myocardial perfusion SPECT (QPS™) **A.** Myocardial contours displaying endocardial and epicardial surfaces overlying the end-diastolic (ED) and end-systolic (ES) frames, three short-axis images, a midcavity horizontal, and a midcavity vertical long axis. **B.** Quantitative polar plots measuring regional myocardial wall perfusion (B1, B2) , motion (B3) and wall thickening (B4) from gated SPECT. **C.** Three-dimensional display of the endocardial (solid) and epicardial (grid) left ventricular surfaces calculated by the automatic algorithm. **D.** Endocardial time–volume curve and calculated LVEF from end-systolic and end-diastolic volumes.

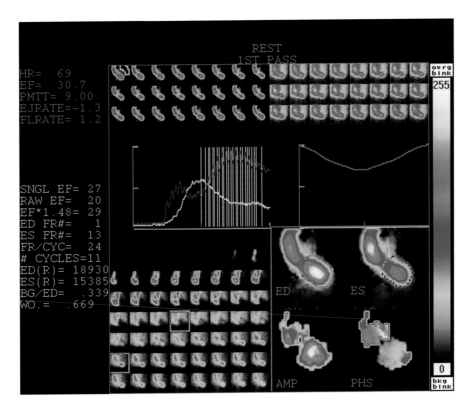

Figure 23-1. FPRNA (anterior projection) images are shown, with the serial images at the lower left, demonstrating tracer transit from the superior vena cava, to right atrium, to right ventricle to the pulmonary phase, left heart phase, and systemic circulation. Using regions of interest (ROIs) drawn over the LV and left lung (far upper left image, also blue and green), histograms are obtained (shown above serial images, in blue and green, respectively), which show overlapping RV counts with systoles (curve valleys) and diastoles (curve peaks) from which the cardiac cycles (CYC) are derived which comprise the representative cycle. Each cardiac cycle is marked (red for diastole, green for systole). The pulmonary curve is used to compute the pulmonary mean transit time (PMTT). The length of the representative cycle in frames (FR) is used to derive the heart rate (HR). The images of the raw representative cycle are shown at upper right. This is subjected to the frame method of background subtraction (i.e., using the background to end-diastolic image ratio (BG/ED) and the washout factor (WO) needed to set the pulmonary area to zero counts), in order to derive the corrected representative cycle (upper left images) from which single ROI ejection fraction (SNGL EF), which is higher than the raw EF, but lower than the dual ROI derived EF, which is used to account for valve plane motion. The Fourier amplitude (AMP) and phase (PHS) images at the lower right demonstrate reduced apical amplitude and delayed contraction of the apex, respectively.

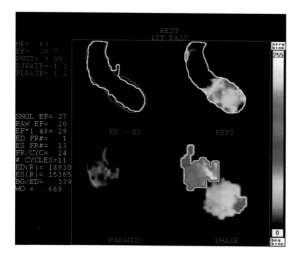

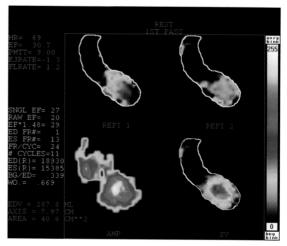

Figure 23-2. FPRNA (anterior projection) functional images are shown, with end-diastolic and end-systolic perimeter image at the upper left (ED-ES), a paradox image (lower left), regional ejection fraction index (REFI, upper right), and Fourier phase images (lower right) shown. The Fourier phase image demonstrates delayed contraction of the majority of the apex, with a small area of paradoxical movement (aneurysmal) evident at the apex on the PARADOX (ES counts − ED counts) image. These functional images allow assessment of regional function without the need for visual interpretation of cine images.

Figure 23-3. Additional FPRNA (anterior projection) functional images are shown, with regional ejection fraction index for the first and second halves of systole (REFI1 and REFI2, upper frames), an alternative method of determining the presence of delayed contraction. Note that the apical region has more ejection fraction in the latter half of systole, compared with the inferobasal wall. Fourier amplitude (AMP, lower left) and stroke volume (SV, ED − ES, lower right) images are shown. The graphic extending from the valve plane to the apex on the SV image is used to compute the LV volume using the Sandler and Dodge equation for the anterior projection.

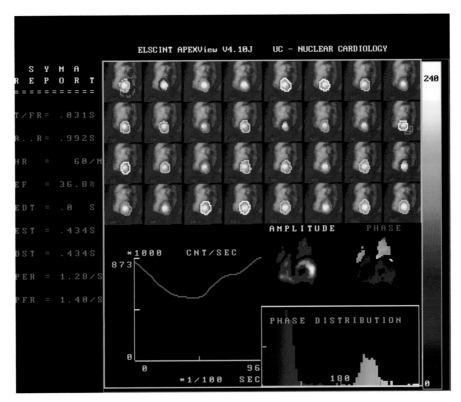

Figure 23-4. ERNA analysis is shown for images obtained in the left anterior oblique 45-degree projection. The 32 ECG-gated frames are analyzed using a guiding region of interest (ROI, frame 1) obtained either manually or using Fourier phase and amplitude images to automatically locate and outline the LV. Automated LV edge detection is performed using a combination of first and second derivative of count profiles inside the guiding or master ROI. Background correction is performed based on the counts per pixel within a small periventricular ROI (frame 16) drawn carefully to avoid the ventricle or the spleen. The counts within the 32 ROIs are shown after background correction in the lower left histogram. The first derivative of this ventricular volume curve is used to compute the peak filling and emptying rates (PFR and PER). The Fourier phase and amplitude functional images demonstrate inferoapical and septal hypokinesis with late contraction, when compared with the RV and the basal lateral portion of the LV.

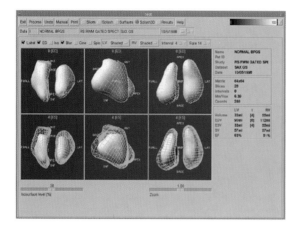

Figure 23-5. Gated tomographic ERNA analysis is shown after three-dimensional reconstruction of the left and right ventricles and surface rendering. This display (BPQS, Cedars Sinai, Los Angeles) is termed *Splash3D*. All three synchronized pairs of 3D views are displayed. The lower views can be gated, and each of these views can be rotated interactively. It is also possible to superimpose an isosurface in this mode for rapid display of regional wall motion.

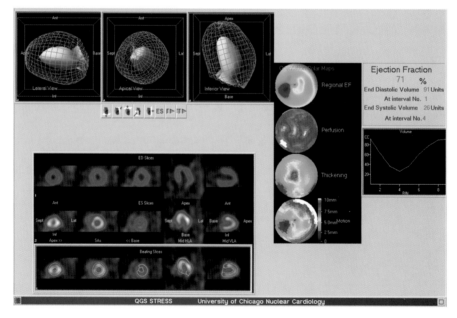

Figure 23-6. Gated SPECT myocardial perfusion images are shown analyzed with the commercially available QGS program (Cedars-Sinai) used for display and automated calculation of ejection fraction and volume. Changes in volume are tracked from ED to ES, for calculation of wall motion and regional thickening, displayed in polar map format. Three-dimensional surface rendered diagrams (above) and actual SPECT slices with fitted edges (below) are also shown. These images were obtained with Tl-201 in a normal patient.

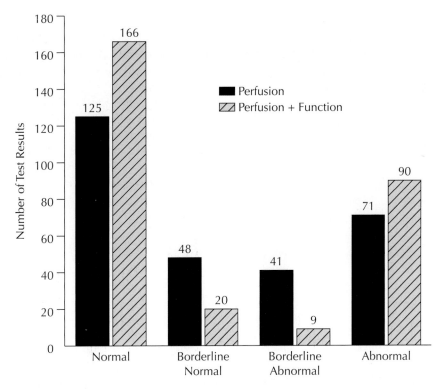

Figure 13-2. Changes in test interpretations after interpretation of perfusion and function images (hatched bars) compared with stress and rest perfusion images alone (solid bars) for all 285 patients in the study referred for evaluation for coronary artery disease (CAD). Adapted from Smanio et al.[4]

by the time of imaging. In both ED and stress-only imaging, a reference image must be obtained for comparison. Reversible perfusion abnormalities must be considered abnormal.

Evaluation of Gated SPECT Imaging to Distinguish Etiology of Dilated Cardiomyopathies

It has been estimated that over 4 million Americans have dilated cardiomyopathies, LV dysfunction, and heart failure. These conditions often are related to myocardial infarction from CAD. However, many patients have no evidence of CAD but rather cardiomyopathies and heart failure due to non–CAD-related conditions such as viral myocarditis, sarcoidosis, valvular dysfunction, and the like. A determination of the etiol-

ogy of dilated cardiomyopathies is of considerable clinical importance. Previous data examining the value of stress MPI alone or ventriculography (echocardiography) has not shown distinction of these etiologies to be useful. However, combining perfusion and function in the assessment of dilated cardiomyopathies may be of clinical benefit.[5] This may be particularly true of the presence of patterns consistent with ischemic cardiomyopathy etiology. Table 13-3 demonstrates findings consistent with either ischemic or nonischemic cardiomyopathies.

Ischemic cardiomyopathies are generally related to similar multiple past MIs. Thus, perfusion patterns should demonstrate moderate to severe either fixed or partially reversible perfusion abnormalities consistent with this diagnosis. Assessment of ventricular function by gated

Table 13-3

Imaging Patterns in Patients
with Dilated Cardiomyopathies

Condition	Imaging Pattern
Ischemic cardiomyopathy	
Myocardial perfusion	Large fixed or reversible defect
Myocardial function	Marked regional dysfunction
Nonischemic cardiomyopathy	
Myocardial perfusion	Small fixed defect
Myocardial function	Global dysfunction

SPECT imaging should also demonstrate regional wall motion abnormalities. In addition, the entire left ventricle may also be hypokinetic, but at least some component of regional abnormalities should be present. In contrast, patients with nonischemic cardiomyopathy demonstrate mild, generally fixed perfusion abnormalities most often in the inferior wall. In contrast to ischemic cardiomyopathies where regional wall motion abnormalities are typical, wall motion in nonischemic cardiomyopathies is uniformly abnormal. The study by Danias et al.[5] demonstrates clear differences in regional wall motion variability (Figure 13-3).

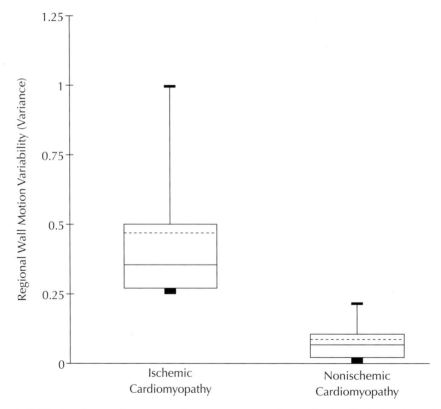

Figure 13-3. Individual patient wall motion variance among vascular territories, for ischemic and nonischemic cardiomyopathy groups. The horizontal solid lines inside the boxes represent the median values. The dotted lines represent the mean group values. The upper and lower box borders indicate the 75th and 25th percentiles, respectively. The whisker caps represent the 95th and 5th percentiles. Adapted from Danias et al.[5]

Use of ECG-Gated SPECT Imaging in the Assessment of Viability

The appropriate selection of patients with CAD and LV dysfunction for surgical revascularization is of utmost importance in cardiology. For patients with moderate to severe LV dysfunction, the operative risk is higher than in patients with normal ventricular function. However, in select patients the outcomes after revascularization are improved over medical therapy alone. The determination of myocardial viability in the areas of damaged myocardium is of considerable importance. Patients who demonstrate myocardial viability preoperatively can improve outcomes with surgical revascularization, while those with no evidence of myocardial viability do not and may suffer morbidity/mortality from the surgical procedure.[6,7] The determination of myocardial viability can be made using various modalities such as echocardiography, magnetic resonance imaging (MRI), dobutamine echocardiography, MPI, positron emission tomography (PET) imaging, and radiolabeled free fatty acid imaging. Recent data suggests comparability among many of these methods in regard to predicting outcomes.[6] Often, the determination of myocardial viability involves use of multiple pieces of information. MPI with ECG-gated SPECT offers that possibility.

The use of ECG-gated SPECT imaging has been documented to enhance the evaluation of myocardial viability. Studies such as Levine et al.[8] demonstrated improvement in SPECT sensitivity and negative predictive value using a combination of ventricular perfusion and function (Figure 13-4). Physicians seek information regarding myocardial viability in their patients with ventricular function < 35%. The assessment of myocardial viability using MPI has been demonstrated to be successful with all three available radiopharmaceuticals, including thallium 201 (Tl-201), technetium 99m (Tc-99m) sestamibi, and Tc-99m tetrofosmin. The Tl-201 data have shown improved assessment of viability using a rest redistribution model with a separate second acquisition at 4 or 24 hours. Recent data have demonstrated similar viability assessment with resting Tc-99 sestamibi or tetrofosmin.[9] In general, using any of these radiopharmaceuticals, in order for a patient to demonstrate myocardial viability there must be radio tracer activity of $\geq 50\%$ in the area under consideration in relation to perfusion in a normal region. Using these criteria, improvement of ventricular function, perfusion, and outcomes all are measures of viability.[6,7]

Evaluation of Right Ventricular Function

A distinct advantage of ECG-gated SPECT imaging is the ability to evaluate both left and right ventricular function. In certain disease processes, LV perfusion and function may be entirely normal but right ventricular (RV) function may be markedly abnormal such as in pulmonary hypertension and the like. In other circumstances, biventricular dysfunction is present. The evaluation of RV function in conjunction with LV function may be of considerable use in distinguishing ischemic from nonischemic cardiomyopathies.[5] An example of both left and right ventricular enlargement in a 35-year-old diabetic patient with diabetic cardiomyopathy and no evidence of CAD is shown in Figure 13-5. Both left and right ventricular cavities were markedly dilated. ECG-gated SPECT imaging demonstrated severe global hypokinesis of both ventricles. The presence of RV dysfunction in this patient was helpful to distinguish ischemic from nonischemic etiology of the patient's ventricular dysfunction.

Evaluation of RV function should be made on every patient and mentioned in the report. Although RV dysfunction is rare, the exercise of evaluation will ensure that RV dysfunction is not missed. RV evaluation is best made with multiple short-axis slices as well as the horizontal long-axis views. Increasing the gain after evaluation of LV function may be important because the RV wall is thinner than the LV; therefore, fewer counts are present for visualization. RV perfusion abnormalities have been noticed in patients with inferior MI, although special processing is necessary.[10]

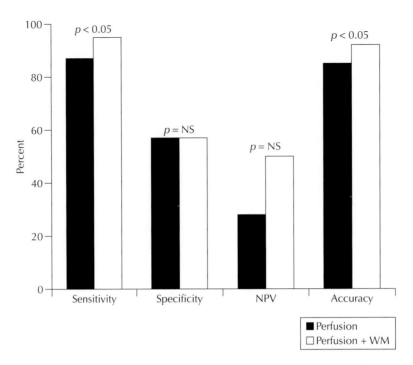

Figure 13-4. Comparison of perfusion alone with perfusion + wall motion for prediction of viability: the addition of ECG gating significantly improved sensitivity. Negative predictive value, odds ratio, and accuracy also improved, whereas specificity and positive predictive value did not change. Overall, perfusion + wall motion was significantly better than perfusion alone for the prediction of viability. Adapted from Levine et al.[8]

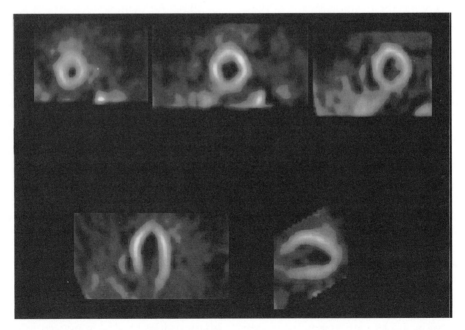

Figure 13-5. Gated-SPECT in 35-year-old female with diabetic cardiomyopathy. Both left and right ventricular cavities were markedly dilated. ECG-gated SPECT imaging demonstrated severe global hypokinesis of both ventricles. (**See also Color Insert**).

Evaluation of Myocardial Stunning During ECG-gated SPECT Imaging

Until recently, it has been assumed that wall motion evaluation of patients undergoing stress MPI represents resting conditions since acquisition begins within 15 to 45 minutes after the stress has been completed. However, recent evidence has suggested the contrary. Johnson et al.[11] first suggested that regional changes between exercise stress imaging and rest imaging on the same patients occasionally occurs in the presence of severe ischemia. In that study, several patients with exercise-induced myocardial perfusion abnormalities also had transient regional wall motion abnormalities associated with the stress imaging. Thus, the rest study demonstrated normal ventricular function in the same area. The authors suggest this may be related to continued wall motion abnormalities and continued LV dysfunction beyond exercise, which may persist for up to 1 hour.

Since this study, several other manuscripts have evaluated the value of gated SPECT during both rest and stress conditions. The presence of regional wall motion abnormalities has been associated with high-grade stenosis and worse outcome. Thus, there is benefit to performing gated SPECT imaging for both rest and stress studies.[12,13]

Value of Ventricular Function in Risk Stratification

The prognostic value of stress MPI has been well documented over the past 20 years. More recently, however, several studies have demonstrated an incremental value to a combination of perfusion and function, which complement each other. Sharir et al.[14] demonstrated that the prediction of cardiac death is heavily weighted in favor of ventricular function (ejection fraction over perfusion alone) (Figure 13-6). However, in an-

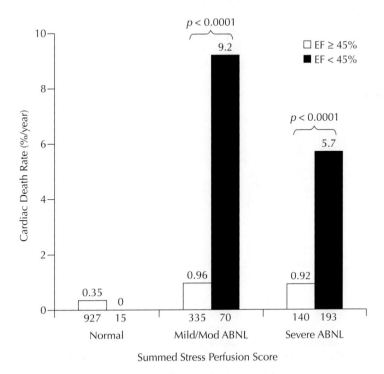

Figure 13-6.   Cardiac death rate (%/year) as a function of perfusion abnormality and EF. The number of patients within each category is indicated below each column. Mod indicates moderate, and ABNL, abnormality. Adapted from Sharir et al.[14]

other model in which the event was myocardial infarction, myocardial perfusion was a better predictor than myocardial function[15] (Figure 13-7).

CONCLUSION

The ability to simultaneously evaluate LV function along with myocardial perfusion with gated SPECT imaging has been one of the most remarkable advances in the field of nuclear cardiology. Acquisition of the functional data is simple and inexpensive. It can be done using the same

infrastructure as required for standard perfusion imaging and requires only an additional 2 to 3 minutes of acquisition time. It provides information that adds significantly to that obtained from evaluation of perfusion alone. There is a wealth of data which show that combined assessment of myocardial perfusion and function has incremental value over assessment of individual parameters alone. Thus, gated SPECT, which adds little to the cost of the procedure, will likely improve the cost-effectiveness of nuclear imaging.

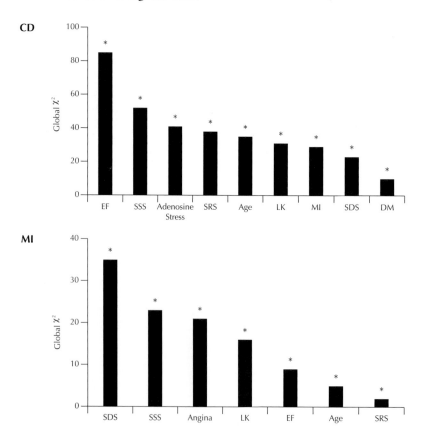

Figure 13-7. Univariate Cox regression analysis for prediction of cardiac death (CD) and nonfatal myocardial infarction (MI). LK = prescan likelihood of coronary disease; DM = diabetes mellitus. EF = ejection fraction. SSS = summed stress score. SDS = summed difference in scores. SRS = summed rest score. *P < 0.02. The best predictor of cardiac death was EF, while the best predictor of MI was the degree of ischemia (SDS). Reprinted by permission of the Society of Nuclear Medicine from: Sharir, T. et al., Prediction of Myocardial Infarction Versus Cardiac Death by Gated Myocardial Perfusion SPECT: Risk Stratification by the Amount of Stress-Induced Ischemia and the Poststress Ejection Fraction. *J. Nucl. Med.* 2001;42:831–837.

REFERENCES

1. Cerqueira MD, Weissman NJ, Dilsizian V, et al. Standardized myocardial segmentation and nomenclature for tomographic imaging of the heart: A statement for healthcare professionals from the Cardiac Imaging Committee of the Council on Clinical Cardiology of the American Heart Association. *J Nucl Cardiol* 2002;9:240–245.

2. DePuey EG, Rozanski A. Using gated Tc-99m sestamibi SPECT to characterize fixed myocardial defects as infarct or artifact. *J Nucl Med* 1995;37:952–955.

3. Taillefer R, DePuey EG, Udelson JE, et al. Comparative diagnostic accuracy of Tl-201 and Tc-99m sestamibi SPECT imaging (perfusion and ECG-gated SPECT) in detecting coronary artery disease in women. *J Am Coll Cardiol* 1997;29:69–77.

4. Smanio PEP, Watson DD, Segalla DL, et al. Value of gating of technetium-99m sestamibi single-photon emission computed tomographic imaging. *J Am Coll Cardiol* 1997;30:1687–1692.

5. Danias PG, Ahlberg AW, Clark BA, et al. Combined assessment of myocardial perfusion and left ventricular function with exercise technetium-99m sestamibi gated single-photon emission computed tomography can differentiate between ischemic and nonischemic dilated cardiomyopathy. *Am J Cardiol* 1998;82:1253–1258.

6. Allman KC, Shaw LJ, Hachamovitch R, Udelson JE. Myocardial viability testing and impact of revascularization on prognosis in patients with coronary artery disease and left ventricular dysfunction: a meta-analysis. *J Am Coll Cardiol* 2002;39:1151–1158.

7. Bax JJ, Poldermans D, Elhendy A, et al. Improvement of left ventricular ejection fraction, heart failure symptoms and prognosis after revascularization in patients with chronic coronary artery disease and viable myocardium detected by dobutamine stress echocardiography. *J Am Coll Cardiol* 1999;34:163–169.

8. Levine MG, McGill CC, Ahlberg AW, et al. Functional assessment with electrocardiographic gated single-photon emission computed tomography improves the ability of technetium-99m sestamibi myocardial perfusion imaging to predict myocardial viability in patients undergoing revascularization. *Am J Cardiol* 1999;83:1–5.

9. Udelson JE, Coleman PS, Metherall J, et al. Predicting recovery of severe regional ventricular dysfunction. Comparison of resting scintigraphy with ^{201}Tl and ^{99m}Tc-sestamibi. *Circulation* 1994;89:2552–2561.

10. Travin MI, Malkin RD, Garber CE, et al. Prevalence of right ventricular perfusion defects after inferior myocardial infarction assessed by low-level exercise with technetium 99m sestamibi tomographic myocardial imaging. *Am Heart J* 1994;127:797–804.

11. Johnson LL, Verdesca SA, Aude WY, et al. Postischemic stunning can affect left ventricular ejection fraction and regional wall motion on post-stress gated sestamibi tomograms. *J Am Coll Cardiol* 1997;30:1641–1648.

12. Emmett L, Iwanochko RM, Freeman MR, et al. Reversible regional wall motion abnormalities on exercise technetium-99m-gated cardiac single photon emission computed tomography predict high-grade angiographic stenoses. *J Am Coll Cardiol* 2002;39:991–998.

13. Sharir T, Bacher-Stier C, Dhar S, et al. Identification of severe and extensive coronary artery disease by postexercise regional wall motion abnormalities in Tc-99m sestamibi gated single-photon emission computed tomography. *Am J Cardiol* 2000;86:1171–1175.

14. Sharir T, Germano G, Kavanagh PB, et al. Incremental prognostic value of post-stress left ventricular ejection fraction and volume by gated myocardial perfusion single photon emission computed tomography. *Circulation* 1999;100:1035–1042.

15. Sharir T, Germano G, Kang X, et al. Prediction of myocardial infarction versus cardiac death by gated myocardial perfusion SPECT: Risk stratification by the amount of stress-induced ischemia and the poststress ejection fraction. *J Nucl Med* 2001;42:831–837.

CHAPTER 14

Clinically Relevant Report Writing

Robert C. Hendel

INTRODUCTION

The final product of a nuclear cardiology procedure is the report. This directly reflects not only on the performance of the imaging study performed, but also on its interpretation. It is ultimately the critical piece of information that guides patient management. As such, it is essential that the report be inclusive yet clear in its meaning. The quality of the report reflects not only on the interpreting physician, but also on the nuclear cardiology laboratory and on the field of nuclear cardiology itself.

Many current nuclear cardiology reports fall far short of the mark of clarity. Words such as *suggestive of, possible,* and other qualifiers should be avoided. Additionally, the unique descriptions of perfusion abnormalities such as describing the severity as "2+" or the use of words such as *paradoxical* should be removed. While the intent of the reader may be well known within one institution, significant problems may arise should the report migrate out of the individual laboratory's usual realm. In describing the location of various perfusion abnormalities, consistency must be present and words such as *posterior* are now not recommended. Finally, ubiquitous and somewhat insulting comments, such as "clinical correlation is suggested," should be avoided. The latter phrase need not be included, as the correlation of all imaging results should be performed with regard to the clinical history. Finally, descriptions such as "of unknown significance" or "equivocal" should be restricted to the most extreme of circumstances.

A number of publications have delineated the importance of a nuclear cardiology report,[1–3] and recently guidelines have been proposed to support the components of the content of this report.[2] Obviously, individuality is critical, and reports will need to be adjusted to suit the laboratory as well as the individual nuclear cardiologist. However, some standardization is critical so as to optimize the information and to provide the most clinically relevant data to the referring physician.

Currently, reports are often variable in content and in form. While this is acceptable, ambiguity and a lack of an impression are not helpful to the patient, to the referring physician, or to nuclear cardiology. The most important goal of a nuclear cardiology report should be the communication of critical findings to the referring physician and their clinical implications. Additionally, the report should serve to document information that is pertinent to reimbursement and accreditation licensure. The latter includes drug management and radiation safety. Finally, certification and accreditation is based often on nuclear cardiology reports and such bodies such as the Intersocietal Commission for the Accreditation of Nuclear Medicine Laboratories (ICANL) will review these reports to make sure that they are consistent with what is felt to be the standard of nuclear cardiology.

CRITICAL COMPONENTS OF THE NUCLEAR CARDIOLOGY REPORT

Patient Data

Information that is important to not only the interpretation of the study but also to provide clinical relevance must be included in the report (Table 14-1). This includes the age, gender, and body habitus of the patient. Height, weight, body surface area, and chest circumference are

Table 14-1
Required Clinical Information

- Demographics (age, gender, race)
- Body habitus (height, weight)
- Symptoms
- Medications
- Cardiac risk factors
- Prior cardiac events
- Prior diagnostic tests
- Therapeutic cardiac procedures

items that may be included. Relevant clinical information including past cardiac history such as myocardial infarction (MI) or the performance of revascularization should be included. Additionally, major cardiac risk factors should be noted. The patient's current medications should be included, as they may impact on the interpretation of the results. They also provide documentation of the current clinical status of the subject.

Indications

The indication for the procedure should be fairly delineated. Ideally, this should be obtained from the report as well as from patient history. Several critical indications for the procedure include:

- Diagnosis
- Assessment of the extent and severity of known coronary artery disease (CAD)
- Risk assessment
- Determination of myocardial viability
- Evaluation of acute chest pain syndrome

The actual indication may also be referenced to a specific diagnostic code to assist in matters related to reimbursement. Many laboratories include the ICD9-CD codes directly in the report.

Procedures

Procedures should be well delineated so as to provide a frame of reference for subsequent comparisons as well as to explain the testing results directly to the referring physician (Table 14-2). The mode of stress should be noted. If exercise, the specific protocol such as Naughton or Bruce should be noted. The duration of exercise should be stated as well as the protocol stage achieved. Finally, the number of metabolic equivalents (METS) should be specified. The adequacy of the test results should be stated, such as the target heart rate achieved in terms of the maximum predicted heart rate and the reasons for test termination. If pharmacologic stress testing is performed, the agent and dose should be specified. In addition, whether adjunctive exercise was performed and its type should be mentioned.

Table 14-2
Procedure

- Type and protocol of stress procedure
- Adequacy of results
- Symptoms during protocol
- Hemodynamic response (heart rate, blood pressure)
- ECG changes
- Radiopharmaceuticals utilized (with dose)
- Imaging protocol
- Functional data
- Attenuation/scatter correction

The presence of symptoms as well as the hemodynamic responses should be well delineated. The heart rate as well as blood pressure changes should be noted. Electrocardiographic changes, including those that deviate from the baseline electrocardiogram (ECG) should be mentioned. The resting ECG should be stated, especially if there are abnormalities noted such as left bundle branch block (LBBB), left ventricular hypertrophy (LVH), or nonspecific ST/T wave abnormalities.

The perfusion imaging agent and dose administered at peak stress should be mentioned. If the stress is continued after the radiopharmaceutical injection, the duration of the continuation of stress should be mentioned. The actual imaging protocol should also be stated. For example, planar or single photon emission computed tomography (SPECT) should be stated as well as whether the imaging was performed in a supine or prone position. A 1- or 2-day protocol should be specified and single or double isotope studies should be noted. If gated or SPECT or first-pass imaging was performed, again this should be well described and noted whether it was performed at stress or rest. Finally, advanced imaging techniques such as attenuation correction should be noted.

Findings

The results or findings portion of the report should provide an in-depth discussion of all find-

ings noted upon review of the nuclear cardiology study. It should be comprehensive and attempt to describe all pertinent findings (Table 14-3).

The first portion of the results section should deal with image quality. This should be stated as either excellent, good, fair, or poor. Extracardiac activity should also be well described and correlated with any potential clinical information.

The perfusion defect characteristic should be carefully described. This includes the size (small, moderate, large), type (ischemic, reversible, persistent, mixed), and severity (mild, moderate, severe). The location of the abnormality in terms of segmentation and vascular territory should also be described to the best of the interpreter's abilities and using standard nomenclature.[4] Clear delineation between single- and multivessel disease should be performed.

Markers of extensive disease, such as multivessel distribution or the presence of abnormal tracer distribution in the lungs, should be carefully noted. Additionally, the presence of cavity enlargement, either immediately following stress or on both stress and rest images, should be present. If transient ischemic cavity dilation (TID) is noted, the TID ratio should be described. Left ventricular (LV) function assessment is now a mainstay of myocardial perfusion imaging (MPI). Both global and regional function should be described qualitatively as well as quantitatively. The left ventricular ejection fraction (LVEF) should be stated. If the LVEF is > 60%, the interpreter may describe this as normal or simply " > 60% or > 70%." This is in recognition of the fact that it is

Table 14-3
Results

- Study quality
- Defect description (size, reversibility, severity, location)
- Extensiveness (TID, lung activity, right ventricular activity)
- Left ventricular function (global, regional)
- Extracardiac activity

common to see artifactually increased LVEFs in patients with small LV cavities, and it is somewhat nonsensical to report an LVEF of 91%. Both the rest and poststress function should be noted, if available. Regional defects should be carefully described as either hypokinetic, akinetic, or diskinetic, and the location given.

Impression

The impression is frequently the only portion of the report read by the referring physician. It is critical that it be crisp in its meaning, and the final diagnosis must be clear. Most reports should begin the impression section with a statement that perfusion imaging is either normal or abnormal. A study may still be interpreted as normal even if there are perfusion abnormalities noted in the results section. This discrepancy should be explained in the impression section briefly by commenting on whether or not this was believed to be due to an artifact, such as soft tissue, LBBB, or patient motion. The functional information should be incorporated in a brief manner describing whether LV function is reduced and whether regional wall motion abnormalities are present. The amount of LV dysfunction should be semiquantitated, such as stating that there is moderately reduced LV systolic function.

The impression section is also the place for correlation of the perfusion imaging data with clinical information, data from the results of the stress test, and any correlation with angiographic data as it is known. A comparison to prior studies should be undertaken, and a direct statement regarding any significant changes should be made. As the diagnostic accuracy of perfusion imaging is superior to that of ECG stress testing, an abnormal ECG response to exercise with normal perfusion images should be considered to be a false positive, especially in the setting of resting ST-segment abnormalities. Of note, however, is that ECG changes occurring during a vasodilator infusion may portend a worse prognosis, even in the setting of normal SPECT images.[5]

Finally, the impression must directly address the question that was asked. Therefore, specific comments should be made regarding the indications and reasons for performing the procedure. For example, many laboratories performing a diagnostic study will comment directly on the likelihood of CAD. Some practitioners, however, are concerned about the legal ramifications of such a statement and opt not to include this type of language. If the study is ordered for the delineation of risk, the prognostic value should be stipulated in the report. Following an MI, the findings of a second vascular distribution or peri-infarction ischemia should be noted and equated with an increased risk of subsequent cardiac events. Likewise, perioperative assessments should comment specifically in the report on whether an increased risk for perioperative cardiac complications is present based on the study. For acute imaging procedures, the interpreter should note whether there is any evidence of ongoing ischemia or MI.

LOGISTICS

Once the report is prepared, it is critical that this information be disseminated to the referring physician as soon as possible. Preliminary results are often discouraged, in deference to the viewpoint that the final results should be available within the same day of the study. If this is not feasible, then some form of preliminary communication should likely ensue. Same-day reporting, however, is strongly encouraged.

The report may be transmitted to the referring physician by means of facsimile, e-mail, or intranet transfer. It may also be obtainable through hospital records. Telephone notification should occur, especially in the setting of high-risk findings. Many laboratories choose to notify the referring physician of all abnormal results. In fact, some laboratories contact all physicians with the results by telephone.

The final report should be prepared in a rapid manner and be "signed off" as soon as possible—ideally, within 24 hours. The final report may include copies of the images either embedded within the report or as an add-on. This provides for subsequent reference to future reports.

Finally, the report should be data based and provided as an electronic record for rapid recall. Quality assurance information also may be obtained in this fashion.

SUMMARY

In conclusion, reporting should incorporate the "Five C's":

- **Clarity.** Ambiguity must be minimized, and the overall message or the report should come through loudly.
- **Completeness.** Symptoms, stress test results, perfusion data, and functional information should all be described within the report. Additionally, it should be related to the clinical scenario as well as any additional cardiac testing data available.
- **Consistency.** The report should be consistent in terms of the individual readers' daily patterns as well as within a given laboratory. Group reading sessions should be undertaken so that all readers within a given laboratory adopt a similar manner of reading. This is critical, as a given reader is often not available to interpret a study on a subsequent visit.
- **Clinical relevancy.** The question that is asked should be directly answered.
- **Communication.** Rapid reporting of all results is critical to the performance of a successful laboratory. All physicians should be notified of critical values such as patients with multivessel disease or severe ischemia. Telephone contact or facsimile transmission of reports to physicians with patients who possess high-risk findings is highly encouraged.

As described throughout this chapter, the report is probably the most critical aspect of the nuclear cardiology procedure. It provides a direct reflection of nuclear cardiology. Without a high-quality report, the value of the overall procedure may be negated. Therefore, all laboratories and individual readers should strive for the highest-quality report possible, conveying the maximum amount of clinical information. This will ensure continued referrals and the further development and growth of nuclear cardiology.

REFERENCES

1. Cerqueira MD. The user-friendly nuclear cardiology report: What needs to be considered and what is included. *J Nucl Cardiol* 1996;4:350–355.
2. Port SC. Imaging guidelines for nuclear cardiology procedures, part II. *J Nucl Cardiol* 1999;6:G48–84.
3. Wackers FJ. Intersocietal Commission for the Accreditation of Nuclear Medicine Laboratories (ICANL) position statement on standardization and optimization of nuclear cardiology reports. *J Nucl Cardiol* 2000;7:397–400.
4. Cerqueira MD, Weissman NJ, Dilsizian V, et al. Standardized myocardial segmentation and nomenclature for tomographic imaging of the heart: A statement for healthcare professionals from the Cardiac Imaging Committee of the Council on Clinical Cardiology of the American Heart Association. *J Nucl Cardiol* 2002;9:240–245.
5. Abbott BG, Afshar M, Berger AK, Wackers FJ. Prognostic significance of ischemic electrocardiographic changes during adenosine infusion in patients with normal perfusion imaging. *J Nucl Cardiol* 2003;10:9–16.

CHAPTER 15

Electron Beam Computed Tomography

Kourosh Mastali
Robert C. Hendel

CALCIUM AND ATHEROSCLEROSIS

Atherosclerotic calcification starts around the second decade of life following the formation of fatty streaks[1] and it appears to be a regulated process,[2] not simply a marker of aging. The abundance of calcium in coronary trees among the elderly is a reflection of the fact that the presence of coronary atherosclerosis is more common in this population. Blakenhorn et al[3] demonstrated the association of calcium with intimal atherosclerosis and luminal narrowing in a study of 3,500 segments of coronary trees collected from 76 postmortem specimens which was confirmed by subsequent studies.[4–7] The extent of coronary calcification may be a marker of "physiologic" age and may in and of itself have importance as a risk factor. Several risk algorithms now include coronary calcification scores as a variable used to calculate an individual's risk for developing obstructive coronary artery disease (CAD).

Calcium is an important part of atherosclerotic plaque, and there is an inverse association between the extent of coronary artery calcification and the risk of plaque rupture and thrombosis,[8,9] as calcification appears to stabilize the plaque. Unstable or "soft" plaques consist of a lipid rich core with a thin fibrotic covering. In contrast, stable or "hard" plaques have thicker caps and a decreased lipid core. The early atherosclerotic events, such as incomplete layering of calcium, make the plaque more prone to rupture, in contrast to heavily calcified plaques, which are more stable.[10] This might be due to increased stress near the junction of calcific cap and adjacent intima, which in part is due to their different physical properties.[11]

ELECTRON BEAM COMPUTED TOMOGRAPHY AND CORONARY CALCIUM IMAGING

X-ray techniques, including computed tomography (CT) scanning, primarily look at the differences in tissue densities, including the presence and extent of calcification. Electron beam computed tomography (EBCT) allows for the rapid acquisition of three-dimensional images of the heart, which can be accomplished in one or two breath-holds.[12] This cross-sectional technique uses an electron e-ray source and stationary tungsten targets. To minimize the motion artifact, images are acquired close to end of diastole, triggered by electrocardiogram (ECG) signals corresponding to 80% of the RR interval. The scan slice is approximately 3 mm thick (range 1.5–6 mm), and usually 30 to 40 adjacent slices are needed to image the heart. Overall, EBCT is fast (subsecond scanning times, with total acquisitions of < 15 minutes), simple to use, does not require provocative (stress) testing, and is operator independent. An example of an EBCT image is shown in Figure 15-1.

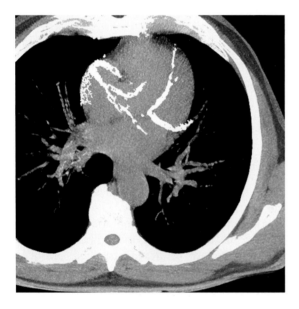

Figure 15-1. EBCT transaxial image of an asymptomatic 51-year-old man with a history of hyperlipidemia. The linear white regions within the heart represent extensive calcification of the coronary arteries. The patient subsequently underwent an exercise test which was strongly positive, with 2 to 3 mm of ST-segment depression. Dual-isotope imaging revealed a large area of ischemia in the distribution of the proximal left anterior descending coronary artery, which was later confirmed by coronary angiography.

Agatston et al[13] described a method in which a calcium score can be calculated by multiplying the lesion area times a density factor derived from the maximal Hounsfield units within the area of interest. Figure 15-2 shows the calculation of coronary calcium score by Agatston method. A calcium score can be calculated for a given coronary segment, coronary artery, or the entire epicardial coronary tree. An alternative method to determine calcium score by measuring the actual volume of the plaque has been evaluated by Callister et al,[14] which has a smaller variability compare to the traditional Agatston method. A normal distribution of calcium scores based on age and gender has been established by scanning 9,728 asymptomatic individuals (Table 15-1),[15] which provides a reference for interpretation of a specific calcium score with EBCT, thereby defining groups with the highest levels (percentile) of coronary calcification.

There is a linear correlation of the EBCT-derived calcium coronary score and the extent of coronary artery plaque based on histologic studies in which EBCT scans were performed on dissected coronary arteries from autopsied hearts.[16–18] It has been reported that total coronary tree calcium area detected by EBCT is about 20% of the total atherosclerotic plaque area.[16] Overall, the reproducibility of coronary artery calcification measurements appears high, with most of the differences due to patient motion and the misregistration of images.[19] However, some authors have shown that the quantification of coronary calcium by EBCT, although reliable, has substantial interest variability, up to about 20% variations with repeated scanning.[20] Therefore, the thresholds for disease extent are unlikely to be rigid and monitoring of disease progress may have some limitations.

There have been significant technological advances in multislice CT (MSCT—helical or spiral CT) in recent years, allowing the imaging of coronary arteries with improved resolution using this new method for detecting coronary artery calcification. This technique incorporates fast rotational speeds with thin "slices" to reduce the

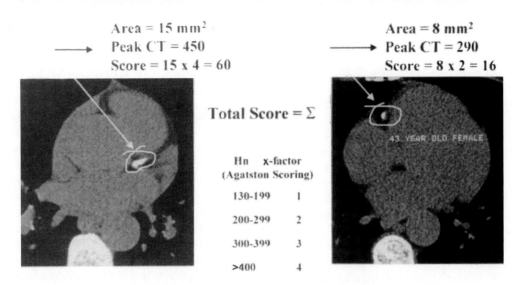

Area = 15 mm² → Peak CT = 450 Score = 15 x 4 = 60

Area = 8 mm² → Peak CT = 290 Score = 8 x 2 = 16

Total Score = Σ

Hn (Agatston Scoring)	x-factor
130-199	1
200-299	2
300-399	3
>400	4

Figure 15-2. Representative method of coronary calcium scoring by EBCT with use of the Agatston method. Area surrounding calcification is identified by a standardized computer program that determines the total area of calcification by using threshold > 130 Hounsfield units. Peak x-ray density (Hounsfield unit) is then determined, and a multiplier of the calcium area is determined. For image on left (left anterior descending coronary artery), calcium score is 60. For image on right (right coronary artery), calcium score is 16. For these two slices, score would be 76. Total calcium score is the sum of all individual tomographic calcium scores for the entire epicardial coronary artery system. (Adapted from Rumberger et al.[35] with permission.)

Table 15-1

Calcium Score Nomogram

	Age, years						
	35–39	40–44	45–49	50–54	55–59	60–64	65–70
Men (5,433)	(479)	(859)	(1,066)	(1,085)	(853)	(613)	(478)
25th percentile	0	0	0	0	3	14	28
50th percentile	0	0	3	16	41	118	151
75th percentile	2	11	44	101	187	434	569
90th percentile	21	64	176	320	502	804	1178
Women (4,297)	(288)	(859)	(822)	(903)	(693)	(515)	(485)
25th percentile	0	0	0	0	0	0	0
50th percentile	0	0	0	0	0	4	24
75th percentile	0	0	0	10	33	87	123
90th percentile	4	9	23	66	140	310	362

The number of patients in each group is in parentheses.
From Raggi et al.[15] with permission.

time of acquisition and minimize motion artifact. The spatial resolution of these devices is superior to that of EBCT, but overall image quality is more compromised by increased heart rates. Figure 15-3 shows an MSCT angiogram, which shows an obstructed left descending coronary artery. MSCT detectors allow for the acquisition of four simultaneous slices, and with reconstruction algorithms and ECG gating create high-quality images with little cardiac motion, especially when the heart rate is < 70 beats per minute (the image quality of MSCT is highly dependent on heart rate). However, the literature addressing the clinical relevance of this technique is very limited, but suggests the comparable results for detecting coronary calcification when compared with EBCT.[21] Noninvasive coronary angiography appears to be a growing possibility with the use of MSCT.[21]

DETECTION OF CORONARY ARTERY DISEASE

Like traditional cardiac risk factors, including diabetes mellitus, hypertension, and hyperlipidemia, an abnormal EBCT has been associated with an increased risk for the development of CAD.[22-29] The presence of abnormal coronary artery calcification increases the likelihood of obstructive CAD by more than 10-fold, which is substantially larger than the risk noted with the presence of traditional risk factors.[22] Guerci et al.[23] reported an increased risk for CAD associated with specific levels of calcification, as evidenced by the finding that as the coronary calcium score rose, so did the risk of obstructive CAD.[23] In a similar fashion, an increased coronary calcium score with EBCT is associated with the presence of an abnormal single photon emis-

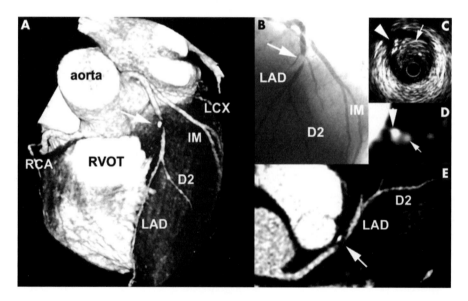

Figure 15-3. Multislice computed tomography angiogram of an obstructed left anterior descending (LAD) coronary artery and a heart rate of 49 beats per minute. A significant stenosis (arrow) can be observed in the LAD. The three-dimensional volume rendered overview **A.** shows the lesion just distal to small diagonal branch, which is confirmed by conventional angiography **B.** The cross-sectional **D.** and longitudinal reconstruction **E.** show a partially calcified lesion, which is confirmed by intracoronary ultrasound **C.** D2, second diagonal branch; IM, intermediate branch; LCX, left circumflex coronary artery; RCA, right coronary artery; RVOT, right ventricular outflow tract. (Adapted from Nieman K, et al. *Heart* 2002;88:470–474.)

sion computed tomography (SPECT) study, irrespective of age and gender, with the EBCT findings being the best predictor of perfusion abnormalities on a SPECT examination.[24]

Several meta-analyses have been performed examining the diagnostic value of EBCT. One such analysis, shown in Table 15-2, reveals a sensitivity of 91% for the detection of CAD.[25] This is at least as high as other diagnostic methods and appears to be superior to several other noninvasive techniques. However, the specificity of EBCT is quite low (49%), perhaps due to its inability to detect noncalcified stenoses (plaque). Another meta-analysis demonstrated that the summary receiver operator characteristic curves demonstrated comparable diagnostic accuracy of EBCT to exercise stress testing, with a pooled sensitivity of 92.3% and a low pooled specificity of 51.2%.[30] The explanation for the diagnostic properties of EBCT is offered in the study by Baumgart,[26] who demonstrated that EBCT was abnormal in 97% of patients with a hard plaque

noted on intravascular ultrasound (IVUS), but was substantially less (47%) when only soft plaque was present.

The close association of coronary artery calcification and calcium scores obtained with EBCT likely serves as the basis for the high sensitivity of EBCT for the detection of CAD[31] and makes it unlikely that a flow-limiting coronary stenosis would be present in the absence of coronary artery calcification, as assessed by EBCT. The specificity of EBCT is also impacted by the coronary artery calcium score. Budoff et al.[32] reported that specificity of EBCT for detecting CAD increases as the calcium score rises and also correlates with the number of coronary arteries involved.

The diagnostic value of EBCT, as reflected by its sensitivity and specificity, may have dramatic impact on the clinical use of the technique and its role in patient management. Due to the low specificity of EBCT, additional diagnostic testing is often indicated to confirm the presence or ab-

Table 15-2

Comparison of Exercise Testing and Adds-on or Other Test Modalities

Grouping	No. of Studies	Total No. of Patients	Sensitivity, %	Specificity, %	Predictive Accuracy, %
Meta-analysis of standard exercise ECG	147	24,047	68	77	73
Excluding MI patients	41	11,691	67	74	69
Limiting workup bias	2	2,350	50	90	69
Meta-analysis of exercise test scores	24	11,788			80
Perfusion scintigraphy	2	28,751	89	80	89
Exercise echocardiography	58	5,000	85	79	83
Nonexercise stress test					
Pharmacologic stress scintigraphy	11	< 1,000	85	91	87
Dobutamine echocardiography	5	< 1,000	88	84	86
EBCT	16	3,683	91	49	70

From O'Rourke et al.[25] with permission.

sence of physiologically important CAD. Many of these subsequent tests may be normal and fail to confirm the presence of obstructive CAD, thereby increasing health care costs and potentially the risk to an individual patient. The concern about the low specificity of EBCT has led the American College of Cardiology/American Hospital Association (ACC/AHA) Expert Consensus Panel to conclude "EBCT appears not to be superior to other currently available diagnostic procedures for diagnosis of angiographic coronary heart disease."[25] However, it is critical to realize that atherosclerotic disease is still present and may still indicate a marker of clinical risk, even in the absence of an abnormal stress test or coronary angiogram.

Few studies have directly compared myocardial perfusion imaging (MPI) with EBCT. Overall, the sensitivity of EBCT appears to be slightly higher than that of thallium 201 (Tl-201) or technetium 99m (Tc-99m) sestamibi imaging, but the specificity of EBCT is usually reported as being substantially lower than with SPECT imaging.[33–35] The relative risk of obstructive CAD is higher with EBCT than with perfusion imaging, however (149 vs. 3.4[33] or 4.5 vs. 2.0.[34] These studies were limited, however, by being performed in the era prior to the routine use of gated SPECT imaging, which has significantly improved specificity.

RISK STRATIFICATION

Although the detection of coronary artery calcium and significant CAD may have clinical relevance, a key factor in patient management is whether or not a patient is at risk for cardiac events. Therefore, the ability of a test such as EBCT to predict nonfatal myocardial infarction (MI), or cardiac death has important clinical ramifications. The prognostic implications of EBCT and the imaging of coronary artery calcification is based on the complete extent of atherosclerosis, both hard and soft plaques. It is well recognized that the even soft plaques are more prevalent with high calcification scores. Additionally, the ability

of EBCT not only to detect calcification but to quantitate the atherosclerotic burden offers a supplemental tool for risk assessment.

Several studies are now available that demonstrate the prognostic utility of EBCT.[36–43] In fact, the majority of studies have shown EBCT to be a superior predictor of cardiac events than the usual risk factors. Detrano et al.[36] followed 491 patients for follow-up period of 30 ± 13, and reported that a calcium score ≥ 75.3 was associated with a sixfold increase in number of subsequent cardiac events, with the vast majority of events occurring in patients with a calcium score ≥ 100. After including age, sex, number of diseased vessels based on angiography, and calcium score in a logistic regression model, it was noted that calcium score was the only independent predictor of cardiac events. The level of coronary artery calcium score was also shown to correlate with subsequent cardiac events by Arad and colleagues, who demonstrated that among 1,173 patients, a coronary artery calcium score > 160 was associated with a risk 35 times that of normal studies for the development of MI, death, cerebrovascular accident (CVA), or revascularization (Table 15-3).[37] A similar study of 600 men and women revealed a threefold increase of cardiac death or nonfatal MI when significant coronary calcium was present on EBCT.[38] Therefore, EBCT provides incremental prognostic value to the usual clinical information.

Recently, there has been interest in using calcium score in conjunction with newly defined risk factors to predict subsequent cardiac events. Park et al.[44] reported that calcium and C-reactive protein (CRP) appear to be complementary but independent for the prediction of cardiovascular events. He reported using the combination of coronary calcium score tertiles and elevated CRP levels (defined by the 75th quartile) identified a sixfold difference in risk of MI and cardiac death, and a sevenfold difference in the risk of any cardiovascular event between the lowest risk (lowest tertile calcium score and normal CRP) and the highest risk (highest tertile of calcium score and elevated CRP level).

Table 15-3

Coronary Artery Calcification Score and Diagnostic Accuracy

CAC Score Threshold	Sensitivity	Specificity	PPV	NPV	OR	95% CI	p
≥ 100	0.89	0.77	0.055	0.998	25.8	5.9–113	< 0.00001
≥ 160	0.89	0.82	0.071	0.998	35.4	8.1–155	< 0.00001
≥ 680	0.50	0.95	0.140	0.992	20.0	7.6–52	< 0.00001

CAC = coronary artery calcification; PPV = positive predictive value; NPV = negative predictive value; OR = odds ratio.
CAC threshold of 100 and 680 were previously found to correlate with worst stenosis of 20% and 50%, respectively, on quantitative coronary angiography. CAC of 160 represent the maximum of sensitivity plus specificity.
From Arad et al[37] with permission.

Based of these studies, coronary calcium appears to be more than a radiologic finding, and has significant clinical relevance. In fact, calcium score detected by EBCT is highly correlated with subsequent cardiac events.

ASYMPTOMATIC PATIENTS: EBCT AS A SCREENING TEST

EBCT has excellent potential to serve as a screening test for CAD, not only to detect significant obstructive disease but also to provide risk assessment for potential cardiac patients. The fact that the test is noninvasive, quick to perform, associated with minimal risk, and relatively inexpensive makes EBCT an attractive option for individuals at risk for CAD. Due to its high sensitivity, EBCT has been advocated by many to be used as screening test for the presence of CAD, although the ACC/AHA Expert Consensus did not recommend such an application. Due to the low specificity of EBCT, caution should be applied when considered for use as a screening tool in the general public, especially in a population with low likelihood of CAD. The risk is not due to the EBCT itself, as the procedural risk is negligible and the direct cost is moderate ($250–$400). However, an abnormal EBCT may trigger additional diagnostic testing, including stress testing or angiography, with resultant patient risk and expense.

However, EBCT may also be useful in guiding medical therapy, especially when the exact risk for the patient is borderline and the management strategy unclear. A high calcium score may encourage the practitioner to assume a more aggressive approach to risk factor modification. Additionally, the knowledge of an abnormal EBCT may promote patient compliance.

Beyond just a diagnostic tool for asymptomatic subjects, EBCT has substantial prognostic value even among asymptomatic individuals. In a trial of 1,289 asymptomatic patients, it was shown that a calcium score ≥ 50 was associated with 6.9-fold increase in cardiac death and nonfatal myocardial infarction.[39] As shown in Table 15-4, these findings were confirmed in other studies on asymptomatic patients, clearly demonstrating an increased risk for subsequent cardiac events (cardiac death, nonfatal MI, revascularization) as the coronary artery calcium score rises.[37,39,41–43] A recent meta-analysis with 4,348 asymptomatic individuals demonstrated an 8.7-fold (95% CI 2.7–28) increase in risk for future cardiac events.[42]

CONCLUSION

Based of available clinical evidence, it appears that the detection and quantification of coronary artery calcification has important clinical ramifications. It is clear that coronary calcification cor-

Table 15-4

Risk Stratification with Coronary Calcium Score Derived from EBCT

Study	n	Follow-up Duration	Calcium Definition	Event Definition	Event Rate
Agatston et al.,[41] 1996	367	36–72 m	CCS > 50	Angina, MI, revascularization	6.89 (OR)
Arad et al.,[37] 1996	1,173	19 m	CCS > 160	Cardiac death, MI	35.4 (OR)
Detrano et al.,[39] 1997	1,289	19 m	CCS > 50	Cardiac death, MI	6.9 (OR)
O'Malley et al.,[42] 2000 (meta-analysis)	4,348	42 m	CCS: 3.1–50	Death, MI	4.2 (RR)
Wong et al.,[43] 2000	926	39 m	CCS ≥ 271	MI, CVA, revascularization	8.8 (RR)

CCS = coronary calcium score; n = number of patients; OR = odds ratio; RR = relative risk.

relates well with the presence of ischemic heart disease. Additionally, this calcification, as detected by EBCT is predictive of cardiac events including cardiac death and nonfatal MI. However, it is unclear whether this noninvasive detection of coronary artery calcification should be applied to all patients, including asymptomatic ones with few risk factors. The AHA/ACC summarized the state of the art regarding EBCT in an Expert Consensus Document, with the major conclusion shown in Table 15-5.[25]

It is important to have a cohesive strategy for a patient based on his or her individual risk of future cardiovascular event. Based on a number of studies, the presence of coronary calcium is a strong independent risk factor for future cardiac event. Furthermore, EBCT may be a cost-effective screening tool in asymptomatic individuals, especially if it is used in subjects with higher risk for cardiac events.[45] A negative or very low (< 10) calcium score is associated with very low risk of significant CAD. In this group of individuals, general public guidelines for primary prevention seem to be sufficient. However, there are a minority of individuals, particularly in the younger age group, who have cardiac events even with low coronary calcium score.

Individuals with a low calcium score (10–100) have mild atherosclerosis, and risk factor modification, including NCEP step 2 diet

Table 15-5

ACC/AHA Consensus Conclusions Regarding EBCT

1. A negative EBCT test makes the presence of atherosclerotic plaque, including unstable plaque, very unlikely.

2. A negative test is highly unlikely in the presence of significant luminal obstructive disease.

3. Negative tests occur in the majority of patients who have angiographically normal coronary arteries.

4. A negative test may be consistent with a low risk of a cardiovascular event in the next 2 to 5 years.

5. A positive EBCT confirms the presence of a coronary atherosclerotic plaque.

6. The greater the amount of calcium, the greater the likelihood of occlusive CAD, but there is not a one to one relationship, and findings may not be site specific.

7. The total amount of calcium correlates best with the total amount of atherosclerotic plaque, although the true "plaque burden" is underestimated.

8. A high calcium score may be consistent with moderate to high risk of a cardiovascular event within the next 2 to 5 years.

Adapted from ACC/AHA expert consensus document[25] with permission.

and daily aspirin, may be an appropriate course of action. In individuals with a moderate calcium score (101–400), nonobstructive atherosclerotic coronary disease is likely, and in this group aggressive risk factor modification, daily aspirin, and probably exercise stress test are the appropriate course of action. A high calcium score (> 400) indicates a high likelihood of significant CAD, with a specificity of approximately 90%. In this group of patients, very aggressive risk factor modification, daily aspirin, and a noninvasive stress test to evaluate for ischemia are an appropriate course of action.[35]

In summary, EBCT and multislice CT are exquisitely sensitive for the detection of coronary artery calcification and are able to approximate the extent of coronary artery atherosclerosis. Additionally, the calcification score also correlates with future cardiac event, enabling this technique to risk stratify even asymptomatic individuals. EBCT has a potential to monitor the progression of CAD through serial imaging, especially to monitor the response to treatment. However, the reproducibility of EBCT calcium score must be high before EBCT can be used routinely for the purpose of monitoring of the disease progression. Currently, methods have a limitation in this regard due to moderately high variability among serial testing[20] Finally, there are data to suggest that coronary calcification imaging, especially with EBCT, may be a very cost-effective approach to patients with suspected CAD and has been shown to be superior to other diagnostic/prognostic techniques in this regard.[35]

REFERENCES

1. Stray HC. The sequence of cell and matrix changes in atherosclerotic lesions of coronary arteries in the first forty years of life. *Eur Heart J* 1990;11(Suppl E):3–19.
2. Doherty TM, Detrano RC. Coronary arterial calcification as an active process: A new perspective on an old problem. *Calcif Tissue Int* 1994;54:224–230.
3. Blankenhorn DH. Coronary artery calcification: A review. *Am J Med Sci* 1961;242:41–49.
4. Eggen DA, Strong JP, McGill HC. Coronary calcification: Relationship to clinically significant coronary lesions and race, sex and topographic distribution. *Circulation* 1965;32:948–955.
5. Warburton RK, Tampas JP, Soule AB, et al. Coronary artery calcification: Its relationship to coronary artery stenosis and myocardial infarction. *Radiology* 196;91:109–115.
6. Frink RJ, Achor RWP, Brown AL, et al. Significance of calcification of the coronary arteries. *Am J Cardiol* 1970;26:241–247.
7. McCarthy JH, Palmer FJ: Incidence and significance of coronary artery calcification. *Br Heart J* 1974; 36:499–506.
8. Margolis JR, Chen JT, Kong Y, et al. The diagnostic significance of coronary artery calcification: A report of 800 cases. *Radiology* 1980;137:609–616.
9. Deterano RC, Wong ND, Tang W, et al. Prognostic significance of cardiac cinefluoroscopy for coronary calcific deposits in asymptomatic high-risk subjects. *J Am Coll Cardiol* 1994;24:354–358.
10. Fitzgerald PJ, Ports TA, Yock PG. Contribution of localized calcium deposits to dissection after angioplasty: An observational study using intravascular ultrasound. *Circulation* 1992;86:64–70.
11. Sharma SK, Israel PH, Kamean, et al. Clinical angiographic, and procedural determinants of major and minor coronary dissection during angioplasty. *Am Heart J* 1993;126:39–47.
12. Lipton M, Brundage BH, Higgins CB, et al. Clinical applications of dynamic computed tomography. *Prog Cardiovas Dis* 1986;28:349–366.
13. Agatston AS, Janowitz WR, Hildner FJ, et al. Quantification of coronary artery calcium using ulrafast computed tomography. *J Am Coll Cardiol* 1990; 15:827–832.
14. Callister TQ, Cooil B, Raya SP, et al. Coronary artery disease: Improved reproducibility of calcium scoring with and electron beam CT volumetric method. *Radiology* 1998;208:807–814.
15. Raggi P, Callister TQ, Cooil B, et al. Identification of patients at increased risk of first unheralded acute myocardial infarction by electron-beam computed tomography. *Circulation* 2000;101:850–855.
16. Rumberger JA, Simons DB, Fitzpatrick LA, et al. Coronary artery calcium area by electron beam computed tomography and coronary atherosclerotic plaque area: A histopathologic correlative study. *Circulation* 1995;92:2157–2162.
17. Mautner GC, Mautner SL, Froelich J, et al. Coronary artery calcification: Assessment with electron beam CT and histomorphometric correlation. *Radiology* 1994;192:619–623.
18. Janowitz WR, Agatston AS, Kaplan G, et al. Differences in prevalence and extent of coronary calcium detected by ultrafast computed tomography in asymptomatic men and women. *Am J Cardiol* 1993;72:247–254.

19. Rich S, McLaughlin VV. Detection of subclinical cardiovascular disease: The emerging role of electron beam computed tomography. *Prev Medicine* 2002;34:1–10.

20. Achenbach S, Ropers D, Mohlenkamp S, et al. Variability of repeated coronary artery calcium measurements by electron beam tomography. *Am J Cardiol* 2001;87:210–213.

21. Janowitz WR. Current status of mechanical computed tomography in cardiac imaging. *Am J Cardiol* 2001;88(Suppl)35E–8E.

22. Rumberger JA, Sheedy PF II, Breen JF, et al. Electron beam computed tomography and coronary disease: Scanning for coronary calcification. *Mayo Clinic Proc* 1996;71:369–377.

23. Guerci AD, Spadaro LA, Gerdman KJ, et al. Comparison of electron beam computed tomography scanning and conventional risk factor assessment for the prediction of angiographic coronary artery disease. *J Am Coll Cardiol* 1998;32:673–679.

24. Zuo-Xiang HE, Hendrick TD, Pratt CM, et al. Severity of coronary artery calcification by electron beam computed tomography predicts silent myocardial ischemia. *Circulation* 2000;101:244–251.

25. O'Rourke RA, Brundage BH, Froelicher VF, et al. ACC/AHA expert consensus document on electron-beam computed tomography for the diagnosis and prognosis of coronary artery disease. *Circulation* 2000;102:126–140.

26. Baumgart D, Schmermund A, George G, et al. Comparison of electron beam computed tomography with intracoronary ultrasound and coronary angiography for detection of coronary atherosclerosis. *J Am Coll Cardiol* 1997;30:57–64.

27. Bielak LF, Kaufmann RB, Moll PP, et al. Small lesions identified by electron beam computed tomographic exams of the heart: Calcification or noise? *Radiology* 1994;192:631–636.

28. Breen JF, Sheedy PF, Schwartz RS, et al. Coronary artery calcification detected with ultrafast CT as an indication of coronary artery disease. *Radiology* 1992;185:435–439.

29. Mauthner SI, Mautner GC, Froehlich J, et al. Coronary artery disease: Prediction with in vitro election beam CT. *Radiology* 1994;192:625–630.

30. Nallamothu BK, Saint S, Bielak L, et al. Electron-beam computed tomography in the diagnosis of coronary artery disease. *Arch Intern Med* 2001;161:833–838.

31. Rumberger JA, Sheedy PF II, Breen JF, et al. Coronary calcium, as determined by electron beam computed tomography, and coronary disease on arteriogram: Effect of patient's sex on diagnosis. *Circulation* 1995;91:1363–1367.

32. Budoff MJ, Georgiou D, Brody AS, et al. The value of receiver operating characteristic (ROC) curve analysis to detect coronary artery disease by coronary calcification on ultrafast CT: A multicenter study (Abstract). *J Am Coll Cardiol* 1994;23:210A.

33. Spadaro L, Sherman S, Roth M, et al. Comparison of thallium stress testing and electron beam computed tomography in the prediction of coronary artery disease (Abstract). *J Am Coll Cardiol* 1996;27 Suppl:175A.

34. Shavell DM, Burdoff MJ, LaMont DH, et al. Exercise testing and electron beam computed tomography in the evaluation of coronary artery disease. *J Am Coll Cardiol* 2000;36:32–38.

35. Rumberger JA, Brundage BH, Rader DJ, Kondos G. Electron beam computed tomographic coronary calcium scanning: A review and guidelines for use in asymptomatic persons. *Mayo Clin Proc* 1999; 74:243–252.

36. Detrano R, Hsiai T, Wang S, et al. Prognostic value of coronary calcification and angiographic stenosis in patients undergoing coronary angiography. *J Am Coll Cardiol* 1996;27:285–290.

37. Arad Y, Spardaro LA, Goodman K, et al. Predictive value of electron beam CT of the coronary arteries: 19 month follow up of 1,173 asymptomatic subjects. *Circulation* 1996;93:1951–1953.

38. Puentes G, Detrano R, Tang W, et al. Estimation of coronary calcium mass using electron beam computed tomography: A promising approach for predicting coronary events? *Circulation* 1995;92(Suppl 1):313.

39. Detrano R, Schwendener C, Doherty T, et al. Coronary calcium results predict coronary heart disease deaths in high risk asymptomatic adults (Abstract). *J Am Coll Cardiol* 1997;29:128A.

40. Guerci AD, Spadaro LA, Popma JJ, et al. Electron beam tomography of the coronary arteries: Relationship of coronary calcium score to angiographic findings in asymptomatic adults (abstract). *Am J Card Imaging* 1995;9:5A.

41. Agatston AS, Janowitz WR, Kaplan GS, et al. Electron beam CT predicts future coronary events. *Circulation* 1996;94(Suppl 1):360.

42. O'Malley PG, Taylor AJ, Jackson JL, et al. Prognostic value of coronary electron-beam computed tomography for coronary heart disease events in asymptomatic populations. *Am J Cardiol* 2000;85:945–948.

43. Wong ND, Hsu JC, Detrano RC, et al. Coronary artery calcium evaluation by electron beam computed tomography and its relation to new cardiovascular events. *Am J Cardiol* 2000;86:495–498.

44. Park R, Detrano R, Xiang M, et al. Combined use of computed tomography coronary calcium scores and C-reactive protein levels in predicting cardiovascular events in nondiabetic individuals. *Circulation* 2002; 106:2073–2077.

45. Liberman SM, Wolkiel CJ, Freels S, et al. Use of electron beam tomography to develop cost-effective treatments for primary prevention of coronary artery disease. *Circulation* 1995;92 (Suppl 1):512.

CHAPTER 16

Echocardiography

Philip R. Liebson
Thomas T. Kason

INTRODUCTION

This chapter will focus on the use of echocardiography (ECHO) in diagnosis and prognosis. It will consist of a presentation of the general scope of ECHO, including the newer techniques of contrast ECHO and tissue Doppler. It will conclude with a discussion of complementary use of single photon emission computed tomography (SPECT) imaging and ECHO in diagnostic and prognostic approaches to coronary heart disease (CHD), with comments on the cost-effectiveness of ECHO.

GENERAL SCOPE OF ECHOCARDIOGRAPHY

Ultrasound is used to assess structural and functional properties of the heart and proximate blood vessels. Structural components assessed include the pericardium, heart valves, cardiac chambers and walls, the thoracic aorta, proximal pulmonary arteries, pulmonary veins entering the heart, and the proximate superior and inferior vena cava. Functional properties evaluated include systolic and diastolic performance characteristics of the ventricles, presence and degree of intracardiac or proximal vascular shunts, presence and degree of valvular stenosis or regurgitation, and, particularly in regard to coronary artery disease (CAD), the presence of segmental wall motion abnormalities of the left ventricle. Recent adaptation of power Doppler techniques have facilitated the development of myocardial perfusion analysis.

An echocardiograph machine is portable and can be used on patient evaluations at any location. Newer handheld instruments may revolutionize diagnostic assessment during routine rounding in the hospital. Ultrasound is safe, does not use radiation, and in comparison with other imaging technologies, provides rapid diagnostic information. It is also less expensive than many other diagnostic imaging studies.

A study of 542 echocardiograms performed on 500 inpatients over a period of 5 months revealed that the main indications for study were left ventricular function (54%) and valve function (16%).[1] Significantly, 89% of ordering physicians felt that echocardiography was ordered to guide future treatment. Chart review validated changes in treatment on the basis of ECHO occurred in 38% of patients, especially in the intensive care unit.

ECHO has been used serially routinely in heart transplant patients in conjunction with myocardial biopsy, especially follow-up stress testing using dobutamine infusion. Aside from underlying changes suggesting myocardial ischemia, serial studies are useful to determine serial changes in right ventricular function, pulmonary pressures, tricuspid regurgitation, and development of pericardial effusion.[2] Diastolic compliance studies using inflow Doppler evaluation may be useful in early detection of allograft rejection.

Echocardiographic Modalities: M-mode, 2D, Doppler

The modalities of echocardiographic study for structural properties include M-mode (M = motion) and 2D. M-mode is based on reflection of transducer-transmitted ultrasound signals from boundaries with differing acoustic impedances, such as the endocardial–lumen chamber interface. Each returned signal is transduced into an electronic signal and transformed as a moving display of the point signal in time. Thus, the M-mode display shows structural components at different depths (Y axis) and the motion of these structural components in time (X axis) (Figure 16-1). Essentially, these components are points of structural moving in time to form lines. 2D, on the other hand, is a sector scan of an array of M-mode signals (usually phased array) electronically sweeping over an area of the heart 30 to 60 times a second to produce a sequence of real-time structures in apparent continuous motion. It is in effect a tomographic view of a section of the heart. The M-mode scan is guided by a mobile cursor displayed on the 2D image.

The modality for many of the functional properties of the cardiac structures is Doppler. This consists of a transmitted ultrasound frequency from the same transducer used for 2D/M-mode. However, the return signal to the transducer that is selectively evaluated is that of a changed frequency based on the Doppler shift of the transmitted signal produced by reflection from a moving structure, primarily red blood cells. The Doppler signal obtained is displayed

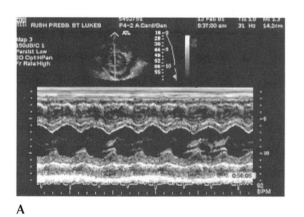

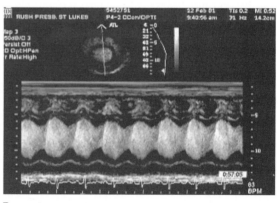

A   B

Figure 16-1.   M-mode evaluation of LV wall thicknesses and dimensions. **A.** Second harmonics imaging without contrast. IV septum is seen above and pLV posterior wall below with lumen between. **B.** Use of contrast highlights the endocardial–lumen interface. X axis = time; Y axis = distance (1 cm markings). (***See also Color Insert***).

on a moving sweep showing signals above or below a baseline depending on the direction of blood flow (toward or away from the transducer) and the velocity of blood flow (amplitude of the deflection). The Y axis displays the amplitude and direction of the Doppler signal, the X axis the change in the Doppler signal in time. The amplitude is proportional to the frequency shift and calculated as a velocity in cm/sec or m/sec. The Doppler signal discussed is similar to M-mode in that it is derived from a mobile cursor displayed on the 2D sector scan. Two types of Doppler signals can thus be evaluated: pulsed-wave (PW) Doppler, which interrogates a limited locus on the line, and continuous-wave (CW) Doppler, which displays all the returned signals from the entire line. PW Doppler is useful in evaluating blood flow signals from normal valves and is spatially specific but is limited in peak amplitudes obtained. CW, on the other hand, is not spatially specific to one point on the cursor, but allows assessment of high-velocity signals such as those present with valvular stenosis or regurgitation. A third Doppler approach is colorflow Doppler, analogous to CW and PW as 2D is to M-mode. The colorflow Doppler signal is derived from a sweeping array of Doppler interrogations across the 2D sector scan and is seen as a moving color pattern superimposed on the 2D display, primarily in the cardiac chambers and proximate blood vessels. Blood flow moving toward the transducer is characteristically red, and flow moving away from the transducer is displayed as a blue color. Signals of varying frequencies or high frequencies, as would be obtained by turbulent flow, especially with valvular regurgitation and stenosis, are displayed as heterogeneous color patterns with speckled appearances.

Techniques of Echocardiography: Transthoracic, Transesophageal, Stress Testing

The two primary techniques used in echocardiography include transthoracic echocardiography (TTE) and transesophageal echocardiography (TEE). A summary of the evaluations is provided

in Table 16-1. TTE is accomplished by placing a transducer in several locations on the chest, primarily the left parasternal, apical, subcostal, and suprasternal positions. Transesophageal study is accomplished by having the patient swallow a flexible endoscopic probe with a transducer at its tip, following local oropharyngeal analgesic spray and conscious sedation. The probe can be guided to provide 180 degrees electronic rotation, flexed in four directions by manual rotating gears, or moved up and down to allow visualization from

Table 16-1
Application of Echocardiography

Transthoracic Echo (TEE)
Structural:
1. Appearance of atria, ventricles, valves, pericardium
2. Appearance of aortic root, proximal pulmonary artery, proximal inferior vena cava
3. Calculation of LV wall mass
Functional:
1. LV performance measures:
2. Stroke volume, cardiac output, wall stress, ejection fraction, segmental wall motion
3. Calculation of degrees of valve stenosis and regurgitation
4. Estimation of peak pulmonary artery pressure (with tricuspid regurgitation)
5. Estimation of left ventricular end-diastolic pressure (with mitral regurgitation)
6. Calculation of shunts

Transesophageal Echo (TTE)
Structural
1. Vegetations, abscesses, especially prosthetic valves, adherence of masses
2. Appearance of mitral valve for surgical repair
3. Assessment of interatrial septal defects
4. Evaluation for anomalous prosthetic valve drainage
5. Evaluation of most of thoracic aorta
6. Evaluation of atrial appendages for thrombi

various points in the esophagus or proximal gastric region. With the probe in the upper part of the stomach, a cross-sectional view of the left ventricle is obtained and the chamber dimension and wall motion can be continuously observed for blood volume and systolic performance, respectively.

The use of TTE is the standard approach to any initial study, with perhaps the exception of the evaluation for thoracic aortic dissection, prosthetic valve endocarditis, or source of embolus in the older patient, in which it may be more cost-effective to initiate a TEE study. The most common reasons for a TTE are assessment of left ventricular (LV) function, evaluation for pericardial effusion, interrogation for valvular stenosis or regurgitation, and, frequently, for vegetation. A comprehensive evaluation of the heart for structural and functional abnormalities includes many diagnostic possibilities. Aortic root size and proximal pulmonary artery appearance can also be assessed with Doppler interrogation to rule out patent ductus arteriosus. TTE is usually not helpful for evaluation of the atrial appendages, pulmonary veins, or thoracic aorta except for the suprasternal view of the aortic arch.

TEE provides for definite evaluation for vegetation, interrogation of the interatrial septum for patent foramen ovale and atrial septal defect, especially sinus venosus defects, and thoracic aorta visualization for aneurysms, dissections, and hematomas. It is more sensitive than TTE for diagnosis of smaller vegetations and prosthetic valve vegetations and abscesses. Prosthetic valve mitral regurgitation is easily assessed by TEE but may not be assessed by TTE because of acoustic shadowing of the left atrium due to the structural components of the prosthesis.

Evaluation for valvular stenosis is more readily accomplished by TTE, especially for aortic stenosis. The atrial sizes and appearances of the ventricular apices are also better visualized by TTE. In most cases, TEE is selected only if TTE does not provide adequate diagnostic findings with the exceptions indicated above.

With the development of newer contrast agents that can be injected intravenously and pass through the pulmonary system, the left ventricular chamber can be opacified so that virtually every ECHO study can visualize endocardial surfaces. Our laboratory uses contrast with every stress ECHO study, although most other laboratories are more selective. The use of contrast in our laboratory has decreased the percentage of poorly visualized studies from 30% to less than 1%.

Selected functional information obtained by ECHO (Table 16-2) includes left ventricular ejection fraction (LVEF), stroke volume, diastolic function abnormalities, shunt ratios and volumes, estimated pulmonary artery pressures, end-diastolic LV pressures, stenotic valve areas, regurgitant volume, and regurgitant orifice areas. ECHO is useful for assessment of LV wall mass, an important prognostic indicator for cardiovascular events.

STRESS ECHOCARDIOGRAPHY

General

Stress modalities used in the assessment of left ventricular wall motion abnormalities attributable to CAD include exercise, pharmacologic stress testing, and pacing. The principle of these approaches rests on evidence that increased myocardial oxygen needs associated with stress testing will decrease segmental wall motion in the ischemic area. A second principle, that of viability, rests on the evidence that a segment of noncontracting myocardium during the resting state will, if viable, begin to contract with stress testing but eventually cease contracting at maximal stress. A variety of applications may be assessed with stress ECHO (Table 16-3).

The stress test results are usually graded by direct observation by the reader based on a score for each myocardial segment from normal (1) through hypokinetic, akinetic, and dyskinetic (2–4). Therefore, summation of wall motion scores of each segment (usually 16 segments are evaluated) (Figure 16-2) provides a global assessment of abnormality, the higher scores reflecting more severe global abnormalities. Note that there is no gradation of hypokinesis per se.

Table 16-2

Some Functional Assessments by Echocardiography

General Hemodynamic Assessment

Cardiac Output (systemic): LVOT (VTI × CSA) × HR[a]

Cardiac Output (pulmonary): PA (VTI × CSA) × HR[a]

Shunt: Pulmonary output − Systemic output[a]

Extrinsic Left Ventricular Performance

Stroke volume = LVOT (VTI × CSA)

$\qquad$ = LVEDV − LVESV[a]

LV volume = (LVID)3 (M-mode)

$\qquad$ = π/4 Σ ai bi L/n (Modified Simpson's Rule–2D)[a]

Ejection fraction = (LVEDV − LVESV)/LVEDV (M-mode, 2D- AQ)

Diastolic Left Ventricular Characteristics

Decreased relaxation: (1) Mitral Doppler A > E (2) E DT > 250 msec[a]

Increased stiffness: (1) Mitral Doppler E >> A (2) E DT < 130 msec

(3) PV Diastolic velocity >> Systolic velocity[a]

Estimated Left Atrial Pressure (with Mitral Regurgitation)

LAP = Peak aortic pressure − 4V² (mitral regurgitation velocity)

Mitral Regurgitant Volume (V)

1. V = Mitral inflow (VTI × CSA) − LVOT (VTI × CSA)

2. V = Regurgitant orifice area (derived from PISA × mitral regurgitant VTI)

Mitral Valve Area (A)

1. A by planimetry in the parasternal short axis 2D view (TTE).[a]

2. A = 220/pressure ½ times of regression of Doppler mitral inflow velocity[a]

3. A = LVOT CSA × 0.785 (LVOT VTI/MV VTI) (Continuity Equation)

Aortic (Ao)Valve Area

1. A by planimetry using TEE

2. A = LVOT CSA × LVOT VTI/Ao VTI (Continuity Equation)

Aortic Regurgitant Volume

1. V = LVOT (VTI × CSA) − mitral inflow (VTI × CSA)

Pulmonary Artery Peak Pressure (Tricuspid Regurgitation [TR] Necessary for Assessment)[a]

P = 4V² + Estimated RA pressure, V = Peak TR velocity (Bernoulli Equation)

CSA = cross-sectional area; VTI = velocity time integral (area under a Doppler parabolic velocity profile); LVOT = left ventricular outflow tract; LVEDV = left ventricular end diastolic volume; LVESV = left ventricular end systolic volume; LVID = left ventricular internal dimension (M-mode); PV = pulmonary vein; Doppler E and A = peak early (E) and atrial (A) velocities of mitral Doppler inflow; E DT = deceleration time of mitral inflow E velocity extrapolated to baseline.

[a] Standard in routine clinical echocardiography. Interpretations: Simpson's rule = area determined by integration of disks in LV chamber using internal computerized techniques; AQ = Acoustic quantification = internal computerized method for display of LVEF from computerized LV area change; 4V² = Bernoulli formula for estimation of interchamber gradient from peak Doppler velocity (V). PISA = technique of determining a regurgitant orifice area using colorflow Doppler display just above the regurgitant orifice (Proximal Isovelocity Surface Area).

Table 16-3

Stress Echocardiography

1. LV wall motion abnormalities
2. Changes in LV dimension
3. LV myocardial perfusion (with power Doppler contrast)
4. Changes in LV ejection fraction
5. Pliability of stenotic aortic valve
6. Changes in dynamic LV outflow gradients

The test is carried out until a target heart rate is reached, preferably at least 85% of predicted heart rate for age, adjusted for sex, unless ECHO evidence for ischemia develops or side effects or patient discomfort supervene.

Exercise Stress Echocardiography

Exercise is carried out using a treadmill or by bicycle test. With either type of study, ECHO views are acquired at rest, immediately after exercise, and at recovery. In treadmill testing, a bed is placed near the treadmill and the patient placed back on the bed within a short time interval after

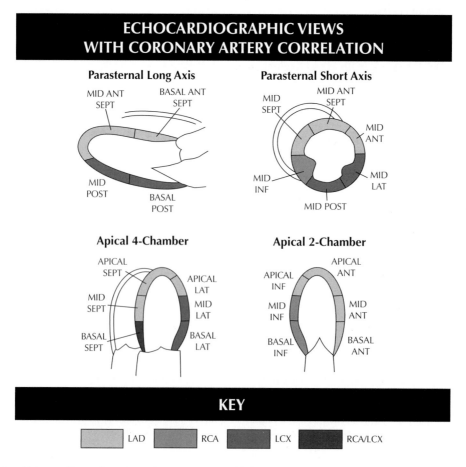

Figure 16-2. Echocardiographic views for assessment of left ventricular regional wall motion. Colors indicate usual distribution of major coronary arteries.

the end of peak exercise, usually within 15 to 20 seconds, with the expectation that comprehensive echocardiographic acquisition of the four standard views will be accomplished within 1 minute. Bicycle exercise may either be upright or supine. With bicycle exercise, ECHO views may be obtained after each level of exercise, unlike treadmill stress testing.

Compared with electrocardiographic stress testing per se, echocardiography increases the sensitivity and specificity of the test, evaluates wall thickening rather than electrophysiologic phenomena while remaining a low-risk procedure. The disadvantage is that, in our experience, only about 70% of studies are of excellent visualization and that study results are based on qualitative assessment of wall motion changes. The treadmill stress test may utilize one of the several choices of standard treadmill protocols.

There are some differences between treadmill and bicycle stress testing. The advantages of bicycle stress testing include the acquisition of ECHO views at each level of exercise and improved sensitivity. With treadmill imaging, higher workloads can be reached, specificity is somewhat higher, and leg fatigue is less. Treadmill testing is also better tolerated by most patients. Bicycle testing with ECHO is more commonly used in Europe than in the United States. In a randomized crossover trial of supine bicycle exercise versus treadmill stress testing, while a similar double product (heart rate × blood pressure) was reached, the detection of ischemia by ECHO was more frequent with bicycle exercise (47/57 vs. 38/57).[3]

The accuracy of exercise ECHO has been evaluated by comparison with coronary arteriography based on > 50% stenosis of one or more major coronary vessels. The overall accuracy in larger series is between 80% and 90%, with sensitivity ranging between 80% and 97% and specificity averaging 85 to 90%. Sensitivity for single-vessel disease is somewhat lower, ranging in large series between 64% and 92%. In terms of relative risk for a cardiac event, Marwick et al.,[4] for example, evaluated 463 consecutive patients over an average of 44 months after an exercise ECHO

test, after excluding those undergoing revascularization or lost to follow-up (an additional 37). The relative risk for a cardiac event with a positive test was 5.06. In a longer follow-up study, Marwick et al.[5] evaluated clinical, exercise testing, and ECHO data in 5,375 patients of both sexes. Over a 6-year follow-up, those with normal exercise echocardiograms had a mortality of 1%. Using the Duke treadmill score to determine prognosis, the investigators determined that exercise ECHO results were able to substratify those patients with intermediate-risk Duke scores into groups with varying yearly mortality (2–7%).

The location of wall motion abnormality may provide independent prognostic value. Elhendy et al.[6] studied 4,347 patients with known or suspected CAD using exercise ECHO. Using multivariate analysis, the investigators found that the percentage of ischemic segments at peak exercise and the presence of abnormalities in the left anterior descending (LAD) coronary artery distribution independently predicted cardiac events.

Recently, three-dimensional (3D) real-time acquisition of ECHO has been investigated for stress testing. One example is a device that uses a matrix phased-array transducer in a 600 pyramidal volume.[7] Volume sets were obtained from apical and parasternal windows, resulting in visualization of 98% of segments at peak exercise. Acquisition time at peak exercise averaged 35 seconds from the apical window and 50 seconds from the parasternal window. In a study of 279 consecutive patients evaluated by 2D and 3D studies, interobserver agreements on detection of ischemia at peak dosage was 93% with 3D compared with 85% with 2D, and mean scanning time was 58% shorter.[8] Unfortunately, the frame rate is somewhat slow for rapid heart rates obtained during exercise, and image quality is somewhat inferior to that of some commercially available digital machines.

Pharmacologic Stress Echocardiography

Although dipyridamole and adenosine ECHO stress testing have been utilized in some laboratories, especially in Europe, the predominant mode of pharmacologic ECHO stress testing in the United States uses dobutamine. This modality is utilized to determine both the presence of myocardial ischemia and myocardial viability. The protocol for myocardial ischemia involves graded-dose infusions of dobutamine from 5 μg/kg/min up to 40 μg/kg/min in 3-minute stages until the target heart rate is reached. Atropine is added if the heart rate fails to reach target. ECHO images are acquired at the lowest dose and peak dose, in addition to baseline and recovery. In some large studies, approximately 5% of patients do not have an adequate acoustic window.[9] In our laboratory, up to 30% have segments that are not adequately visualized by usual techniques. Therefore, we use contrast injection with all stress studies and achieve 99% adequate visualization. In regard to the increase in myocardial blood flow developed in dobutamine stress echocardiography (DSE), comparison with dipyridamole infusion indicated that near maximal coronary vasodilation caused by dipyridamole was attainable using dobutamine and atropine evaluated in young healthy volunteers.[10]

Sensitivity, specificity, and predictive accuracy of DSE for diagnosing CAD averages 80 to 85% with sensitivity increasing from approximately 75% with one-vessel disease to over 90% with three-vessel disease.[9] Sensitivity for detection of isolated left circumflex disease is lower than that for isolated LAD or right coronary artery disease (approximately 55% vs. 75%). Serious side effects are rare, being less than 1:1000 studies.[9] In approximately 5 to 8% of patients the study may be stopped prematurely because of side effects including ventricular and supraventricular dysrhythmias (< 1%), severe hypertension (< 1%), paradoxic hypotension, or LV outflow tract obstruction (3 to 4%).[11,12] In comparison with exercise stress testing, paradoxical hypotension with DSE is rarely a consequence of ischemia and related to beta$_2$ receptor–mediated vasodilatation. Severe ischemia by ECHO is an unusual reason for stopping the test before the target heart rate is reached (< 1%). Approximately 85%

of studies result in the maximal predicted heart rate being reached.[11]

Because of the increase in blood pressure due to dobutamine, it is not advised to perform DSE on patients with baseline systolic pressures > 170 mm Hg. Although there is some concern about the safety of dobutamine stress testing in the presence of ventricular mural thrombi, because of the possibility of emboli, one study evaluating safety in 55 patients with apical thrombi demonstrated no such complication.[13]

Various techniques have recently been tested to improve the accuracy of DSE. These include the use of transpulmonary contrast, color kinesis of the myocardial wall, three-dimensional techniques, automated detection, and analysis of coronary artery flow.

Acoustic quantification is a technique of automated endocardial tracking available in selected equipment that is used for quantification of LV volume and performance (Figure 16-3). The tracking system automatically outlines endocardial–lumen borders, outlining the inner LV wall. Real-time estimations of LV volume are obtained from the four-chamber view of the LV and converted to digital loops. Instantaneous and continuous waveforms of the LV volume

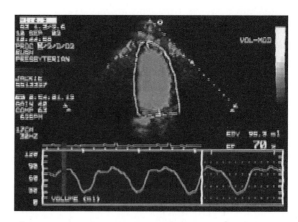

Figure 16-3. Acoustic quantification and online delineation of LV ejection fraction. Note the LVEF of 70% derived from the change in identified endocardium-lumen interface. (Courtesy of Philips Ultrasound.) (*See also Color Insert*).

throughout the cardiac cycle are displayed providing readouts of end-diastolic and end-systolic volumes and LVEF. Transpulmonary contrast injection enhances this approach.[14] The automated technique shows no significant difference from the more laborious and time-consuming hand-traced ejection fraction.[14]

Color kinesis imaging is a new technique based on acoustic quantification to evaluate endocardial motion (Figure 16-4). The technique applies ultrasound information received by the transducer from the myocardial–blood interface between successive acoustic frames and encodes transitions as color overlays on the 2D images.[15] The technique provides an objective approach to evaluation of segmental wall motion, allowing quantification of fractional area change of segments of the LV wall. This method has the capability of allowing a more quantitative assessment of LV motion, especially with dobutamine stress testing.[15]

Color kinesis imaging of the myocardium using automated detection of stress-induced wall motion improved accuracy compared with the usual analysis by expert readers of gray-scale images (93% vs. 82%).[16]

Dobutamine stress testing has been used early

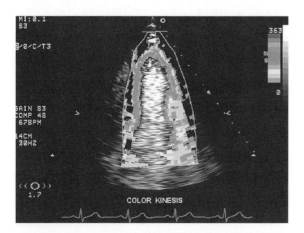

Figure 16-4. Kinesis of the left ventricle. This technique is useful for assessment of relative regional endocardial motion using analysis of the coded segments. (Courtesy of Philips Ultrasound.) (***See also Color Insert***).

after acute myocardial infarction (AMI) just before discharge, with dosage dobutamine up to 40 µg/kg/min. In a study of 178 patients with first uncomplicated AMI, negative predictive values of DSE compared with exercise electrocardiography were similar for all death or nonfatal MI events (95 to 98%).[17] A positive DSE had independent prognostic value for all these events (relative risk = 6.6) compared with those having a negative dobutamine study, whereas positive exercise electrocardiogram was not predictive.[17] For dobutamine stress testing in general, a study of 860 patients with known or suspected CAD, with follow-up averaging 24 months, 4% of those with negative tests developed cardiac events, compared with 14% of those with positive dobutamine studies.[18] The relative risk of a positive test was 3.9. Interestingly, event rates for those with a fixed wall defect were not significantly different from those with developed wall motion abnormalities during stress testing. In multivariate analysis, a history of congestive heart failure (CHF), percentage of abnormal segments at peak stress, and an abnormal LV end-systolic volume were independent predictors of cardiac events.

LV remodeling patterns may influence sensitivity of DSE. Yuda et al.[19] demonstrated a decreased accuracy of testing results for patients with concentric remodeling (normal LV mass with increased wall thickness/chamber dimension ratio) and eccentric hypertrophy (left ventricular hypertrophy [LVH] with normal or decreased thickness/radius ratio) than in those with normal geometry of concentic hypertrophy (LVH with increased thickness/radius ratio) (61–64% vs. 85%). A low calculated wall stress at peak dosage also was associated with decreased sensitivity and accuracy.

Dobutamine stress testing appears to induce less of an ischemic burden than exercise stress testing on the basis of heart rate–blood pressure product, associated with higher peak wall motion abnormality scores with exercise testing.[20]

Right ventricular (RV) function has also been tested using DSE in patients with isolated right CAD. The anterior, lateral, inferior walls and wall of the RV outflow tract are evaluated in standard views including the subcostal views, and peak stress views are selected based on adequacy of baseline visualization. In one study, adequate visualization was 80%.[21] RV asynergy developed in 68% of those with right CAD, preponderantly in the anterior segment and never in the anterior segment.

DSE has been used to evaluate viability of myocardial segments and contractile reserve. Hibernating myocardium, a reversible dysfunctional condition resulting from persistently low coronary perfusion, is asynergic or poorly contracting at rest. It should be remembered that asynergy may develop from subendocardial infarct alone, since most of myocardial thickening develops from subendocardial thickening. Hibernating myocardium cannot be differentiated at rest from infarcted myocardium. However, low-dosage infusion of dobutamine causes developed or improved contraction of the myocardial segment that again becomes asynergic with higher dosage. This is termed the *biphasic response*, indicating viability.[22] This evaluation may be used to guide efficacy of revascularization.

Sustained improvement of regional function during dobutamine infusion, unlike the biphasic response, may be a poor marker of functional recovery because the supplying artery is not flow limiting in the former case.[22] Follow-up DSE studies of potentially viable myocardium after revascularization indicated that a biphasic response was predictive of recovery in 63% at 3 months and 75% at late follow-up.[23] The positive predictive value was greatest with the most initially severe dyssynergic segments (90% vs. 67%). In some walls even without apparent contractile reserve before revascularization, improvement may occur after revascularization.[24] It is possible that collateralization after reperfusion may have perfused viable tissue in infarct zones previously unable to respond to inotropic stimulation.

Dipyridamole or adenosine stress echocardiography offers an alternative to DSE especially when blood pressure or heart rate considerations preclude the latter, although atropine is frequently co-administered for a heart rate increase in order to improve sensitivity. The principle of the test, unlike DSE, is unequal distribution of coronary vasodilatation with relatively fixed flow in the stenosed artery, leading to an ischemic wall motion response. This technique is also safe and effective in risk stratification, especially for hypertensives with chest pain.[25]

Pacing Stress Echocardiography

Pacing stress echocardiography is another technique that avoids effects on blood pressure while providing a controlled heart rate effect. The sensitivity, specificity, and accuracy for the diagnosis of significant CAD is found to be high, with one study showing sensitivity of 95%, specificity of 87%, and accuracy of 92%.[26] The ability to immediately terminate pacing is an added advantage.

NEW ECHOCARDIOGRAPHIC TECHNIQUES

Contrast Echocardiography

Endocardial–Lumen Visualization   Over 30 years ago, agitated saline and indocyanine green were shown to produce significant echogenicity in blood, normally lacking echogenicity due to microbubbles of air. Agitated saline is still used routinely by intravenous injection with standard TTE to demonstrate right-to-left intracardiac shunting. Over the past decade, several generations of more stable contrast agents have been employed, progressing from albumin microspheres containing air to contrast agents containing perfluorocarbons. Sonication of microspheres produces microcavities producing microbubbles, which disintegrate. At present, these contrast agents have been made smaller, more stable, and more uniform, allowing passage through the pulmonary capillary system and increased visualization of both the left ventricular cavity and the myocardium.[27]

Its application has been primarily in enhancing visualization of the endocardial–cavity interface in routine TTE evaluation of the LV and during stress testing, especially in conjunction with second harmonic imaging.[28] Other uses include enhancement of diagnosis of aortic dissection with transesophageal study by identification of true and false lumens, assessment for space-occupying masses within cardiac chambers as with thrombi in the left atrial appendage with TEE.

Second harmonic imaging is based on the principle of selective reception of twice the emitted ultrasound frequency by the transducer, producing an image from the second harmonic component of the ultrasound signal (Figure 16-5). This significantly improves definition of endocardial borders, compared with the fundamental (primary frequency) mode. It is now becoming standard in state-of-the art ECHO equipment. It is useful, and indeed had initially been developed

to enhance visualization of transpulmonary contrast agents. The use of second harmonic imaging in TTE in association with contrast agents has been shown to improve the detection of atrial right-to-left shunting in patients with suspected cardiac sources of cerebral emboli, and may preclude the necessity of TEE.

In regard to accuracy and reader variation, the addition of contrast to second harmonic imaging alone improved interreader variability and provided closer correlation with EBCT results.[29] Harmonic imaging and/or contrast can significantly enhance visualization compared with the previous fundamental imaging technology (Figure 16-6). In studies of second harmonic imaging alone versus addition of contrast in patients

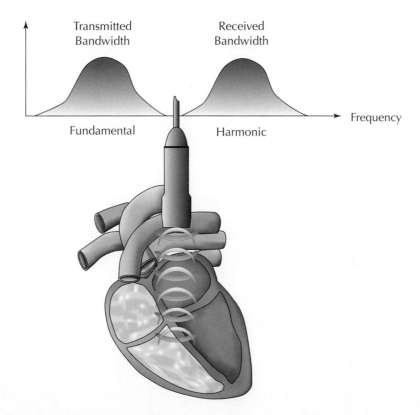

Figure 16-5. Illustration of harmonic imaging principles. The fundamental frequency is transmitted but only the second harmonic frequency reflected bandwidth is selected for display. In this way, signals arising from contrast within cardiac structures can be differentiated from signals reflected by structures themselves. (Courtesy of Philips Ultrasound and Dr. Sandeep Nathan.)

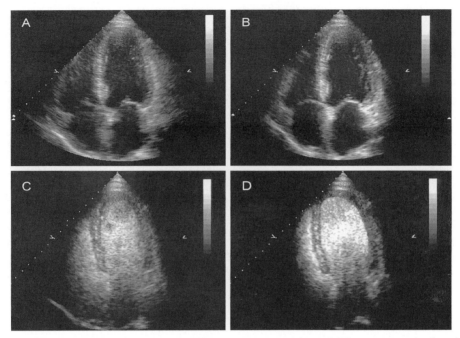

Figure 16-6. Illustration of the use of contrast and harmonics. **A.** Fundamental frequency is displayed. **B.** Second harmonics frequency display. **C.** Fundamental frequency with contrast. **D.** Second harmonics frequency with contrast.

in an intensive care unit, in which suboptimal visualization of the LV is frequent, interpretability of wall motion improved significantly with contrast.[30] Contrast may also be useful in identifying apical thrombi or confirming their presence (Figure 16-7). In dobutamine stress testing, intravenous contrast improved the visualization of wall segments at rest and during exercise.[31]

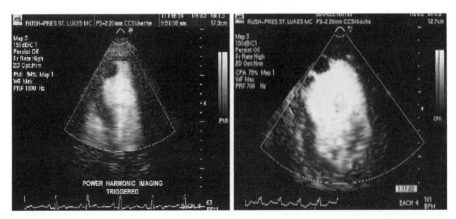

Figure 16-7. Use of contrast to delineate a left ventricular thrombus. **Left:** Power harmonic imaging triggered to the ECG allows delineation of thrombus and myocardial perfusion. **Right:** Harmonic contrast imaging without power allows delineation of thrombus without evaluation of myocardial perfusion. **(See also Color Insert).**

Myocardial Perfusion   The use of harmonic power Doppler with contrast has led to investigation of myocardial perfusion (Figure 16-8). Contrast enhances myocardial blood flow signals and power Doppler enhances lower-amplitude Doppler shifts from the myocardial blood flow. This technique allows study of the area at risk after a coronary occlusion, regional coronary flow reserve during stress testing, evidence of collateral myocardial flow, and myocardial viability.

The appearance of contrast in the myocardium is color coded related to the amount of contrast appearance (Figure 16-9). For example, black indicates nonperfusion of a segment, purple, low perfusion, and orange normal perfusion. The cardiac chamber itself is bright yellow. In comparisons with SPECT imaging using technetium 99m (Tc-99m) sestamibi at rest, segmental sensitivity in patients with moderate or severe SPECT defects ranged from 14 to 65% and specificity from 78 to 95%, depending on the dose of contrast agent.[32] Combination of wall motion assessment and myocardial perfusion increased the sensitivity to 46 to 55% with specificity of 82 to 83%. Thus, at present, although specificity of contrast myocardial perfusion is high, its sensitivity remains low, especially in evaluation of apical perfusion.

Recently, myocardial contrast has been used for delineating the vascular territory of the septum in preparation for nonsurgical reduction

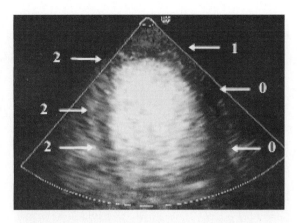

Figure 16-9.   Power contrast harmonic imaging perfusion grading scale from 0 (no perfusion) to 2 (normal perfusion). (***See also Color Insert***).

therapy with alcohol in patients with hypertrophic obstructive cardiomyopathy.[33] Myocardial contrast echocardiography (MCE) correlated well with SPECT imaged area ($r = 0.7$) without statistically significant difference.

Tissue Doppler Imaging

Tissue Doppler imaging applies left ventricular myocardial velocities, assisting in the evaluation of myocardial ischemia and diastolic abnormalities (Figure 16-10). This requires the elimination of high-velocity signals from blood flow by a high-pass filter so that the low-velocity signals from

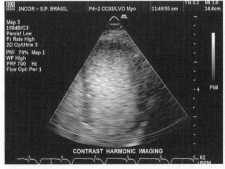
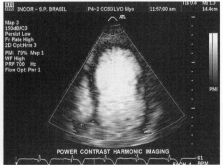

Figure 16-8.   Contrast harmonic imaging (**left**) and power contrast harmonic imaging (**right**). The latter allows evaluation of perfusion in the myocardium, and also enhances quantification of LV ejection fraction when used in conjunction with ECG gating and border detection algorithms. (***See also Color Insert***).

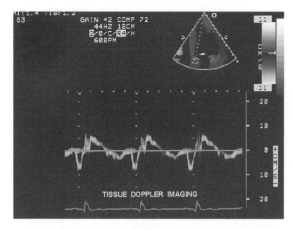

Figure 16-10. Tissue Doppler imaging. The 2D image coding of general myocardial motion during on time frame (**top**) and pulsed Doppler assessment of regional myocardial motion throughout the cardiac cycle (**bottom**). (Courtesy of Philips Ultrasound.) (*See also Color Insert*).

moving valves and myocardium can be displayed. Both pulse wave and color-coded tissue Doppler imaging (TDI) can be accomplished. Because Doppler signals generated by wall motions are of high energy, examination can be accomplished when with poor 2D imaging windows.[34] Pulsed TDI can be useful for quantifying systolic and diastolic events even during isovolumic periods.

In comparing pulsed TDI versus color-coded TDI, among the advantages of pulsed TDI are real-time velocity interrogation with improved temporal resolution. Offline analysis is not required, and peak myocardial velocities rather than mean velocities can be ascertained.[35] Disadvantages of pulsed TDI include inability to localize sampling to endocardium or epicardium, limited spatial resolution, and no correction for normal cardiac translational motion during sampling.

APPLICATIONS OF ECHOCARDIOGRAPHY

Detection of Coronary Artery Disease

Stress testing is an important noninvasive technique to evaluate CAD. The range of stress testing includes exercise electrocardiogram (ECG),

exercise ECG with an additional imaging modality (echocardiography or SPECT scanning), or pharmacologic echocardiography or SPECT. Exercise is preferred to pharmacologic stress primarily because it gives prognostic information as well. Imaging has been added to ECG because of the lower sensitivity and specificity of the former. A key question, however, is what is the ideal imaging modality: echocardiography or SPECT scanning?

The advantages of exercise stress ECHO over SPECT include the lack of radiation exposure, shorter duration of examination, relatively lower cost, ability to evaluate structure, and virtual online examination results. On the basis of meta-analyses, the overall sensitivity of ECHO is similar to SPECT (85–87%) but the specificity of ECHO may be slightly higher (77% vs. 64%).[36]

There are limitations, however, in comparison with nuclear imaging. Images are accomplished only after rather than during exercise, and rapid recovery of wall motion may ensue with single-vessel disease. Post-exercise images are difficult because of respiratory excursions and translational motion of the heart. Resting segmental akinesis may obfuscate residual ischemia in the segment. ECHO is in large part operator dependent, and good images may be obtained in only 70 to 75% of patients without the use of contrast. Interreader variability may be high because of the subjective evaluation of wall motion changes. Evaluation of myocardial perfusion is becoming possible but is in its early stages of development.

SPECT imaging evaluates flow reserve rather than an ischemic response, which is not necessary for assessment as with stress ECHO. Evaluations are obtained during peak exercise, and the sensitivity may be somewhat higher with single-vessel disease. However, SPECT imaging also has a lower sensitivity with single-vessel versus two- or three-vessel disease, as with exercise ECHO, and may be diminished in isolated circumflex coronary artery stenosis.[37] Other advantages of SPECT include less operator dependency, visualization is almost 100%, and the resting ejection fraction is measured objectively with computerized applications. Limitations in comparison with ECHO, aside from those previously listed, include attenuation artifacts, the lack of a real-time approach, and lower spatial resolution.

Myocardial perfusion imaging during exercise stress testing may now be accomplished using power harmonic Doppler with contrast injection. In a study of 100 patients undergoing exercise stress testing, myocardial contrast ECHO results agreed with SPECT evaluation in 76% of patients.[38] Compared with quantitative angiography, sensitivity of all three modalities (SPECT and the two ECHO evaluations) was 75%. The combination of ECHO wall motion assessment and ECHO myocardial contrast increased ECHO accuracy to 86%. The results suggest that this combination may increase the reliability of ECHO assessment of underlying CAD.

For pharmacological stress testing, similar results between ECHO and SPECT imaging obtain. For example, Smart et al.[39] evaluated 183 patients using dobutamine–atropine stress ECHO and dipyridamole SPECT imaging. Sensitivities were similar (87% and 80%, respectively) based on coronary angiography results. Dobutamine stress ECHO was more specific however (91% vs. 73%). It should be noted that concordance between ECHO and SPECT for type of abnormality in terms of fixed or reversible defects of CAD was significant but low (kappa 0.35).

Myocardial perfusion studies comparing pharmacologic ECHO vs. SPECT have demonstrated similar results. For example, with the use of dipyridamole in 30 patients, evaluation of concordance between segmental scores for reversible ischemia was high (92%).[40] A similar study using adenosine stress testing in 123 patients yielded a concordance of 72 to 81% in the individual three coronary territories, the highest concordance involving the LAD coronary artery distribution.[41] Coronary flow reserve has also been compared between the two techniques using adenosine with contrast enhancement for ECHO studies when needed.[42] TTE assessment of the distal LAD coronary flow reserve was measured in 33 patients, calculated as ratio of hyperemic to basal peak or mean diastolic flow velocities. This yielded a sensitivity of 92% and specificity of 90% for predicting perfusion defects with SPECT, suggesting the possible utilization of such a measurement in situations in which exercise ECHO cannot be performed.

In summary, for both exercise and pharmacologic stress testing for the diagnosis of underlying CAD, sensitivities of ECHO and SPECT are similar, but specificity of ECHO may be somewhat higher. ECHO appears to be similar to SPECT in assessment of myocardial perfusion and coronary flow reserve, but the technique is not yet routinely used in ECHO laboratories.

Risk Stratification

Although there is a wealth of experience with SPECT imaging regarding risk assessment, the data are convincing that both nuclear cardiology and ECHO modalities can sufficiently be used interchangeably to determine prognosis once the diagnosis of CAD is made.[43,44] Although most of these studies evaluate the prognostic efficacy of these imaging techniques in separate studies, few studies have provided direct comparisons in the same patient. In a comparison of exercise testing with ECG, SPECT, and ECHO in 248 patients, Olmos et al.[45] demonstrated that both imaging techniques provided comparable results in predicting cardiac events. For exercise ECHO, the best predictors were wall motion score and induction of ischemia during exercise, while for SPECT, it was percentage of perfusion defects.

Many patients cannot be studied with exercise techniques; and pharmacologic stress testing is therefore performed to assess risk. An evaluation of records of over 1,000 patients undergoing DSE with follow-up for cardiac events demonstrated that the mortality rate over 12 months was 8% with a positive DSE and 3% with a negative DSE.[46] MI developed in 10% and 3%, respectively. Similarly, dobutamine SPECT imaging demonstrated that the incidence of cardiac death or nonfatal MI increased progressively from just under 1% for normal studies to over 11% for those with fixed and reversible defects, with intermediate event rates for fixed and reversible defects alone.[47] A similar study by these investigators revealed no differences in prognostic values for SPECT and DSE.[48]

Dipyridamole or adenosine SPECT imaging is more common than dobutamine imaging in many institutions. Therefore, a comparison with DSE for prognostic significance would be salient for most institutional testing. Shaw et al.[49] reviewed 10 reports on such nuclear stress testing and 5 on dobutamine ECHO involving 1,994 patients and 445 patients, respectively, in preoperative risk assessment for vascular surgery. Odds ratios for death, MI, and secondary cardiac end points were higher for ECHO abnormalities (14–27-fold increase) than for nuclear redistribution perfusion defects (fourfold) compared with negative tests. However, wider confidence intervals were found for ECHO studies. These results indicate that both pharmacologic imaging techniques are reliable for preoperative cardiac risk prediction.

Imaging studies may be performed in the postinfarction period with either resting studies or low-level stress testing. They provide information on the size of infarction, prediction of both short-term and long-term prognosis, and assessment of viability of apparently nonmoving segments. For example, SPECT imaging has been useful in determination of infarct size.[50] In the past, exercise stress testing was contraindicated within 3 to 5 days after an AMI. However, studies have shown that exercise testing can safely be done with a low-level protocol within 3 days of hospital admission for an AMI.[51] DSE can also be used to determine the size of the infarction, residual stenosis of the involved artery, multivessel disease, and viable myocardium.[39] In fact, patients shown to do poorly after MI are patients in whom the DSE reveals large MI, poor global LV function, lack of response to low-dose dobutamine, and ischemia distant from the area of infarct.[52]

Viability studies using nuclear imaging indicate that viability can be assessed by the identification of a reversible defect on stress testing in an asynergic region, with functional recovery in over 80% of these regions.[53] DSE is also used to determine viability. If a segment is initially akinetic at rest, begins to contract with low-dose infusion, and becomes akinetic with higher doses, it is considered viable. Both DSE and SPECT imaging viability evaluation was assessed by Baumgartner et al.[54] in 12 patients with CAD and severely reduced LV function who were to undergo cardiac transplantation. Nuclear techniques appeared to be more sensitive for segments with < 50% viable myocytes (by histologic study after transplantation) than DSE. For example, the sensitivity for detection of viability in segments with > 25% viable myocytes was 81% for SPECT but only 66% for DSE. Specificities were lower with SPECT, however. In segments with > 50% viable myocytes, sensitivities for viability were similar, but specificity was much higher for DSE (82% vs. 49%). An overall comparison of ECHO and nuclear imaging is difficult due to the differences in the evaluation. One comparison of four studies published before 1998, including the same patients with both techniques, indicated that, in summary, nuclear imaging identified jeopardized myocardium in 38% versus 26% with echocardiography.[55]

In patients entering the emergency room with chest pain syndromes, imaging is frequently used to assess the possibility of significant underlying CAD, especially in those with low to moderate probability of MI. SPECT imaging in this setting was associated with a 93% sensitivity for MI, a negative predictive value of over 99% for identifying or excluding MI.[56] Selected studies of resting ECHO in patient triage to rule out MI have sensitivities of 88 to 95% and specificities in the 85 to 95% range.[57] The use of dobutamine stress testing increases the sensitivity and in our institution, is used in emergency room patients with low to moderate suspicion of chest pain with normal baseline echocardiograms. Access to ECHO stress testing has some advantage over nuclear techniques because of the immediate determination of results.

A summary of the results of ECHO and nuclear studies in the evaluation of CAD diagnosis, prognosis, and evaluation of myocardial viability is found in Table 16-4.

Coronary Artery Disease in Women

Because exercise electrocardiography has been determined to have lower sensitivity and specificity in women and in men, the use of ECHO or SPECT imaging during stress testing provides increased predictive accuracy. Unfortunately, breast attenuation artifacts may provide some difficulty in nuclear imaging. There appears to be a 10% lower sensitivity in women than men, with similar specificity, whatever the technique. With DSE, for one-vessel disease, sensitivity of ECHO stress testing is 40%, increasing to 60% with multivessel disease (> 50% stenosis).

In a large study of over 3,700 men and women evaluating CAD, exercise ECHO showed a similar lower positive predictive value in women than in men (66% vs. 84%), with lower sensitivity in women but similar specificity.[58] However, the study demonstrated that test verification bias can increase the sensitivity and decrease the specificity of the test substantially. This relates to evaluation based on referral patterns for coronary angiography, the "gold standard" for evaluation of sensitivity and specificity. Another consideration in noninvasive testing in women is the decreased positive predictive value of a test because of the lower prevalence of CAD in women.

If exercise ECG testing is used with evaluation of the Duke Treadmill Score (DTS) without any further imaging, the DTS is more reliable in women than in men for excluding the diagnosis of CAD. In fact, according to Alexander et al.,[59] fewer women are found to have significant CAD (more than one vessel with higher than 75% stenosis: women 20% vs. men 47%) or severe disease (triple vessel or left main stenosis: women 3.5% vs. men 11.4%) when the DTS is employed.

A meta-analysis evaluating exercise electrocardiography, echocardiography, and SPECT imaging detecting CAD in women demonstrated an increased sensitivity of both imaging techniques over ECG (61%, 86% and 78% respectively), with a somewhat higher specificity of ECHO in comparison with ECG and nuclear imaging (ECHO 79%, ECG 70%, nuclear 64%).[60] The sensitivities and specificities were therefore only moderate.

The WISE trial (Women's Ischemia Syndrome Evaluation) demonstrated that DSE reliably detected multivessel CAD in women but was usually negative in women with single-vessel CAD.[61] For women with multivessel disease, the sensitivity was 81.8%. DSE reliably detects multivessel stenosis in women, but sensitivity and specificity appear lower than in men. In one series of 92 women with suspected CAD, overall sensitivity with an adequate heart rate response was 50% overall and 82% with multivessel disease.[61] Exercise ECHO also provides important prognostic information after a cardiac event, as the presence of ischemia by exercise ECHO was a powerful predictor of future events in women with known CAD.[62]

In summary, nuclear imaging and ECHO increase the sensitivity of detection of CAD in women compared with ECG stress testing. However, the predictive accuracy may be lower than in men because of lower prevalence of CAD in women. There is no conclusive evidence that one imaging modality is superior to the other in evaluation of women.

Left Ventricular Ejection Fraction

LV volumes and ejection fraction are important in prognostic evaluation and for therapeutic protocols. One of the most important objectives of the noninvasive tests is to accurately delineate the LV border and measure the end-diastolic and end-systolic volumes, and from these values estimate the LVEF. There is good evidence that the LVEF calculated from a gated SPECT study compares well to radionuclide ventriculography.[63]

For ECHO, accurate assessment of LVEF is accomplished by computerized offline analysis with nuclear imaging. However, it is the standard practice to estimate LVEF by ECHO based on

Table 16-4
Echocardiography versus Nuclear Imaging in CAD Evaluation

CAD Diagnosis
Echocardiography

Smart	[58]	183	DSE	All	87 (se)	91 (sp)		
				1 V	84 (se)			
				2,3V	91 (se)			
Fleischmann	[55]	44 studies {MA} Ex			85 (se)	77 (sp)		
Atar	[28]	54	Pacing		95 (se)	87 (sp)	95 (+ pv)	87 (− pv)
Geleijnse	[11]	28 studies {MA} DSE			80 (se)	84 (sp)	81 (pa)	
			(se):	1V 74	2V 86	3V 92		

Nuclear

Smart	[58]	183	DipyTcSPECT	All 80(se)	73 (sp)	
			(se):	1V 74	2,3V 86	
Fleischmann	[55]	44 Studies {MA} Ex Th/TcSPECT		87(se)	64 (sp)	

Prognostic Significance
Echocardiography

Odds Ratio of Positive Test

Shaw	[68]	445	DSE	Death/MI	14–27		
Krivokapich	[65]	1183	DSE	Death/MI	3		
			DSE + ECG	Death/MI	6		
Steinberg	[62]	120	DSE	Death/MI/ Revasc	79 (se)	52 (sp)	67 (+ pv) 67 (− pv)
Olmos	[64]	248	Ex	Event-Free Survival (5Y)			Normal > 90% Fixed WMA > 50% Ischemia > 30% Mixed 10%
Greco	[19]	178	DSE Post-MI MI/Death/UA	− pv	98%		
			Ex	− pv	95%		
			Event Free Survival (4Y)	DSE	+ 84%	− 95%	
			For "Hard Events"	Ex	+ 88%	− 90%	

Nuclear

Shaw	[68]	1994	DipyTh Death/MI	4 [OR]	
Calnon	[63]	308	DobTcSPECT Death/MI	5 [OR]	
Olmos	[64]	248	Ex Th SPECTEvent-Free Survival (5Y)	Normal	90%
				Fixed defect	60%
				Ischemia	> 30%
				Mixed	0

Table 16-4 (continued)

Echocardiography versus Nuclear Imaging in CAD Evaluation

Evaluation of Viability

Echocardiography

Baumgartner	[73]	12	DSE	(> 75%)[a]	78 (se)		
				(50–75%)	71 (se)		
				(25–50%)	15 (se)		
				(< 25%)	19 (se)		
Cornel	[25]	61	DSE		89 (se)	81 (sp)	75 (pa)
Senior	[24]	504 {MA}	DSE		84 (se)	81 (sp)	82 (pa)

Nuclear

Baumgartner	[73]	12	SPECT	(75%)	87 (se)	
				(50–75%)	87 (se)	
				(25–50%)	82 (se)	
				(< 25%)	38 (se)	
Senior	[24]	207	Tc-99 MIBI		83 (se)	69 (sp)
		209	Tl-201 reinjection		86 (se)	47 (sp)
		145	Tl-201 rest–redistribution		90 (se)	54 (sp)

[a] % segment myocyte viability by histology after heart transplant; [ ] = reference; (se) = sensitivity; (sp) = specificity; (pa) = predictive accuracy; (+ pv) = positive predictive value; (– pv) = negative predictive value; {MA} = meta-analysis; DSE = dobutamine stress echocardiography; ex = exercise study; dipy = dipyridamole; V = coronary vessel disease.

semiquantitative evaluation by the ECHO reader, utilizing M-mode assessment of LV fractional shortening in ventricles without geometric distortion. Although various laborious geometric models have been used to evaluate LVEF with 2D imaging (Figure 16-11), they are rarely applied in routine clinical evaluation. One of the concerns about ECHO visualization is the difficulty with endocardial border detection in many patients. The use of contrast harmonic imaging has improved such border detection to allow quantitative assessment of LVEF (see Figure 16-8). Application of this technique in patients with technically difficult studies by fundamental imaging improved visualization to such a degree that quantitative ECHO correlated closely with nuclear imaging assessment of LVEF ($r = 0.95$).[64]

Gorge et al.[65] showed that modern, high-resolution two-dimensional echocardiography pro-duced an LVEF determination that compared favorably with the value from cardiac catheterization. In fact, the method of determining the LVEF seems less important than the technique used. Chuang et al.[66] showed that volumetric methods (i.e., cardiac magnetic resonance imaging [MRI] and three-dimensional ECHO) produced values in agreement with each other more often than biplane methods (i.e., biplane MRI or two-dimensional ECHO). It thus appears that volumetric methods are more accurate than biplanar methods. Also, in ECHO, technological advancements allow more accurate determinations of the LVEF. For example, acoustic quantification using automated border detection can allow fairly reliable beat-to-beat online assessment of changes in ejection fraction (see Figure 16-3), applying a geometric equation to the 2D depiction of the left ventricular structure in the apical view.

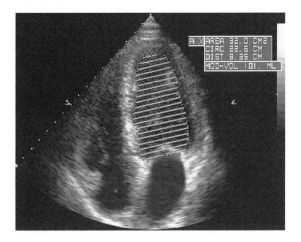

Figure 16-11. Use of internal computer in commercial echocardiography equipment to calculate LV ejection fraction. End diastolic and end systolic frames are chosen for measurements in two planes. This illustrates Simpson's method (biplane method of disks) in one of the tomographic views. (**See also Color Insert**).

The use of this technology has not been routinely used in most of the clinical laboratories. The accurate determination of LV function, however, has important prognostic significance, even independent of exercise capacity.[67] Such predictors include initial LV dimension and LVEF, and changes in dimension and LVEF with exercise, in addition to segmental wall motion abnormalities. In summary, in the current practice of clinical medicine, nuclear techniques probably more readily allow accurate determination of LVEF, although semiquantitative ECHO techniques are routinely used to estimate LVEF on routine studies with accuracy of within 5 to 10% of the true LVEF.

Cost-Effectiveness and Convenience

The use of contrast greatly adds to the diagnosis in nondiagnostic or inconclusive stress ECHO exams. The cost-effectiveness of contrast ECHO has been assessed in several recent publications. One study evaluated all patients undergoing stress ECHO[68,69] and found that of those with baseline suboptimal images undergoing stress

ECHO, 53% subsequently had nuclear stress tests compared with only 3% if they received contrast enhancement. This represented a saving of $238 a patient (1998 charges) after deducting the cost of the contrast agent.

There is increasing interest in the possibility of limited transthoracic studies, especially in regard to cost-effectiveness. An example of its use could be the limited assessment for LVH, a significant risk factor in hypertensive patients. However, a limited study provided a diagnostic yield of only 47% of outpatients and 75% of inpatients.[70] The authors concluded that limited imaging strategy is most cost-effective in young outpatients.

A major development in the field of echocardiography is the miniaturization of the ECHO machine. Whereas most ECHO machines are large and located in the ECHO lab, there are new machines emerging that typically weigh less than 6 pounds and are portable. These hand-carried ultrasounds (HCUs) have the advantage of being at the point of patient care and adding to the physical exam. However, these machines lack some important features of standard ECHO machines, namely spectral Doppler, electrocardiographic, or M-mode capabilities. The machines need to be operated by someone skilled in cardiac ultrasonography, and the data interpreted by a cardiologist trained to read echocardiograms. Unfortunately, the studies provided by these machines are not as accurate as a full study produced by a standard ECHO machine and can miss some major cardiovascular diagnoses. However, the HCUs do add to the physical exam. In one study, physical examination by a board-certified cardiologist failed to detect 59% of cardiovascular pathology, but this was reduced to 29% when the cardiologist used an HCU.[71]

Although the American Society of Echocardiography does not yet recognize the HCU as meeting the requirements for a complete ECHO examination, it recommends appropriate user-specific training to use these handheld devices.[72] Increasing level of training would be dependent on whether use is for a brief extension of the physical examination, goal-directed follow-up, or goal-directed complete examination.[72] Handheld devices are much less expensive than larger state-of-the-art devices. Although the expanded role of these devices will probably mean an increase in their technologic complexity, it is expected that the cost of the technology will decline with increased production.

CONCLUSION

Both echocardiography and nuclear imaging are valuable tools to evaluate LV function and for assessing CAD. They have demonstrated efficacy in prognostic evaluation for cardiac events and in evaluating myocardial viability. Although variations in predictive accuracy have been demonstrated between these techniques in some cases, the main impact of the availability of these modalities is in bolstering clinical diagnosis and prognosis through somewhat different interrogations. Both technologies are undergoing major advancements, and it is conceivable that their combined availabilities in one noninvasive laboratory could improve to the efficiency, cost-effectiveness, and clinical capabilities of cardiac studies.

REFERENCES

1. Tam JW, Nichol J, MacDiarmid AL, et al. What is the real clinical utility of echocardiography? A prospective observational study. *J Am Soc Echocardiogr* 1999; 12:689–697.
2. Burgess MJ, Bhattacharyya A, Rey SG. Echocardiography after cardiac transplantation. *J Am Soc Echocardiogr* 2002;15:917–925.
3. Badruddin SM, Ahmad A, Mickelson J, et al. Supine bicycle versus post-treadmill exercise echocardiography in the detection of myocardial ischemia: A randomized single-blind crossover trial. *J Am Coll Cardiol* 1999;33:1485–1490.
4. Marwick TH, Mehta R, Arheart K, et al. Use of exercise echocardiography for prognostic evaluation of patients with known or suspected coronary artery disease. *J Am Coll Cardiol* 1997;30:83–90.
5. Marwick TH, Cased C, Vasey C, et al. Prediction of mortality by exercise echocardiography. *Circulation* 2001;103:2566–2571.
6. Elhendy A, Mahoney DW, Khanderia BK, et al. Prognostic significance of the location of wall motion abnormalities during exercise echocardiography. *J Am Coll Cardiol* 2002;40:1623–1629.
7. Zwas DR, Takuma S, Mullis-Jansson S, et al. Feasibility of real-time 3-dimensional treadmill stress echocardiography. *J Am Soc Echocardiogr* 1999; 12:285–289.
8. Ahmad M, Xie T, McCulloch M, et al. Real-time three-dimensional dobutamine stress echocardiography in assessment of ischemia: Comparison with two-dimensional dobutamine stress echocardiography. *J Am Coll Cardiol* 2001;37:1303–1309.
9. Geleijnse ML, Fioretti PM, Roelandt JRTC. Methodology, feasibility, safety and diagnostic accuracy of dobutamine stress echocardiography. *J Am Coll Cardiol* 1997;30:595–606.
10. Tadamura E, Iida H, Matsumoto K, et al. Comparison of myocardial blood flow during dobutamine–atropine infusion with that after dipyridamole administration in normal men. *J Am Coll Cardiol* 2001;37:130–136.
11. Secknus M-A, Marwick TH. Evolution of dobutamine echocardiography protocols and indications: Safety and side effects in 3,011 studies over 5 years. *J Am Coll Cardiol* 1997;29:1234–1240.
12. Lee C-Y, Pellikka PA, Shub C, et al. Hypertensive response during dobutamine stress echocardiography. *Am J Cardiol* 1997;80:970–971.
13. Cusick DA, Bonow RO, Chaudry FA. Safety of dobutamine stress echocardiography in patients with left ventricular apical thrombus. *Am J Cardiol* 1997; 80:1252–1254.
14. Spencer KT, Bednarz J, Mor-Avi V, et al. Automated endocardial border detection and evaluation of left ventricular function from contrast-enhanced images using modified acoustic quantification. *J Am Soc Echocardiogr* 2002;15:777–781.
15. Mor-Avi V, Vignon P, Koch R, et al. Segmental analysis of color kinesis images. *Circulation* 1997; 95:2082–2097.
16. Koch R, Lang RM, Garcia M-J, et al. Objective evaluation of regional left ventricular wall motion during dobutamine stress echocardiographic studies using segmental analysis of color kinesis images. *J Am Coll Cardiol* 1999;34:409–419.
17. Greco CA, Salustri A, Seccareccia F, et al. Prognostic value of dobutamine echocardiography early after uncomplicated acute myocardial infarction: A comparison with exercise electrocardiography. *J Am Coll Cardiol* 1997;29:261–267.
18. Chuah S-C, Pellikka PA, Roger VL, et al. Role of dobutamine stress echocardiography in predicting outcome in 860 patients with known or suspected coronary artery disease. *Circulation* 1998; 97:1474–1480.
19. Yuda S, Khoury V, Marwick TH. Influence of wall stress and left ventricular geometry on the accuracy of

dobutamine stress echocardiography. *J Am Coll Cardiol* 2002;40:1311–1319.

20. Rallidis L, Cokkinos P, Tousoulis D, et al. Comparison of dobutamine and treadmill exercise echocardiography in inducing ischemia in patients with coronary artery disease. *J Am Coll Cardiol* 1997;30:1660–1668.

21. San Román JA, Vilacosta I, Rollán MJ, et al. Right ventricular asynergy during dobutamine–atropine echocardiography. *J Am Coll Cardiol* 1997;30:430–435.

22. Senior R, Lahiri S. Role of dobutamine echocardiography in detection of myocardial viability for predicting outcome after revascularization in ischemic cardiomyopathy. *J Am Soc Echocardiogr* 2001; 14:140–248.

23. Cornel JH, Bax JJ, Elhendy A, et al. Biphasic response to dobutamine predicts improvement of global left ventricular function after surgical revascularization in patients with stable coronary artery disease. *J Am Coll Cardiol* 1998;31:1002–1010.

24. Lombardo A, Loperfido F, Trani C, et al. Contractile reserve of dysfunctional myocardium after revascularization: A dobutamine stress echocardiography study. *J Am Coll Cardiol* 1997;30:633–640.

25. Cortigiani L, Paolini EA, Nannini E. Dipyridamole stress echocardiography for risk stratification in hypertensive patients with chest pain. *Circulation* 1998;98:2855–2859.

26. Atar S, Nagai T, Cercek B, et al. Pacing stress echocardiography: An alternative to pharmacologic stress testing. *J Am Coll Cardiol* 2000;36:1935–1941.

27. Cheng S-C, Dy TC, Feinstein SB. Contrast echocardiography: Review and future directions. *Am J Cardiol* 1998;81(12A):41G–48G.

28. American Society of Echocardiography Task Force on Standards and Guidelines for the Use of Ultrasonic Contrast in Echocardiography. Contrast echocardiography: Current and future applications. *J Am Soc Echocardiogr* 2000;13:331–342.

29. Thomson HL, Basmadjian A-J, Rainbird AJ, et al. Contrast echocardiography improves the accuracy and reproducibility of left ventricular remodeling measurements. *J Am Coll Cardiol* 2001;38:867–875.

30. Reilly JP, Tunick PA, Timmermans RJ, et al. Contrast echocardiography clarifies uninterpretable wall motion in intensive care unit patients. *J Am Coll Cardiol* 2000;35:485–490.

31. Rainbird AJ, Mulvagh SL, Oh JK, et al. Contrast dobutamine stress echocardiography: Clinical practice assessment in 300 consecutive patients. *J Am Soc Echocardiogr* 2001;14:378–385.

32. Marwick TH, Brunken R, Meland N, et al. Accuracy and feasibility of contrast echocardiography for detection of perfusion defects in routine practice. *J Am Coll Cardiol* 1998;32:1260–1269.

33. Nagueh SF, Lakkis NM, He Z-X, et al. Role of myocardial contrast echocardiography during nonsurgical septal reduction therapy for hypertrophic obstructive cardiomyopathy. *J Am Coll Cardiol* 1998;32:225–229.

34. Isaaz I. What are we actually measuring by Doppler tissue imaging? *J Am Coll Cardiol* 2000;36:897–899.

35. Waggoner ADS, Bierig SM. Tissue Doppler imaging: A useful echocardiographic method for the cardiac sonographer to assess systolic and diastolic ventricular function. *J Am Soc Echocardiogr* 2001;14:1143–1152.

36. Fleischmann KE, Hunink MGM, Kuntz KM, et al. Exercise echocardiography or exercise SPECT imaging? A meta-analysis of diagnostic test performance. *J Nucl Cardiol* 2002;9:133–134.

37. Beller GA, Zaret BL. Contributions of nuclear cardiology to diagnosis and prognosis of patients with coronary artery disease. *Circulation* 2000; 101:1465–1478.

38. Shimoni S, Zoghbi WA, Xie F, et al. Real-time assessment of myocardial perfusion and wall motion during bicycle and treadmill exercise echocardiography: Comparison with single photon emission tomography. *J Am Coll Cardiol* 2001;37:741–747.

39. Smart SC, Bhatia A, Hellman R, et al. Dobutamine–atropine stress echocardiography and dipyridamole sestamibi scintigraphy for the detection of coronary artery disease: Limitations and concordance. *J Am Coll Cardiol* 2000;36:1265–1273.

40. Kaul S, Senior R, Dittrich H, et al. Detection of coronary artery disease with myocardial contrast echocardiography. Comparison with ^{99m}Tc-sestamibi single-photon emission computed tomography. *Circulation* 1997;96:785–792.

41. Heinle SK, Noblin J, Gorree-Best P, et al. Assessment of myocardial perfusion by harmonic power Doppler imaging at rest and during adenosine stress: Comparison with ^{99m}Tc-sestamibi SPECT imaging. *Circulation* 2000;102:55–60.

42. Daimon M, Watanabe H, Yamagishi H, et al. Physiologic assessment of coronary artery stenosis by coronary flow reserve measurements with transthoracic Doppler echocardiography: Comparison with exercise thallium-201 single-photon emission computed tomography. *J Am Coll Cardiol* 2001;37:1310–1315.

43. Steinberg EH, Madmon L, Patel CP, et al. Long-term prognostic significance of dobutamine echocardiography in patients with suspected coronary artery disease: Results of a 5-year follow-up study. *J Am Coll Cardiol* 1997;29:969–973.

44. Calnon DA, McGrath PD, Doss AL, et al. Prognostic value of dobutamine stress technitium-99m-sestamibi single-photon emission computed tomography myocardial perfusion imaging: Stratification of a high risk population. *J Am Coll Cardiol* 2001; 38:1511–1517.

45. Olmos LI, Dakik H, Gordon R, et al. Long-term prognostic value of exercise echocardiography compared

with exercise [201]Th, ECG, and clinical variables in patients evaluated for coronary artery disease. *Circulation* 1998;98:2679–2686.

46. Krivokapich J, Child JS, Walter DO, et al. Prognostic value of dobutamine stress echocardiography in predicting cardiac events in patients with known or suspected coronary artery disease. *J Am Coll Cardiol* 1999;33:708–716.

47. Geleijnse ML, Elhandy A, Van Domburg RT, et al. Prognostic value of dobutamine–atropine stress technetium-99m sestamibi perfusion scintigraphy in patients with chest pain. *J Am Coll Cardiol* 1996;28:447–454.

48. Geleijnse ML, Elhendy A, Cornel JH, et al. Cardiac imaging for risk stratification with dobutamine-atropine stress testing in patients with chest pain. Echocardiography, perfusion scintigraphy or both? *Circulation* 1997;96:137–147.

49. Shaw LJ, Eagle KA, Gersh BJ, Miller DD. Meta-analysis of intravenous dipyridamole-thallium-201 imaging (1985–1994) and dobutamine echocardiography (1991–1994) for risk stratification before vascular surgery. *J Am Coll Cardiol* 1996;27:787–798.

50. Gibbons RJ, Miller TD, Christian TF. Infarct size measured by single photon emission computed tomographic imaging with ^{99m}Tc-sestamibi. *Circulation* 2000;101:101–108.

51. Senaratne MPJ, Smith G, Gulamhusein SS. Feasibility and safety of early exercise testing using the Bruce protocol after acute myocardial infarction. *J Am Coll Cardiol* 2000;35:1212–1220.

52. Carlos ME, Smart SC, Wynsen JC, Sagar KB. Dobutamine stress echocardiography for risk stratification after myocardial infarction. *Circulation* 1997;95:1402–1410.

53. Kitsiou AN, Srinivasan G, Quyyumi AA, et al. Stress-induced reversible and mild-to-moderate irreversible thallium defects. *Circulation* 1998;98:501–508.

54. Baumgartner H, Porenta G, Lau Y-K, et al. Assessment of myocardial viability by dobutamine echocardiography, positron emission tomography and thallium-201 SPECT. *J Am Coll Cardiol* 1998;32:1701–1708.

55. Brown KA. Do stress echocardiography and myocardial perfusion imaging have the same ability to identify the low-risk patient with known or suspected coronary artery disease. *Am J Cardiol* 1998;81:1053.

56. Kontos MC, Jesse RL, Schmidt KL, et al. Value of acute rest sestimibi perfusion imaging for evaluation of patients admitted to the emergency department with chest pain. *J Am Coll Cardiol* 1997;30:976–982.

57. Pearlman AS, Otto CM. Roler of echocardiography in evaluating patients presenting to the emergency room with acute chest pain. In CM Otto (Ed.), *The Practice of Clinical Echocardiography*. Philadelphia: Saunders, 1997: Chapter 9, pp. 179–194.

58. Roger VL, Pelikka PA, Bell MR, et al. Sex and verification bias: Impact on the diagnostic value of exercise electrocardiography. *Circulation* 1997; 95:405–410.

59. Alexander KP, Shaw LJ, Delong EB, et al. Value of exercise treadmill testing in women. *J Am Coll Cardiol* 1998;32:1657–1664.

60. Kwok Y, Kim C, Grady D, et al. Meta-analysis of exercise testing to detect coronary artery disease in women. *Am J Cardiol* 1999;83:660–666.

61. Lewis JF, Lin L, McGorray S, et al. Dobutamine stress echocardiography in women with chest pain: Pilot phase from the National Heart, Lung and Blood Institute Women's Ischemia Syndrome Evaluation (WISE). *J Am Coll Cardiol* 1999;33:1462–1468.

62. Heupler S, Mehta R, Lobo A, Leung D, et al. Prognostic implications of exercise echocardiography in women with known or suspected coronary artery disease. *J Am Coll Cardiol* 1997;30:414–420.

63. Bonow RO. Gated myocardial perfusion imaging for measuring left ventricular function. *J Am Coll Cardiol* 1997;30:1649–1650.

64. Nahar T, Shapiro R, Fruchtman S, et al. Comparison of four echocardiographic techniques for measuring left ventricular ejection fraction. *Am J Cardiol* 2000; 86:1358–1362.

65. Gorge G, Erbel R, Brennicke R, et al. High-resolution two-dimensional echocardiography improves the quantification of left ventricular function. *J Am Soc Echocardiogr* 1992;5:125–134.

66. Chuang ML, Hibberd MG, Salton CJ, et al. Importance of imaging method over imaging modality in noninvasive determination of left ventricular volumes and ejection fraction. *J Am Coll Cardiol* 2000; 35:477–484.

67. McCully RB, Roger VL, Mahoney DW, et al. Outcome after abnormal exercise echocardiography for patients with good exercise capactity: Prognostic importance and severity of exercise-related left ventricular dysfunction. *J Am Coll Cardiol* 2002;39:1345–1352.

68. Tardif J-C, Dove A, Chan KL, et al. Economic impact of contrast stress echocardiography on the diagnosis and initial treatment of patients with suspected coronary artery disease. *J Am Soc Echocardiogr* 2002; 15:1335–1345.

69. Thanigaraj S, Naese RF Jr, Schechtman KB, et al. Use of contrast for image enhancement during stress echocardiography is cost-effective and reduces additional diagnostic testing. *Am J Cardiol* 2001;87:1430–1432.

70. Kimura BJ, Blanchard DG, Willis CL, et al. Limited cardiac ultrasound examination for cost-effective echocardiographic referral. *J Am Soc Echocardiogr* 2002;15:640–646.

71. Spencer KT, Anderson AS, Bhargava A, et al. Physician-

performed point-of-care echocardiography using a laptop platform compared with physical examination in the cardiovascular patient. *J Am Coll Cardiol* 2001;37:2013–2018.

72. Seward JB, Douglas PS, Erbel R, et al. American Society of Echocardiography report. Hand-carried ultrasound (HCU) device: Recommendations regarding new technology. A report from the Echocardiography Task Force on New Technology of the Nomenclature and Standards Committee of the American Society of Echocardiography. *J Am Soc Echocardiogr* 2002; 15:369–373.

CHAPTER 17

Cardiac Magnetic Resonance Imaging

Peter G. Danias
Anita Bhandiwad

INTRODUCTION

Magnetic resonance imaging (MRI) is a noninvasive method that allows the anatomic and functional evaluation for practically every organ system of the human body. MRI is performed in a strong homogenous magnetic field (1.0–1.5 Tesla), which is 20,000 to 30,000 times stronger than the earth's magnetic field. Radiofrequency pulses in the frequency modulation (FM) range are used to excite the tissues, transferring energy to the hydrogen nuclei and causing resonance of their precession. Soon after the application of the radiofrequency pulses, the hydrogen nuclei return to their former energy state, releasing electromagnetic energy that can be detected with specially designed antennas (coils). The received signal can be converted to an image through a series of mathematical transformations that convert the phase and frequency of the electromagnetic waves to a spatially localized gray-scale pixel intensity. Depending on the technical characteris-

tics of the imaging sequence, the same tissue may have different appearance. In general, cardiac imaging is performed with "black blood" or "bright blood" sequences in which the flowing blood appears as dark or bright, respectively. The physics principles behind MRI are quite complicated, but their in-depth knowledge is not necessary for the understanding of the clinical utility of the method. This chapter will discuss only the current applications of MRI for imaging of the heart.

ADVANTAGES OF MRI

MRI offers several advantages that make it a unique imaging tool: It is noninvasive and the exposure to the high magnetic field has no known immediate or late side effects. Neither the patient nor the medical staff are exposed to ionizing radiation and there is no need for potentially nephrotoxic contrast media. The contrast agents that are occasionally used for cardiac MRI examinations are gadolinium products that have negligible complications and bear no structural, cross-allergy, or other similarity to the iodinated contrast media used for conventional radiographic imaging. MRI allows for three-dimensional acquisitions in any orientation, plane, and angulation with exquisitely high resolution. It offers high contrast among different tissues (e.g., flowing blood, myocardium, fat, etc.). Furthermore, the same tissue may have different imaging characteristics depending on its pathophysiologic state (e.g., normal myocardium vs. infarcted vs. edematous from myocarditis, etc.). Information about tissue composition may be important for the initial diagnosis and subsequent follow-up for many cardiac diseases. Finally, because of the ability to offer combined structural and functional imaging, cardiac MRI has the potential to noninvasively provide a comprehensive cardiac evaluation in a single examination.

SAFETY ISSUES

In general, MRI is a very safe imaging modality. However, the exposure to high magnetic fields and rapidly applied gradients is contraindicated for certain patients, such as those with implanted pacemakers, defibrillators, or retained pacing wires. Fatalities have been reported when patients with pacemakers inadvertently had an MRI examination, presumably due to erratic sensing or pacing, local heating at the tip of the pacing wire, and/or induced tachyarrhythmias. Similarly, patients with endocranial clips following neurosurgery should not undergo MRI for the fear of displacing the clips, a potentially devastating complication. Finally, patients with ocular, cochlear, or other metallic implants also should not undergo MRI.

CHALLENGES

For evaluation of the heart, MRI has to overcome several limitations that are not encountered with imaging of other parts of the body. These challenges are largely related to the continuous mo-

tion of the heart due to the cardiac contraction and respiratory motion and have delayed the widespread clinical use of cardiac MRI. For certain applications, additional challenges include the small size of the imaged structure (valve leaflets, coronary arteries) and their rapid motion (valve leaflets). In order to address issues related to cardiac contraction, for most cardiac applications it is required to perform electrocardiographic (ECG) gating. Data can then be obtained during a small time period always at the same part of the cardiac cycle, when the heart is at a constant position and contractile state. To address issues related to respiratory motion, images are either acquired during breath-holding or by gating data acquisition to the respiratory cycle. Respiratory gating can be performed with respiratory belts and bellows, coached breathing, and direct monitoring of the diaphragmatic motion. The latter is accomplished with MRI devices called navigators that monitor the position of the diaphragm in real time. The principle of this techniques is similar to M-mode echocardiography (ECHO), although the implementation is entirely different. Information on the diaphragmatic position can be used to guide data acquisition for the heart, retrospectively or prospectively. Recently, real-time acquisitions have been developed and allow imaging without the need for motion compensation. However, with real-time cardiac MRI the spatial resolution remains rather low, compared to "conventional" ECG-gated imaging.

ANATOMY

MRI can demonstrate the structure of the heart and great thoracic vessels with superb detail. Typically, for anatomic studies black blood techniques are used, in which the signal from the flowing blood is lost as it moves outside the plane of interest and field of view (Figure 17-1). Black blood techniques have the advantage of offering exquisite resolution, with high contrast between the blood pool and surrounding tissues. Clinical applications include the evaluation of the aorta for aneurysms (Figure 17-2), dissection

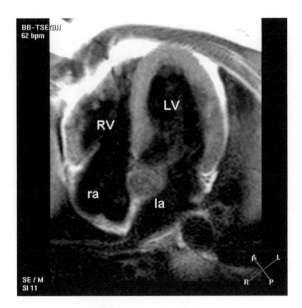

Figure 17-1.   Black blood imaging of the heart in a four-chamber orientation, showing the left and right ventricles (LV and RV, respectively) and the left and right atria (la and ra, respectively). This image, obtained with T1 weighting, shows the fat tissue as bright, the cardiac muscle as gray, and the blood as dark. Anatomic detail of cardiac structure can be obtained.

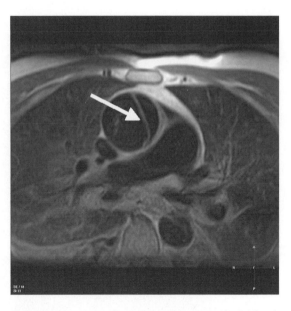

Figure 17-3.   Ascending aortic dissection. Black blood image in the transverse orientation showing clearly the dissection flap (arrow) in the ascending aorta.

(Figure 17-3), and congenital anomalies, such as coarctation, double aortic arch, vascular rings, and so on. In particular with reference to the aortic dissections, since the early and mid 1990s there have been many studies that documented

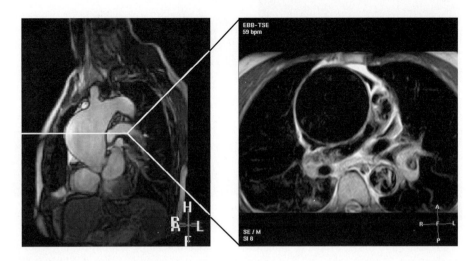

Figure 17-2.   Marked aneurysmal dilatation of the ascending aorta, imaged with a bright blood technique in an oblique saggital orientation (left panel) and dark blood sequence in a transverse orientation (right panel).

that MRI has high sensitivity, specificity, and accuracy for establishing the diagnosis.[1,2] MRI is currently considered equivalent, if not superior, to computed tomography (CT) and transesophageal echocardiography (TEE) as an initial test to diagnose aortic dissection and visualize the entry and exit points of the dissection flap.

Regarding cardiac imaging, MRI is considered as the test of first choice for evaluation of pericardial thickening and constrictive pericarditis. Normally, with black blood sequences the pericardium is a thin dark rim that surrounds the heart, easily delineated from the muscle and epi-

cardial fat.[3] The pericardium is considered abnormal when the thickness exceeds 4 mm, and MRI findings have been shown to be in good agreement with pathology data in patients undergoing surgical pericardial stripping.[4,5]

Anatomic imaging with cardiac MRI is particularly useful in various forms of myocarditides and cardiomyopathies. In hypertrophic cardiomyopathy, MRI (Figure 17-4) is superior to transthoracic echocardiography (TTE) because it can better visualize the apex.[6–8] In acute myocarditis, MRI can show foci of tissue edema with specific imaging approaches (T2-weighted imag-

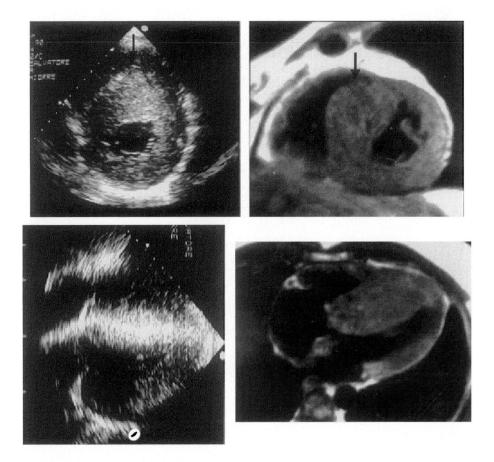

Figure 17-4. Hypertrophic cardiomyopathy, imaged with echocardiography (left panels) and cardiac MRI (right panels), in the short axis (upper panels) and four-chamber (lower panels) orientations. MRI can better quantify the left ventricular hypertrophy and better delineate the apical septal involvement, a region frequently not imaged well with echocardiography. (Modified from Di Cesare[8] with permission.)

ing). The use of paramagnetic contrast agents can also demonstrate areas with increased signal enhancement, suggesting focal inflammation. These changes may have prognostic significance and can be followed over time to monitor disease progression and response to therapy.[9] Arrhythmogenic right ventricular (RV) dysplasia is another form of cardiomyopathy for which cardiac MRI has become the diagnostic noninvasive reference standard.[10] In this disease, the myocardium of the RV free wall is partially substituted by adipose tissue. This results in focal or global systolic dysfunction of the right ventricle and ventricular arrhythmias, which occasionally may be lethal. Cardiac MRI can demonstrate both the fat infiltration, as fat emits bright signal with MRI, and the associated systolic dysfunction. With iron overload (e.g., in patients with hemochromatosis and those with anemias that require frequent transfusions) the imaging characteristics of the myocardium reflect the extent of iron deposition.[11] These data can be used to guide iron chelation therapy and assess patients' prognosis. Finally, in infiltrative diseases of the myocardium such as amyloidosis and sarcoidosis, cardiac MRI can provide clinically useful information regarding the state of the myocardium and be used for assessment of patients' prognosis and guidance of therapy.[12–14]

Primary and secondary tumors that involve the heart, pericardium, or mediastinum can be accurately evaluated with cardiac MRI (Figure 17-5). The vast majority of cardiac tumors in adults are secondary, and they usually originate from surrounding tissues (lung, breast, mediastinum), but in rarer cases through hematogenous dissemination (melanoma). Imaging characteristics that are taken into account to determine whether a cardiac tumor is benign or malignant include the size, shape, and contour; adherence to or infiltration of the myocardium; and pattern of enhancement with contrast. The extent of myocardial involvement frequently determines whether the tumor is respectable or not.

Evaluation of congenital cardiac disease is an-

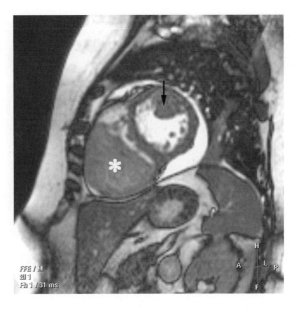

Figure 17-5.   Metastatic sarcoma filling almost the entire right ventricular cavity (asterisk) and infiltrating the anteromedial papillary muscle of the left ventricle (arrow). The image is a single frame from a cine bright blood sequence, obtained in the short-axis orientation. A circumferential pericardial effusion (bright rim surrounding the left ventricle) is also seen.

other area in which cardiac MRI has great clinical value, particularly in adults, before and after surgical correction (Figure 17-6). The ability to image large volumes and reconstruct images in any orientation are unique advantages of cardiac MRI for this indication. As there is no exposure to ionizing radiation, the longitudinal follow-up with serial examinations is possible without risks in this group of patients in whom frequent examinations may be necessary.

FUNCTION

At Rest

Cardiac MRI is the most accurate method for assessment of left and right ventricular function and is considered the reference standard for this evaluation.[15] For functional studies, typically

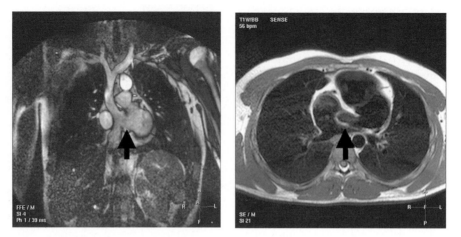

Figure 17-6. Bright blood image in the saggital orientation (left panel) and black blood image in the transverse orientation, in a young adult with transposition of the great arteries surgically corrected with a Senning procedure. The atrial baffle redirecting blood flow at the atrial level is shown (arrow).

bright blood approaches are used, in which the flowing blood has bright signal, hence the name. ECG gating is typically employed, and many phases of the cardiac cycle are obtained, so as to reconstruct a cine loop that spans the entire cardiac cycle. To measure ventricular volumes and ejection fraction, contiguous short-axis images

are obtained, covering the whole heart from apex to base. Then, with image segmentation the endocardial contours can be traced, and using the disk-area method (Simpson's rule) end-diastolic and end-systolic volumes can be measured (Figure 17-7). The ejection fraction can then be easily calculated. Similarly, for measurement of left

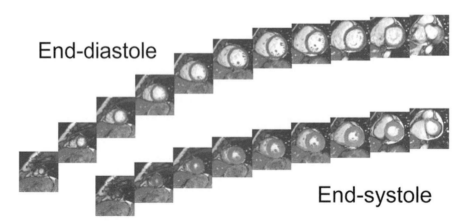

Figure 17-7. Simpson's rule as applied in cardiac MRI. Contiguous short-axis images are obtained to cover the entire left ventricle. The end-diastolic and end-systolic images are selected and the endocardial contours are traced to compute left ventricular volumes. This approach obviates the need for geometric assumptions regarding the shape of the left ventricle.

(and right) ventricular mass, the epicardial contours can be traced; the volume of the heart is included between endocardium and pericardium, and can be used for measurement of myocardial mass. Cardiac MRI is a true volumetric method and, in contrast to the commonly used echocardiography, does not require geometric assumptions regarding the shape of the left ventricle.

Because of combined high spatial and temporal resolution, cardiac MRI can be also used for assessment of RV function.[16] Presently, no other imaging modality can image well the right ventricle, but its size and function may have great prognostic value, in particular for patients with congestive heart failure (CHF) or pulmonary disease.

With Stress

Nonferromagnetic bicycles are available for exercise inside the MRI scanner. These devices have been met with limited acceptance, as supine exercise in the confined environment of the scanner is awkward. Hyperventilation during exercise contributes to significant motion artifacts. To date, very few reports regarding the use of dynamic exercise during cardiac MRI have been presented.[17]

The majority of clinical experience with stress cardiac MRI is with dobutamine as the stress agent. Dobutamine is a beta$_2$ agonist with positive inotropic and chronotropic action, physiological effects similar to exercise and a relatively short half-life (2 min). In a pioneer study by Nagel et al.,[18] 172 patients with suspected coronary artery disease (CAD) (predominantly men) underwent both dobutamine stress ECHO (DSE) with harmonic imaging and dobutamine stress MRI. Coronary angiography was subsequently performed in all patients. Both sensitivity and specificity for detection of significant coronary disease were better for cardiac MRI compared to ECHO (86% vs. 74%, and 86% vs. 70%, for sensitivity and specificity, respectively). Accordingly, the accuracy of dobutamine cardiac MRI (86%) was significantly better than ECHO (73%).[18]

Other investigators have published similar experience with dobutamine MRI.[19] In a study of 153 subjects who could not be adequately assessed with second harmonic ECHO due to poor acoustic windows, dobutamine MRI showed high sensitivity (up to 92% for those with three-vessel disease) with intermediate–high specificity (83%) for detection of significant CAD.

Data regarding the prognostic significance of dobutamine MRI were recently published.[20] In a study of 279 patients, the presence of inducible ischemia, an ejection fraction < 40%, or both, implied a significantly worse prognosis than a normal test. The predictive value of dobutamine MRI for myocardial infarction (MI) and cardiac death were independent of other traditional risk factors.[20]

ASSESSMENT OF VALVULAR FUNCTION

Cardiac MRI is still rather limited in visualizing thin and rapidly moving structures, such as the valve leaflets. Both black blood sequences[21] and bright blood sequences[22] have been described for assessment of valvular structure and function, but usually the qualitative information is inferior to that obtained with ECHO. Turbulence associated with significant valvular stenosis or incompetence presents in bright blood sequences as a signal void, but the size of this jet is heavily dependent on technical factors (namely the ECHO time of the sequence). Thus, it is not appropriate to use the appearance of signal void jets on cardiac MRI as equivalent to turbulence (color mosaic) seen on ECHO.

MRI offers the advantage that it can provide quantitative measurement of blood flow in any orientation. This is possible with a technique named phase contrast, which encodes the velocity of a moving structure into gray-scale pixel intensity. By combining information from conventional and phase images, the flow velocity profile across any large vessel can be accurately measured. This approach can provide a quantitative assessment of valvular regurgitant lesions, right and left heart cardiac output and intra- or extra-cardiac shunts.[23] The phase contrast data can also be combined with volumetric data obtained from the functional assessment (Simpson's rule) of the left and right ventricles, to assess patients with more than one valvular abnormality (Figure 17-7). Though presently clinical decisions regarding management of valvular disease frequently rely on qualitative data, it is likely that a quantitative assessment will be the preferred approach, as our experience with this approach increases and becomes better validated.

ASSESSMENT OF MYOCARDIAL PERFUSION

Current cardiac MRI perfusion techniques measure the alteration of regional myocardial magnetic properties following the intravenous injection of contrast. Gadolinium products are typically used for first-pass imaging, and rapidly diffuse from the intravascular space into the interstitium and remain in the extracellular space when the tissue cell membranes are intact. After a rapid bolus intravenous injection of contrast, there is an abrupt and pronounced signal enhancement sequentially in the RV cavity, the left ventricular (LV) cavity, and then the myocardium. First-pass imaging is completed within 20 to 30 seconds after a bolus injection of the contrast agent, and typically performed during a prolonged breath-hold.

The peak signal intensity is related to the local tissue concentration of the contrast, the myocardial delivery of which is proportional to regional coronary blood flow. In normal volunteers, the first-pass myocardial signal increase is rapid and homogeneous in all myocardial segments. A gradual washout follows several minutes later, and is faster in territories with normal or high blood flow. For standardization, maximum tissue signal intensity is usually described as a percent of the maximal blood pool (LV) signal intensity. The parameters that have been described to quantify myocardial perfusion include the peak signal intensity, the rate of enhancement (slope), the contrast arrival time, and the time to peak signal enhancement. These parameters are typically measured twice, after contrast injection at rest and following vasodilation with dipyridamole or adenosine. With normal epicardial coronary arteries, the rate of signal increase augments following pharmacologic vasodilation, while in regions supplied by stenotic vessels there is no such augmentation and there may even be a decrease in the pattern of signal enhancement. The ratio of signal increase after and before the administration of vasodilators (myocardial perfusion reserve index) has been proposed as the most reliable index of myocardial perfusion.[24]

In studies comparing stress perfusion MRI with radioisotopic scintigraphy, the detection of coronary disease by the two techniques is reported to be similar.[25-30] The addition of MRI wall motion assessment has been reported to further improve the accuracy of MRI for detecting CAD.[30] With newer studies, cardiac MRI has been shown to have diagnostic accuracy comparable to positron emission tomography (PET), with sensitivity of 87% for diagnosis of significant coronary disease.[31] These data are derived from quantitative analyses, which in general are very time consuming and require significant expertise, thereby limiting widespread applicability. Visual assessment of perfusion MRI is also advocated, but in general is less reliable than quantitative approaches.

ASSESSMENT OF VIABILITY

There are several approaches by which cardiac MRI can visualize infarcted myocardium and distinguish it from noninfarcted (viable) myocardium.

1. *T2 signal enhancement.* The acute phase of myocardial perfusion is characterized by myocardial injury and necrosis, associated with a loss of myocyte integrity and gradual development of edema. These changes are manifested as increased T2 signal in acutely or subacutely infarcted tissue.[32,33] In general, though, the specificity of T2 signal changes is poor.[34]

2. *Regional wall thickness and systolic augmentation with dobutamine.* Scar formation gradually occurs in regions of chronic MI. MRI can accurately depict the wall thinning and associated regional systolic dysfunction, and has been shown to correlate well with clinical and histopathologic findings.[35] Augmentation of systolic function with low-dose inotropic stimulation as detected by cardiac MRI correlates well with PET assessment of myocardial viability.[36]

3. *Infarct avid agents.* Experimental contrast agents are being developed to better demarcate viable and nonviable tissue. Various porphyrin-based compounds have been shown to have necrosis-avid properties. In animal models, a gadorphin-2–enhanced zone on MRI correlates very closely with the infarct size as demonstrated by histopathologic examination.[37] However, the use of such agents in humans has not been described due to concerns about toxicity.

4. *^{23}Na imaging.* Scarred areas are characterized by an increase in the concentration of sodium ions and a decrease in the potassium and phosphorous concentration.[38] ^{23}Na imaging has been shown to accurately visualize infarcted territories,[39] but the need for high-field scanners and long imaging times limit the applicability of this approach.

5. *Delayed contrast enhancement.* Delineation and characterization of infarcted tissue can be improved on T1-weighted images by the use of relaxation contrast agents, such as gadolinium DTPA. With myocardial cell death and scar formation, the interstitial space increases, representing an increase in the volume of distribution of gadolinium. Further accumulation of contrast is enhanced by the delayed washout in these regions that usually have decreased blood flow. Equilibrium T1-weighted MRI performed 15 to 25 minutes after contrast administration allows the contrast agent to reach a steady state in the tissue and creates the necessary contrast to differentiate infarcted from viable myocardium. A recently described approach[40] increases the contrast between normal and infarcted myocardium (Figure 17-8) and has been shown to distinguish between ischemic and nonischemic dilated cardiomyopathies[41] and predict improvement of systolic function following revascularization.[42] This imaging strategy was also recently reported to visualize intracavitary clots with high clarity, superior to ECHO and MRI anatomic and functional imaging.[43] This application of cardiac MRI is quickly expanding because it is

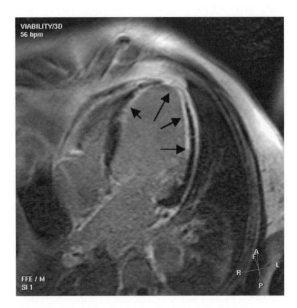

Figure 17-8. Scar imaging with delayed contrast hyperenhancement in a patient with previous myocardial infarction. Using a dual-inversion recovery sequence the signal from normal myocardium is suppressed, and thus noninfarcted myocardium is dark. Gadolinium concentrates in the infarcted regions, making scar appear as bright (arrows). The transmural extent of the scar can be assessed and expressed as a percentage of myocardial wall thickness.

simple to implement, it is validated against many other approaches used for assessment of viability, and has better spatial resolution and image clarity than nuclear techniques, including PET.[44] This MRI assessment of viability is gradually becoming the new reference standard for visualization of infarcted tissue and assessment of viable myocardium.

CORONARY ANGIOGRAPHY

Coronary angiography remains the holy grail of cardiac MRI. However, several factors make coronary imaging challenging. Importantly, the coronaries are a "moving target," as their position varies during the cardiac and respiratory cycles. The coronary tree is a complex 3D structure that deforms during ventricular systole due to the caudal displacement primarily of the base, with simultaneous translation on the horizontal plane and rotation around the long axis of the heart. Besides mechanical contraction, the entire heart is also subject to bulk cardiac motion that follows the diaphragmatic and chest wall respiratory movement. The respiratory component of cardiac motion varies among subjects (diaphragmatic vs. chest wall breathers) and also within each subject, depending on the depth of inspiration. Other technical challenges include the relatively small coronary artery diameter (2–4 mm), the tortuous course of the vessels, and the surrounding epicardial fat. Even with optimal imaging strategies, the interpretation of coronary MRI may be difficult due to deviations of the vessel outside the image plane that cause discontinuities of the vessel lumen and may be misinterpreted as focal stenoses. Visualization of cardiac veins that run parallel and in close proximity to the arteries may also pose additional difficulties to image interpretation.

Since the late 1980s, when the first reports of coronary MRI visualization were published, significant progress has been made. Technical hardware and software developments have allowed "freezing" of the respiratory motion (as previously described) and allowed for submillimeter resolution. Thus, across various implementations, the entire left main, the proximal 3 to 4 cm of the left anterior descending (LAD), the 2 to 3 cm of the left circumflex and the proximal 4 to 5 cm of the right coronary artery can be well visualized in the majority of compliant and motivated volunteers and patients.

Among the first clinical applications of coronary MRI was the evaluation for known of suspected coronary artery anomalies. Initial case reports were followed by comparative studies of series of patients with such anomalies, in which MRI was compared against conventional angiography. In all studies to date,[45–49] coronary MRI has been shown to be equivalent if not superior to x-ray angiography, and has thus become the current gold standard for evaluation of these anomalies (Figure 17-9). Furthermore, in patients with other congenital cardiac anomalies, it is often important to define the course of the proximal coronary arteries to avoid their inadvertent injury during cardiac surgery, when corrective or palliative operations are indicated for the primary cardiac anomaly.

Another unique population in which coronary MRI has particular value is patients with Kawasaki disease. Approximately one third of children affected by this disease develop cardiac complications, the most serious of which are coronary artery aneurysms. The occurrence of coronary aneurysms requires frequent follow-up, which is currently done with ECHO in childhood, but requires x-ray angiography in adolescence and adulthood. MRI has been demonstrated to adequately visualize the size, location, and extent of the coronary aneurysms in these patients (Figure 17-10) and is becoming the preferred modality for serial noninvasive follow-up.[50]

Assessment of patency of bypass grafts is yet another clinically established indication of MRI. Coronary artery bypass grafts (CABGs) are generally easier to image, compared with native coronary arteries, because they are larger in size, have a straighter course, and are less subject to

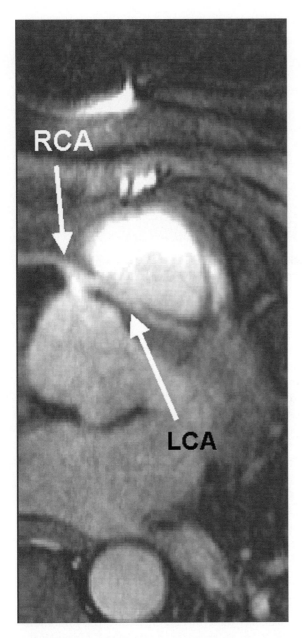

Figure 17-9.   Anomalous coronary artery. Reformatted image demonstrating a single coronary artery originating from the right sinus of Valsalva and then bifurcating to a structurally right coronary artery (RCA) and a left coronary artery (LCA). The latter courses between the aorta and the pulmonary artery, being the "malignant" form of coronary anomaly that has been associated with sudden cardiac death in young adults. (Reprinted from McConnell et al.[54] with permission.)

cardiac motion. Patency is generally determined by visualizing a patent graft lumen in at least two contiguous transverse levels along its expected course (presenting as signal void for spin ECHO techniques and bright signal for gradient ECHO approaches). If a patent graft is not seen at any level, the graft is considered occluded. The sensitivity and specificity of coronary magnetic resonance angiography (CMRA) for assessment of CABG patency is very high for a wide variety of imaging strategies. However, imaging of bypass grafts is hampered by local artifacts from intrathoracic metallic clips, graft markers, and sternal wires. Furthermore, the clinically relevant question is most commonly the assessment of integrity of bypass grafts and the presence of flow-limiting stenoses, rather than patency alone. Recently, interest in imaging of bypass grafts has been resurrected, following a recent report[51] that showed intermediate sensitivity (73%) and intermediate–high specificity (~ 80%) for detection of graft stenoses > 70%.

As the maturity of coronary MRI evolved to allow reliable visualization of the proximal coronary arteries, investigations on the potential utility of coronary MRI for assessment of native coronary atherosclerosis were initiated. More than 30 reports have been published in the Western literature comparing the MRI assessment of coronary stenoses with conventional x-ray angiography. All studies to date have used gradient ECHO approaches in which rapidly moving laminar blood flow appears "bright," while areas of stagnant flow and/or focal turbulence appear "dark" due to local saturation (stagnant flow) or dephasing (turbulence) (Figure 17-11). With bright blood coronary MRI, areas of focal stenoses appear as varying severity of "signal voids" with the severity of the signal loss related to the angiographic stenosis.[52] These studies used various protocols and had different selection criteria. The reported sensitivity and specificity varied widely. Recently, an international multicenter study using common hardware and imaging protocol was published, evaluating 107 patients who were referred for their first diagnos-

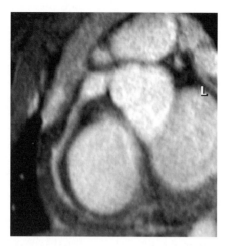 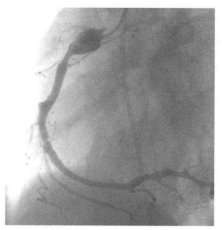

Figure 17-10. Proximal right coronary aneurysm in a patient with Kawasaki disease. Both coronary MRI (left panel) and conventional x-ray angiography (right panel) demonstrate the location and size of the coronary aneurysm. (Reprinted from Greil et al.[50] with permission.)

tic x-ray angiography.[53] Patients were being evaluated for routine clinical indications (e.g., evaluation of known or suspected CAD) and had a typical distribution of coronary risk factors (male predominance; the majority of subjects had hypercholesterolemia, family history of coronary disease, hypertension, and tobacco use), while approximately one quarter had a previous MI. Compared to the quantitative analysis of the x-ray angiogram, which was considered as the reference standard, MRI assessment of the coronaries had high sensitivity and negative predictive value for detecting significant coronary stenoses. The sensitivity for detection of any coronary disease, or left main/three-vessel disease was > 90%, with low–intermediate specificity.[54,55] These data demonstrate a clinical role for MRI evaluation of the coronaries, if the concern is severe/proximal disease. Although data are currently not yet sufficient to support the routine clinical use of coronary MRI for identification of coronary artery stenoses among patients presenting with chest pain or for screening purposes, MRI may have a clinical role for selected populations.

The widespread use of intracoronary metallic stents for elective and emergent interventions is a growing limitation for MRI of the coronaries.

The attractive force and local heating are negligible at 1.5T;[56–59] thus, imaging of patients with intracoronary stents is safe, even shortly after stent implantation. However, as stents are typically made from high-grade stainless steel, nitinol, tantalum, or alloy, they induce local susceptibility artifacts, with signal loss at the site of the stent. This artifact depends on both the stent material and the MRI sequence used, and may be substantial, precluding the direct evaluation of the coronary artery integrity in and around the stent. Assessment of blood flow/direction proximal and distal to the stent using MRI flow methods or spin-labeling methods may provide indirect evidence of a patent stent by documentation of antegrade flow.[60] This approach has the potential to add a physiologic evaluation to the assessment of the coronary arteries and may have particular value in circumventing the limitations posed by stents or surgical clips. Alternatively, the development of MRI-friendly stents[61] may allow better imaging of the stented vessels.

SPECTROSCOPY

Magnetic resonance is one of the very few techniques that allow the direct measurement of me-

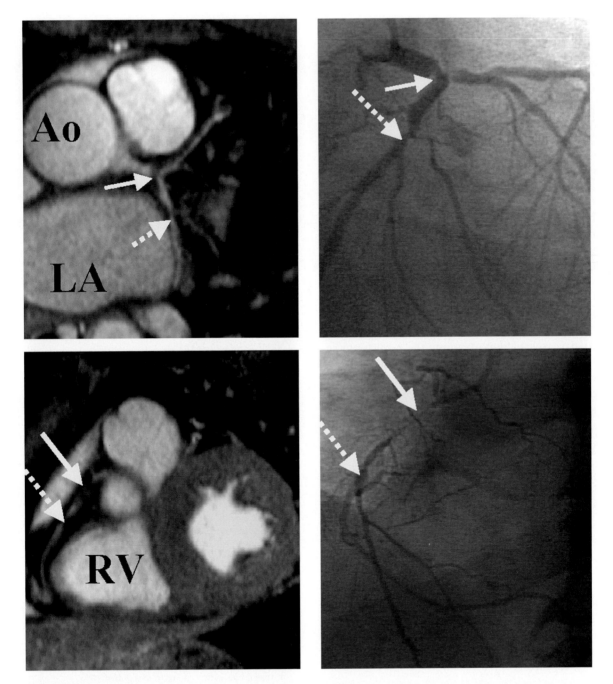

Figure 17-11. Coronary stenoses (arrows) in the left coronary arteries (upper panels) and the right coronary artery (lower panels). The MRI images are shown on the left and the conventional angiographic images are on the right. With bright blood MRI approaches focal coronary stenoses present as signal voids in the coronary vessel. LA = left atrium; RA = right atrium. (Reprinted from Kim et al.[55] with permission.)

tabolism at a cellular and subcellular level. With MR spectroscopy, the relative fractions of inorganic and organic phosphate is possible, and their changes in real time. Spectroscopy relies on the principle that the same atom may emit energy in different spectra, depending on the surrounding atoms in the molecule. Accordingly, the phosphorus spectrum is different for the various forms that phosphorus exists inside the cell (inorganic phosphate; phosphocreatine; and adenosine monophosphate, diphosphate, or triphosphate). The signal from these forms can be measured for a defined tissue sample and used to assess the in vivo energy/metabolic state. In women with syndrome X, an abnormal response to handgrip exercise measured with 32P-MR spectroscopy has been reported.[62] The greatest limitation of this approach, however, particularly for evaluation of the myocardium, is that the recorded signal is extremely weak. Thus, in order to have reliable information, the tissue sample needs to be relatively large (in the order of centimeters), and the recording times are long. For these reasons, MRI spectrometry has not yet taken a role in clinical diagnostic cardiology.

SUMMARY

Cardiac MRI is a noninvasive technology that allows assessment of all aspects of cardiovascular structure and function. It has very high resolution and enables quantitative measurements with great accuracy. Though presently MRI evaluation of cardiac anatomy and function have been extensively validated and have become routine clinical tools, MRI assessment of viability, perfusion, and stress testing are also gaining momentum. These, in combination with MRI coronary angiography may make cardiac MRI the dominant noninvasive modality for cardiac applications in the near future.

BIBLIOGRAPHY

1. Nienaber CA, von Kodolitsch Y, Nicolas V, et al. The diagnosis of thoracic aortic dissection by noninvasive imaging procedures. *N Engl J Med* 1993;328:1–9.

2. Sommer T, Fehske W, Holzknecht N, et al. Aortic dissection: A comparative study of diagnosis with spiral CT, multiplanar transesophageal echocardiography, and MR imaging. *Radiology* 1996;199:347–352.

3. White CS. MR evaluation of the pericardium and cardiac malignancies. *Magn Reson Imaging Clin N Am* 1996;4:237–251.

4. Sechtem U, Tscholakoff D, Higgins CB. MRI of the abnormal pericardium. *Am J Roentgenol* 1986; 147:245–252.

5. Masui T, Finck S, Higgins CB. Constrictive pericarditis and restrictive cardiomyopathy: Evaluation with MR imaging. *Radiology* 1992;182:369–373.

6. Posma JL, Blanksma PK, van der Wall EE, et al. Assessment of quantitative hypertrophy scores in hypertrophic cardiomyopathy: Magnetic resonance imaging versus echocardiography. *Am Heart J* 1996;132:1020–1027.

7. Pons-Llado G, Carreras F, Borras X, et al. Comparison of morphologic assessment of hypertrophic cardiomyopathy by magnetic resonance versus echocardiographic imaging. *Am J Cardiol* 1997;79:1651–1656.

8. Di Cesare E. MRI of the cardiomyopathies. *Eur J Radiol* 2001;38:179–184.

9. Friedrich MG, Strohm O, Schulz-Menger J, et al. Contrast media-enhanced magnetic resonance imaging visualizes myocardial changes in the course of viral myocarditis. *Circulation* 1998;97:1802–1809.

10. van der Wall EE, Kayser HW, Bootsma MM, et al. Arrhythmogenic right ventricular dysplasia: MRI findings. *Herz* 2000;25:356–364.

11. Anderson LJ, Holden S, Davis B, et al. Cardiovascular T2-star (T2*) magnetic resonance for the early diagnosis of myocardial iron overload. *Eur Heart J* 2001;22:2171–2179.

12. Vignaux O, Dhote R, Duboc D, et al. Clinical significance of myocardial magnetic resonance abnormalities in patients with sarcoidosis: A 1-year follow-up study. *Chest* 2002;122:1895–1901.

13. Vignaux O, Dhote R, Duboc D, et al. Detection of myocardial involvement in patients with sarcoidosis applying T2-weighted, contrast-enhanced, and cine magnetic resonance imaging: Initial results of a prospective study. *J Comput Assist Tomogr* 2002;26:762–767.

14. Shimada T, Shimada K, Sakane T, et al. Diagnosis of cardiac sarcoidosis and evaluation of the effects of steroid therapy by gadolinium-DTPA-enhanced magnetic resonance imaging. *Am J Med* 2001; 110:520–527.

15. Sakuma H, Fujita N, Foo TK, et al. Evaluation of left ventricular volume and mass with breath-hold cine MR imaging. *Radiology* 1993;188:377–380.

16. Rominger MB, Bachmann GF, Pabst W, Rau WS. Right ventricular volumes and ejection fraction with fast cine

MR imaging in breath-hold technique: Applicability, normal values from 52 volunteers, and evaluation of 325 adult cardiac patients. *J Magn Reson Imaging* 1999;10:908–918.

17. Roest AA, Kunz P, Lamb HJ, Helbing WA, van der Wall EE, de Roos A. Biventricular response to supine physical exercise in young adults assessed with ultrafast magnetic resonance imaging. *Am J Cardiol* 2001;87:601–605.

18. Nagel E, Lehmkuhl HB, Bocksch W, et al. Noninvasive diagnosis of ischemia-induced wall motion abnormalities with the use of high-dose dobutamine stress MRI: Comparison with dobutamine stress echocardiography. *Circulation* 1999;99:763–770.

19. Hundley WG, Hamilton CA, Thomas MS, et al. Utility of fast cine magnetic resonance imaging and display for the detection of myocardial ischemia in patients not well suited for second harmonic stress echocardiography. *Circulation* 1999;100:1697–1702.

20. Hundley WG, Morgan TM, Neagle CM, et al. Magnetic resonance imaging determination of cardiac prognosis. *Circulation* 2002;106:2328–2333.

21. Arai AE, Epstein FH, Bove KE, Wolff SD. Visualization of aortic valve leaflets using black blood MRI. *J Magn Reson Imaging* 1999;10:771–777.

22. Davis CP, McKinnon GC, Debatin JF, et al. Single-shot versus interleaved echo-planar MR imaging: Application to visualization of cardiac valve leaflets. *J Magn Reson Imaging* 1995;5:107–112.

23. Didier D, Ratib O, Lerch R, Friedli B. Detection and quantification of valvular heart disease with dynamic cardiac MR imaging. *Radiographics* 2000; 20:1279–1299; discussion 1299–1301.

24. Al-Saadi N, Nagel E, Gross M, et al. Noninvasive detection of myocardial ischemia from perfusion reserve based on cardiovascular magnetic resonance. *Circulation* 2000;101:1379–1383.

25. Panting JR, Gatehouse PD, Yang GZ, et al. Echo-planar magnetic resonance myocardial perfusion imaging: Parametric map analysis and comparison with thallium SPECT. *J Magn Reson Imaging* 2001;13:192–200.

26. Keijer JT, van Rossum AC, van Eenige MJ, et al. Magnetic resonance imaging of regional myocardial perfusion in patients with single-vessel coronary artery disease: Quantitative comparison with (201)Thallium-SPECT and coronary angiography. *J Magn Reson Imaging* 2000;11:607–615.

27. Penzkofer H, Wintersperger BJ, Knez A, et al. Assessment of myocardial perfusion using multisection first-pass MRI and color-coded parameter maps: A comparison to 99mTc Sesta MIBI SPECT and systolic myocardial wall thickening analysis. *Magn Reson Imaging* 1999;17:161–170.

28. Matheijssen NA, Louwerenburg HW, van Rugge FP, et al. Comparison of ultrafast dipyridamole magnetic resonance imaging with dipyridamole SestaMIBI SPECT for detection of perfusion abnormalities in patients with one-vessel coronary artery disease: Assessment by quantitative model fitting. *Magn Reson Med* 1996;35:221–228.

29. Klein MA, Collier BD, Hellman RS, Bamrah VS. Detection of chronic coronary artery disease: Value of pharmacologically stressed, dynamically enhanced turbo-fast low-angle shot MR images. *Am J Roentgenol* 1993;161:257–263.

30. Vallee JP, Lazeyras F, Kasuboski L, et al. Quantification of myocardial perfusion with FAST sequence and Gd bolus in patients with normal cardiac function. *J Magn Reson Imaging* 1999;9:197–203.

31. Schwitter J, Nanz D, Kneifel S, et al. Assessment of myocardial perfusion in coronary artery disease by magnetic resonance: A comparison with positron emission tomography and coronary angiography. *Circulation* 2001;103:2230–2235.

32. Wisenberg G, Prato FS, Carroll SE, et al. Serial nuclear magnetic resonance imaging of acute myocardial infarction with and without reperfusion. *Am Heart J* 1988;115:510–518.

33. McNamara MT, Higgins CB, Schechtmann N, et al. Detection and characterization of acute myocardial infarction in man with use of gated magnetic resonance. *Circulation* 1985;71:717–724.

34. Wisenberg G, Finnie KJ, Jablonsky G, et al. Nuclear magnetic resonance and radionuclide angiographic assessment of acute myocardial infarction in a randomized trial of intravenous streptokinase. *Am J Cardiol* 1988;62:1011–1016.

35. Shapiro EP, Rogers WJ, Beyar R, et al. Determination of left ventricular mass by magnetic resonance imaging in hearts deformed by acute infarction. *Circulation* 1989;79:706–711.

36. Baer FM, Voth E, Schneider CA, et al. Comparison of low-dose dobutamine-gradient-echo magnetic resonance imaging and positron emission tomography with [18F]fluorodeoxyglucose in patients with chronic coronary artery disease: A functional and morphological approach to the detection of residual myocardial viability. *Circulation* 1995;91:1006–1015.

37. Pislaru SV, Ni Y, Pislaru C, et al. Noninvasive measurements of infarct size after thrombolysis with a necrosis-avid MRI contrast agent. *Circulation* 1999;99:690–696.

38. Rehwald WG, Fieno DS, Chen EL, et al. Myocardial magnetic resonance imaging contrast agent concentrations after reversible and irreversible ischemic injury. *Circulation* 2002;105:224–229.

39. Kim RJ, Judd RM, Chen EL, et al. Relationship of elevated ^{23}Na magnetic resonance image intensity to infarct size after acute reperfused myocardial infarction. *Circulation* 1999;100:185–192.

40. Simonetti OP, Kim RJ, Fieno DS, et al. An improved MR imaging technique for the visualization of myocardial infarction. *Radiology* 2001;218:215–223.

41. Wu E, Judd RM, Vargas JD, et al. Visualisation of presence, location, and transmural extent of healed Q-wave and non-Q-wave myocardial infarction. *Lancet* 2001;357:21–28.

42. Kim RJ, Wu E, Rafael A, et al. The use of contrast-enhanced magnetic resonance imaging to identify reversible myocardial dysfunction. *N Engl J Med* 2000; 343:1445–1453.

43. Mollet NR, Dymarkowski S, Volders W, et al. Visualization of ventricular thrombi with contrast-enhanced magnetic resonance imaging in patients with ischemic heart disease. *Circulation* 2002; 106:2873–2876.

44. Klein C, Nekolla SG, Bengel FM, et al. Assessment of myocardial viability with contrast-enhanced magnetic resonance imaging: Comparison with positron emission tomography. *Circulation* 2002;105:162–167.

45. Vliegen HW, Doornbos J, de Roos A, et al. Value of fast gradient echo magnetic resonance angiography as an adjunct to coronary arteriography in detecting and confirming the course of clinically significant coronary artery anomalies. *Am J Cardiol* 1997;79:773–776.

46. Post JC, van Rossum AC, Bronzwaer JG, et al. Magnetic resonance angiography of anomalous coronary arteries: A new gold standard for delineating the proximal course? *Circulation* 1995;92:3163–3171.

47. Taylor AM, Thorne SA, Rubens MB, et al. Coronary artery imaging in congenital heart disease: Complementary role of magnetic resonance and x-ray coronary angiography (Abstract). *J Cardiovasc Magn Reson* 1999;1:284–285.

48. McConnell MV, Ganz P, Selwyn AP, et al. Identification of anomalous coronary arteries and their anatomic course by magnetic resonance coronary angiography. *Circulation* 1995;92:3158–3162.

49. Razmi RM, Meduri A, Chun W, et al. Coronary magnetic resonance angiography (CMRA): The gold standard for determining the proximal course of anomalous coronary arteries (Abstract). *J Am Coll Cardiol* 2001;37:380.

50. Greil GF, Stuber M, Botnar RM, et al. Coronary magnetic resonance angiography in adolescents and young adults with kawasaki disease. *Circulation* 2002;105:908–911.

51. Langerak SE, Vliegen HW, de Roos A, et al. Detection of vein graft disease using high-resolution magnetic resonance angiography. *Circulation* 2002;105:328–333.

52. Pennell DJ, Bogren HG, Keegan J, et al. Assessment of coronary artery stenosis by magnetic resonance imaging. *Heart* 1996;75:127–133.

53. Kim WY, Danias PG, Stuber M, et al. Coronary magnetic resonance angiography for the detection of coronary stenoses. *N Engl J Med* 2001;345:1863–1869.

54. McConnell MV, Stuber M, Manning WJ. Clinical role of coronary magnetic resonance angiography in the diagnosis of anomalous coronary arteries. *J Cardiovasc Magn Reson* 2000;2:217–224.

55. Kim WY, Danias PG, Stuber M, et al. Coronary magnetic resonance angiography for the detection of coronary stenoses. *N Engl J Med* 2001;345:1863–1869.

56. Kramer CM, Rogers WJ, Pakstis DL. Absence of adverse outcomes after magnetic resonance imaging early after sent placement for acute myocardial infarction. *J Cardiovasc Magn Reson* 2000;2:257–261.

57. Scott NA, Pettigrew RI. Absence of movement of coronary stents after placement in a magnetic resonance imaging field. *Am J Cardiol* 1994;73:900–901.

58. Hug J, Nagel E, Bornstedt A, et al. Coronary arterial stents: Safety and artifacts during MR imaging. *Radiology* 2000;216:781–787.

59. Strohm O, Kivelitz D, Gross W, et al. Safety of implantable coronary stents during 1H-magnetic resonance imaging at 1.0 and 1.5 T. *J Cardiovasc Magn Reson* 1999;1:239–245.

60. Hundley WG, Hillis LD, Hamilton CA, et al. Assessment of coronary arterial restenosis with phase-contrast magnetic resonance imaging measurements of coronary flow reserve. *Circulation* 2000; 101:2375–2381.

61. Buecker A, Spuentrup E, Ruebben A, Gunther RW. Artifact-free in-stent lumen visualization by standard magnetic resonance angiography using a new metallic magnetic resonance imaging stent. *Circulation* 2002;105:1772–1775.

62. Buchthal SD, den Hollander JA, Merz CN, et al. Abnormal myocardial phosphorus-31 nuclear magnetic resonance spectroscopy in women with chest pain but normal coronary angiograms. *N Engl J Med* 2000;342:829–835

CHAPTER 18

Cardiac Catheterization

R. Jeffrey Snell
Susie Kim

INTRODUCTION

Claude Bernard performed the first documented cardiac catheterization on a horse in 1844. He measured pressures in the right and left ventricles using an antegrade approach from the jugular vein for the right ventricle and a retrograde approach via the carotid artery for the left ventricle. Over 100 years later, selective angiography was first performed by F. Sones. In 1977, Andreas Grüntzig changed the direction of invasive cardiology from a purely diagnostic modality to a therapeutic one by developing the concept of percutaneous transcoronary angioplasty.[1] Scientists and physicians have combined to develop and refine techniques to help quantitate left ventricular (LV) function and the severity of coronary artery disease (CAD). The standard invasive approach to assessing LV function is by performing contrast left ventriculogram. A number of techniques are used to determine lesion severity, divided into methods (1) to visualize the mor-

phology of disease and (2) to perform a hemodynamic assessment of a lesion. Visual estimation, quantitative coronary angiography, intravascular ultrasound, and angioscopy are techniques to visualize and quantify the plaques. The Thrombolysis in Myocardial Infarction Study (TIMI) flow/TIMI frame count, coronary flow reserve, and fractional flow reserve are methods for the hemodynamic assessment of a coronary lesion. This chapter will review the invasive techniques used in the cardiac catheterization laboratory to evaluate LV function and quantify the degree of CAD.

LEFT VENTRICULOGRAPHY

The information obtained by performing a left ventriculogram is an integral part of a comprehensive diagnostic cardiac catheterization. The knowledge of a patient's LV function, the presence of segmental wall motion abnormalities, and valvular function is not only helpful in the assessment of CAD, but it also allows any subsequent interventional procedure to be performed in a safe fashion. A left ventriculogram may also provide additional information regarding the presence of congenital defects, cardiomyopathies, ventricular septal abnormalities, and the presence of a mural thrombus in the left ventricular cavity.

Technique

The most commonly used catheter for left ventriculograms in the modern cardiac catheterization laboratory is a 6 Fr pigtail catheter. The tip of this catheter has a coiled or loop shape and contains multiple side holes permitting contrast to be injected at high pressure without catheter recoil or myocardial perforation, by keeping the catheter away from the myocardium and by distributing the contrast injection in multiple angles. Following the baseline measurement of aortic pressure, the catheter is manipulated into the left ventricle, taking care to ensure that the catheter is not entrapped in the papillary muscles and is in the midportion of the left ventricle. In this position, the contrast is evenly distributed throughout the ventricle and the presence of mitral valve regurgitation (MVR) can be evaluated without being confounded by catheter-induced regurgitation. For patient safety, as well as obtaining an accurate study, the position of the catheter should be manipulated such that no ventricular ectopy is produced. During this time, pressure measurements should be obtained to detect any gradient between the aorta and the left ventricle, suggesting aortic valve disease, or within the left ventricular cavity, suggesting subaortic stenosis or hypertrophic obstructive cardiomyopathy. Fluoroscopy of the left ventricle may be used to detect valvular calcification and the presence of mural thrombus.

Contrast injection generally is performed with the use of a power injector, allowing a large (approximately 20–40cc) amount of contrast to be injected over a short period of time. This improves the acquisition of complete opacification of the left ventricle for a better study.

Ideally, biplane (as opposed to single-plane) ventriculography should be performed. Simultaneous image acquisition with a second camera permits information to be obtained by adding a third dimension rather than just the two-dimensional view of a single plane without exposing the patient to an additional procedure or extra contrast. The drawback of biplane ventriculography is that it is cumbersome and expensive to have an additional camera, there is additional radiation exposure to the catheterization laboratory personnel, and the image acquired from each camera does not have the quality of a single view due to the increased scattering of radiation from opposing cameras. If a single camera is used, the projection should be in an approximately 30-degree right anterior oblique (RAO) projection for the best representative view of the wall segments of the left ventricle and to assess the mitral valve.

Contrast ventriculography is considered the gold standard for LV function and contains two parts: ejection fraction and wall motion. The assessment by ventriculography can be graded by visual estimation or by calculation based on the end-diastolic volume and end-systolic volume and the use of the area–length equation (Simpson's rule). Generally, the ejection fraction is described as normal (50–69%), mildly depressed (35–49%), moderately depressed (26–34%), severely depressed ($\leq 25\%$), or hyperkinetic ($\geq 70\%$). Wall motion is assessed as degree of contraction per segment of the left ventricle. Obviously, if only a single-plane ventriculography is performed, not all of the wall segments will be scored. The values designated for wall motion are normal, mild hypokinesis (contraction of the myocardium but to a lesser degree than a normal segment), moderate hypokinesis (reduced but easily perceived contraction), severe hypokinesis (mild contraction of the myocardium), akinesis (no contraction), dyskinesis (paradoxical movement of the myocardial segment during contraction), and aneurysmal (dilated baseline myocardial segment). The Coronary Artery Surgery Study designated numerical values for wall motion in the single plane view (normal = 1, mild hypokinesis = 2, severe hypokinesis = 3, akinesis = 4, dyskinesis = 5, and aneurysm = 6).[2] The sum of the scores (5 being the lowest attainable score and 30 the highest) was helpful in determining surgical risk of patients undergoing bypass surgery.[3] Wall motion may also be used for the determination of ischemia or viability of the myocardium, although these techniques are not in widespread use.[4–6]

Risks

There are risks to the patient involved with left ventriculography. Although adverse events are rare, the most common complication is inducing arrhythmias, usually during the injection of contrast, due to the irritation of the myocardium to the force of the contrast, or by the catheter itself. However, persistent ventricular tachycardia or fibrillation is rare, but if it were to occur, standard protocol for treatment of these dysrhythmias should ensue. Hemiblocks, due to the position of the fascicle in the outflow tract, may occur rarely due to trauma from the catheter. If the patient has an existing bifascicular block (right bundle branch block and left posterior block), then the patient may require a prophylactic temporary pacemaker. Perforation and endomyocardial staining are rare complications of a left ventriculography and result from the force of the contrast injection or trauma from the catheter itself. Emergent periocardiocentesis and surgery is required for perforations. Generally, endomyocardial staining does not have a high risk of morbid sequelae, but, if large enough, they could become a nidus for arrhythmias. Air or thromboemboli may occur if a fastidious approach is not taken during the procedure. The risk of emboli from thrombus may be reduced by giving heparin or by frequent flushing of the sheath and catheter during the procedure. In the setting of a normal thrombus, the need for a left ventriculogram should be reevaluated, as embolization may occur following catheter manipulation.

The contrast agent also presents a potential risk. Contrast nephropathy will be discussed later in this chapter. Patients with severe LV failure and hemodynamic evidence of decompensation are at risk for acute pulmonary edema from contrast agent intravascular volume expansion. Low-osmolar agents should be used to reduce any myocardial depression and the volume reduced in dilated, dysfunctional ventricles.

MORPHOLOGIC ASSESSMENT OF CORONARY DISEASE

Visual Assessment

The most widely used method to quantify coronary artery stenosis today is by visual estimate. To achieve a high degree of confidence in using this technique, a number of factors must be present. Since contrast angiography gives only a two-dimensional view of a three-dimensional object, the ostium, proximal, midsegment, and distal portions of the coronary arteries must be viewed in multiple orthogonal views. This is particularly important when evaluating a lesion with an indeterminate degree of narrowing, then the lesion morphology becomes an important factor. As lesions are commonly eccentric, the lumen in one projection may not seem to be significantly affected, although in a different view the severity of the lesion would be more pronounced. Frequently, subtle clues, such as haziness, a lesser degree of contrast density of a lesion, or impaired flow, are noted by the experienced angiographer to help estimate the degree of narrowing. The experience and technical skills of the angiographer is another very important factor. Often, coronary arteries are found to be anomalous or quite tortuous in nature, thus limiting the ability of the angiographer to find proper views of coronary segments. Although the visual assessment of a stenosis is the most common method, it is commonly fraught with errors. There have been multiple studies demonstrating wide intraobserver and interobserver variability.[7–8] Postmortem studies of coronary disease have shown that there is a tendency for the underestimation of the degree of narrowing when compared to coronary angiography.[9–12]

Quantitative Coronary Analysis (QCA)

QCA is an adjunctive technique used with coronary angiography to more accurately measure vessel size and degree of stenosis. There are a number of software programs from different manufacturers; however, the general concept is the same. The angiographer chooses a frame from a cineangiogram run that is a good representation of the lesion. The angiogram is digitized into at least a 512 × 512 × 8-bit pixel matrix. Calibration of pixel size must then be performed, often done by measurement of an object on the cineangiogram frame with a known size and expressed as millimeters/pixel. The vessel and lesion in question are outlined either manually or by "edge detection" software. A preprogrammed algorithm then determines the coronary dimensions and degree of stenosis by percentage (Figure 18-1). The reference diameter is determined by an average or extrapolation

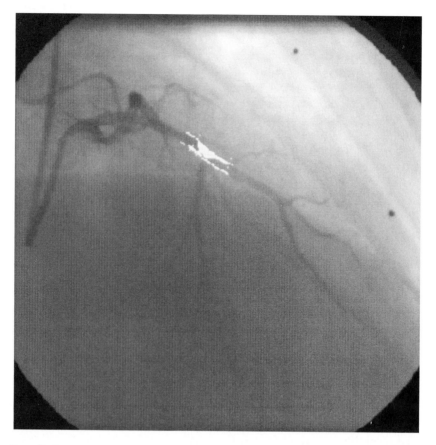

Figure 18-1. Quantitative coronary angiography (QCA). This is an angiogram of a 41-year-old male with recent onset angina and anterolateral ischemia noted on an exercise SPECT study. Angiography revealed a 50 to 70% lesion of the mid LAD. A QCA was performed and calculated the stenoses to be 76%. A PCI was performed on this lesion.

from two points equidistant from the narrowest section. This method of lesion assessment eliminates the subjective nature of visual estimates and reduces interobserver variability.[13–15]

QCA has its own set of limitations. Since the measurement is based on the cineangiogram selected by the angiographer, the measurement can only be as good as the image itself—a foreshortened view of the lesion or a vessel underfilled with contrast may falsely increase the severity of stenosis. A change in vasomotor tone, commonly distal to the lesion, or a lesion out of plane in the cineangiogram can have a variable effect on the degree of stenosis calculated by QCA. To counteract this, intracoronary vasodilators should be given prior to image acquisition. Edge detection can be difficult if there is significant branch overlap or if the disease is so diffuse that there is no "normal" segment from which to mark as the reference vessel.

Angioscopy

Intracoronary angioscopy is a method of evaluating coronary lesions by direct visualization of the vessel wall and its lesion in a blood-free field. The system used for this has two main parts: the imaging network and the delivery device. The imaging network consists of a high-intensity light source, fiber-optic bundle (for imaging and for illumination via the light source), a video monitor, and a recorder for record archiving. The delivery catheter houses some of the imaging equipment and also creates a blood-free field so that images can be obtained. The catheter has a compliant occlusion balloon at its distal end. By inflating this balloon to the point of complete occlusion while injecting saline, a blood-free vessel is created. Care must be taken to monitor the balloon time to avoid unnecessary ischemia and is generally limited to 90 seconds.

The main advantage to angioscopy over coronary angiography is its ability to directly visualize the vessel wall and lesions as well. It is ideal for differentiating among plaque, dissection, and thrombus, which are commonly noted only as a radiolucent area by angiography.[16–18] Even intravascular ultrasound cannot reliably distinguish between a soft plaque and thrombus. This is particularly useful to help determine the successfulness of an angioplasty procedure if there is a question as to dissection or edge after angioplasty. Some have advocated the use of angioscopy in transplanted patients, as their lesion characteristics for allograft vasculopathy tend to be diffuse. On regular cineangiography these might be seen as angiographically normal; however, with angioscopy, the intimal hyperplasia or fibrofatty plaques are easily seen.

Characterization of disease in saphenous vein grafts (SVGs) is another application of angioscopy, determining the extent of thrombus, plaque, or friable tissue that would identify the procedure as high risk and clue the interventionalist to provide precautions that may not otherwise have been done. Finally, there is no better imaging modality available to identify acute thrombosis in the coronary artery and to distinguish which vessel is the culprit vessel.[19]

There are drawbacks or limitations to the use of angioscopy. The catheter itself is bulky; thus, visualization in tortuous vessels or lesions in the distal vessel has a low success rate. Angioscopy is a qualitative measurement of a lesion and does not provide quantification of stenosis. Also, as a blood-free field is needed, aorto-ostial disease cannot be readily assessed due to difficulty in maintaining a saline-filled vessel. Finally, the complications seen with angioscopy contribute to the reluctance for angiographers to use this technique. Although the risk of major complications (myocardial infarction [MI], stroke, death, or serious arrhythmia) is < 2%, the need for subsequent percutaneous transluminal coronary angioplasty (PTCA) after balloon deflation and the risk of no reflow in SVGs are relatively high (9% and 45%, respectively).[20–21]

Intravascular Ultrasound (IVUS)

IVUS is probably the most accurate method of measuring coronary disease today. In this method, a 2.0 Fr catheter with a piezoelectric crystal mounted on the end is advanced over a

0.014-inch guidewire into the coronary artery to a point distal to the lesion. Images are acquired as the catheter is retracted back into the guide, either manually or by an automated approach. The major advantage of the automated pullback device is that the length of a lesion can be measured. This technique may also be used for serial assessments; assuming the same distal landmark is used and the pullback device is set at the same speed, two studies of an artery performed at different times can accurately be compared to each other millimeter by millimeter.

The American College of Cardiology, in collaboration with the European Society of Cardiology and the Society of Cardiac Angiography and Interventions, published a consensus statement to standardize definitions and measurements used in intravascular ultrasound.[22] While making measurements, care must be given to clearly define the leading edge of the intima and adventitia. Extensive calcification cause "shadowing" as the ultrasound beams can detect only the innermost layer of calcium.

IVUS enhances our understanding of the composition the lesion or stenosis in question, which would influence the way lesions are treated. Soft, lipid-filled plaques, fibrous plaques, and calcified lesions each have unique IVUS characteristics. The soft plaques tend to be fairly echolucent, indicative of a high content of lipids,[23–25] whereas calcified lesions are highly echogenic. Fibrous plaques falls somewhere in between. Highly calcified lesions generally are not amenable to balloon angioplasty. Depending on the severity of the calcification, rotoblator atherectomy or cutting balloon angioplasty would be the device of choice in these lesions. Therefore, IVUS can help guide the choice of intervention. IVUS can also help to determine the size and length of a stent needed for a particular lesion. Since the diameter of the vessel is clearly seen with the use of IVUS, the measurement is much more accurate than that of contrast angiography, which reveals only the lumen size of the vessel and could underestimate the vessel caliber in vessels with diffuse disease. Additionally,

as a low minimal-lumen diameter is a predictor for restenosis, it becomes important for an interventionalist to optimize acute luminal gain during the procedure. For example, underdeployed stents, often seen as a haziness (due to thrombus or dissection) at the site of intervention, can negatively influence the outcome of the procedure if not identified and treated properly.

An important application for the use of IVUS in a diagnostic coronary angiography is for the assessment of indeterminate lesions (Figure 18-2), especially those of the left main artery. IVUS imaging of the left main artery enables the angiographer to visualize the disease in relation to the artery free of the limitations faced by contrast angiography. Another use of IVUS is in pa-

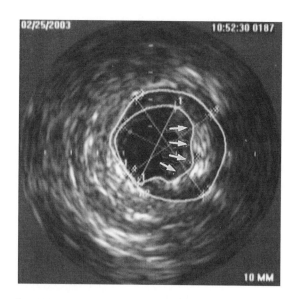

Figure 18-2.   Intravascular ultrasound (IVUS) of the LAD. This is an IVUS of a 52-year-old asymptomatic gentleman who had a positive stress test performed for preoperative clearance. The angiogram revealed an intermediate lesion in the mid LAD. An IVUS was performed. The inner circle represents the lumen of the vessel. The lumen area calculated to be 6.8 mm². The outer circle is the external elastic membrane and represents the reference diameter of the vessel. The reference diameter of the vessel calculated to be 13.6 mm². The area stenosis is 50%. The arrows indicate the crescent-shaped eccentric atheromatous plaque.

tients after cardiac transplants to detect cardiac allograft vasculopathy.[26–27]

HEMODYNAMIC ASSESSMENT OF CORONARY DISEASE

The hemodynamic assessment of a stenosis centers on the concept of coronary flow and the impact of a significant stenosis. While noninvasive methods such as myocardial perfusion imaging (MPI) and echocardiography (ECHO) may be used to indirectly assess coronary flow, this chapter will focus primarily on the invasive measurement of myocardial blood flow.

Determinants of Coronary Vascular Resistance

Myocardial blood flow is primarily regulated at the level of the arteriole by physiologic or pharmacologic factors. The larger epicardial coronary vessels contribute minimally to the total coronary vascular resistance. Autoregulation is the ability for the coronary bed to maintain a constant perfusion despite changes driving pressure.[28] The mechanism of autoregulation has yet to be defined; however, there is strong support for nitric oxide[29,30] and the vascular smooth muscle[31,32] as being the main factors involved. Autoregulation can be seen clinically in humans by epicardial coronary lesions that cause a change in the driving pressure. As the driving pressure drops with a hemodynamically significant lesion, the distal coronary bed dilates to compensate.

Myocardial oxygen consumption is a potent regulator of coronary blood flow. The metabolism of the myocardium is chiefly aerobic. The myocardium has a high oxygen extraction rate,[33] as evidenced by the low coronary venous saturation of 25 to 30%. Increased oxygen demand stimulates vasodilation[34–37] of the coronary bed. A hemodynamically significant epicardial lesion can inhibit blood flow to the distal myocardium, causing a relative hypoxic state to the myocardium it supplies, which in turn stimulates the distal vessel to dilate to enhance oxygen avail-

ability to the area. The vascular endothelium of the coronary bed produces a number of factors that regulate vascular tone by dilatation or constriction. Endothelial-derived relaxing factor (EDRF), now identified as nitric oxide (NO)[38,39] was initially discovered in the early 1980s. EDRF decreases intracellular calcium by stimulating cyclic guanosine monophosphate (cGMP), thus causing dilation of the vascular smooth muscle.[40] EDRF is continuously released by the vascular bed to maintain homeostatic control of blood flow. EDRF release is stimulated by vasoconstrictors. Interestingly, acetylcholine produces an overall vasodilating effect when working in combination with healthy endothelium. Other vasoconstrictors, such as alpha-adrenergic agonists, have a net vasoconstrictive effect; however, their full effect is curtailed by the presence of EDRF. Other stimulants of EDRF include serotonin, adenosine diphosphate (ADP), histamine, bradykinin, increased shear stress, and thrombin.[41] The endothelium is vulnerable to factors that may impair its function. These factors, are related to early atherosclerosis and its risk factors, such as dyslipidemia[42–45] diabetes,[46] and so on. When the endothelium is impaired, the vasomotor response to previously mentioned agents has a net constrictive effect due to loss of EDRF or NO attenuation.[41,42,47] Prostacyclin and endothelium-derived hypoerpolarizing factor (EDHF) are more controversial factors of endothelium-derived vasodilators. EDHF is stimulated by similar factors as EDRF, but it does not play a significant role unless the production of EDRF is impaired.[47,48] Prostacyclin's major influence in vasodilation also seems to occur when NO production is impaired by affecting flow-mediated and metabolic dilation.[41]

Intracoronary Doppler Measurement

The Doppler effect, named for the Austrian scientist Christian Johann Doppler, is the change in the wavelength and frequency as a transmitter changes its distance from the receiver. As the transmitter comes closer to the receiver, the wavelength decreases and thus the frequency increases. The converse is true as the transmitter moves away from the receiver, the wavelength increases, and the frequency decreases. Velocity of red blood cells within a coronary artery may be determined by using a piezoelectric crystal that can both transmit and receive high-frequency sounds and directing its ultrasonic beam toward a target. The Doppler shift represents the difference between the received and transmitted frequency. Velocity also has a direct relationship with blood flow. The difference in Doppler velocities represent changes in coronary blood flow given a constant cross-sectional area (CSA).

Historically, intracoronary Doppler catheters were bulky (3–4 Fr), difficult to use, and could potentially cause false readings by their sheer size obstructing blood flow and encroaching on the CSA of the lumen, especially in smaller or diseased arteries. The latest generation of the Doppler measurement devices has a piezoelectric crystal mounted on a guidewire. This Doppler-tipped 12 to 15-MHz transducer guidewire (0.014–0.018-inch diameter) eliminated most of the limitations of its bulky predecessor. The ultrasound beam is broad providing a large sample size.[49,50] The Doppler signals obtained from the transducer are displayed in real time onto a monitor along with heart rate and other parameters. Technical limitations of the accuracy of Doppler measurement include stenosis geometry and sample volume too small to measure true maximal velocity.[51] A Doppler guidewire can measure the hemodynamics of a lesion in a number of ways.

Coronary blood flow may increase up to fourfold from its resting state in response to physiologic (autoregulation, hypoxia, or neurogenic stimuli) or pharmacologic stimuli (norepinephrine, papaverine, dipyridamole, serotonin, vasopressin, nitroglycerin, adenosine, NO/EDRF). Coronary flow reserve (CFR) is the ratio of hyperemic to resting blood flow velocity. A "normal" ratio is > 2. A hemodynamically significant epicardial lesion causes the postlesion arterioles to dilate to compensate for the reduced perfusion pressure and decreased oxygen supply. When this happens, the response to a pharmacologic agent (e.g., adenosine) is blunted as maximum dilation/velocity postlesion has already been achieved. This would result in an abnormal CFR of < 2. Figure 18-3 contains examples of normal and abnormal CFR measurements.

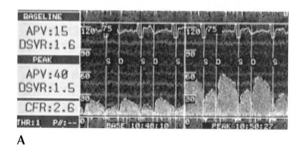
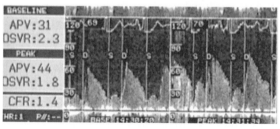

A   B

Figure 18-3.   Coronary flow reserve (CFR). **A.** A CFR was performed on a 52-year-old male with known coronary artery disease and multiple percutaneous coronary interventions (PCI) in the past. He had recurrence of his typical angina. The angiogram revealed a 50 to 60% lesion in the mid RCA. The baseline parameters included an average peak velocity (APV) of 15 cm/sec and a borderline diastolic-to-systolic velocity ratio (DSVR) of APV 1.6. After the administration of intracoronary adenosine, the APV increased to 40 cm/sec, the DSVR was 1.8, and the CFR was normal at 2.6. No intervention was performed. **B.** This patient was a 65-year-old female with a history of a previous PCI who presented with unstable angina. The angiogram revealed a borderline lesion in the proximal circumflex. The baseline parameters included an APV of 31 cm/sec and a DSVR of 2.3. After the administration of intracoronary adenosine, the APV increased only to 44 cm/sec, the DSVR was 1.8, and the CFR abnormal at 1.4. A PCI was therefore performed on this lesion.

There are some important factors that alter the measurement of CFR independent of lesion severity. Changes in the patient's hemodynamic state during the acquisition of data can alter the readings. Tachycardia,[52] increased contractility, and adrenergic stimulation[53,54] will increase CFR. Increased mean arterial pressure may falsely lower the CFR measurement. Abnormalities in the microcirculation could potentially blunt the CFR, giving a "falsely" low reading. Conditions that alter the microcirculation (e.g., syndrome X, hypertension,[52,55,56] diabetes mellitus,[57] infiltrative cardiomyopathy, and myocardial scarring) should be taken into consideration if CFR is measured. Aortic stenosis and left ventricular hypertrophy (LVH) may also give a falsely low CFR.[58–61]

The relative CFR (rCFR) is determined by the ratio of absolute CFR in the targeted coronary artery (i.e., the vessel with a lesion) to the absolute CFR in a coronary artery without disease. rCFR negates the effect of aortic pressure and rate pressure product that plagues absolute CFR as this is thought to be more accurate in determining percent area stenosis and correlates better with other modalities.[59,62–64] However, rCFR can be used only in conditions in which there is a normal coronary artery hyperemic response; those with triple-vessel disease or regional ventricular impairment may have false measurements of rCFR.[65]

The relationship of the velocity of blood flow in a proximal coronary artery segment to its distal counterpart in normal coronary arteries (left anterior descending [LAD], left circumflex, and right coronary artery) has been investigated.[66] An abnormal proximal/distal (P/D) ratio (> 1.7) is due to redistribution of flow to branches of the vessel proximal to the lesion. The value of this test is limited with a low overall sensitivity and specificity for identifying stenoses with significant gradients.[67]

Positron emission tomography (PET) is thought to be the best noninvasive equivalent to CFR and has been shown to correlate well with the intracoronary Doppler flow reserve. PET regional myocardial blood flow and myocardial perfusion reserve were directly compared to Doppler average peak flow velocity (APV) and CFR, respectively, and revealed linear correlation.[68] Perfusion defects seen in exercise 201 thallium (Tl-201) single photon emission computed tomography (SPECT) were also found to correlate well with abnormal intracoronary Doppler assessment[69,70] and was found to be superior to quantitative coronary angiography.[70] The relation of perfusion imaging and CFR is unclear when multivessel disease is present, although a recent study demonstrates that CFR is predictive of outcomes for an indeterminate lesion.[71]

Fractional flow reserve (FFR) is the fraction of normal maximal flow that can be achieved in an artery with a lesion. FFR is measured by the ratio of maximum myocardial blood flow of the artery with a lesion to the theoretical maximum blood flow of the artery if it had no lesion. The FFR in a normal artery is 1.0, because in the absence of a lesion, pressure is constant throughout the coronary bed. In the presence of a significant lesion, the maximal blood flow is reduced and there is a poststenotic pressure drop due to loss of energy and compensatory measures (distal vasodilation) of the coronary bed (< 0.75).[72–76] Ideally, the measurement should be taken under maximal vasodilation by reducing the variability of coronary resistance and improving the accuracy in predicting coronary flow. Figure 18-4 gives examples of FFR assessment of lesions.

Like intracoronary Doppler equipment, catheters used to measure pressure gradients were bulky and had many clinical limitations for use until the more recent advent of pressure wires with similar characteristics to interventional guidewires. Unlike CFR, changes in heart rate, aortic pressure, contractility, or microvascular circulation has no effect on FFR.[77] However, the use of FFR has only been validated for a single or isolated lesion of a coronary artery. Measurements taken in the presence of multiple lesions will overestimate the FFR, as the reading will be a result of the cumulative effect of all the

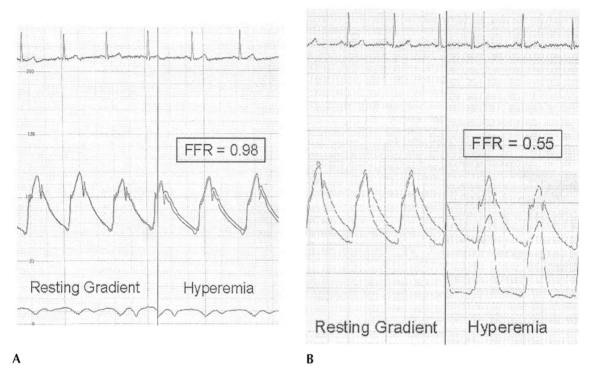

A   **B**

Figure 18-4. Fractional flow reserve (FFR) of the LAD using a Doppler guidewire. **A.** An FFR was performed on a hazy intermediate lesion of the mid LAD. The lesion was crossed with the guidewire mounted with a pressure sensor. At rest, the pressures proximal to the lesion and distal to the lesion are equal, therefore the two safe forms track one another. At maximal hyperemia, there is a slight separation of the two waveforms. The FFR is the mean pressure distal to the lesion divided by the mean pressure proximal to the lesion at maximal hyperemia. In this case it is normal at 0.98, suggesting that this lesion is not hemodynamically significant. **B.** An FFR is performed on this lesion in the mid LAD. After the administration of intracoronary adenosine for maximal hyperemia, there is a significant separation of the waveforms. The FFR was calculated to be 0.55, suggesting a hemodynamically significant stenosis. (Pictures courtesy of JOMED Inc.)

stenoses in question. Microvascular disease, ventricular hypertrophy, and significant collateral blood flow[78–80] will also alter FFR measurement.

TIMI Flow Rates

The TIMI study established a standard classification for grading coronary flow that is easily reproducible and currently widely used.[81] A lesion with TIMI grade 0 flow reveals no evidence of contrast, thus no coronary perfusion, beyond the lesion. TIMI grade 1 flow shows that contrast extends beyond the lesion, but the distal vessel does not opacify. TIMI grade 2 flow represents complete filling of the distal coronary vessel, but at a much slower rate of filling and clearance of contrast than normal (as represented by the filling pattern of the other non–infarct-related coronary vessels or the same vessel proximal to the lesion). TIMI grade 3 flow is normal coronary artery filling and clearance of contrast, thus normal perfusion.

This qualitative method of describing CAD is independent of the degree of stenosis. A severe (90% obstruction) lesion could have normal TIMI 3 coronary flow, and, in contrast, a moderate lesion (50% obstruction) recently involved with an infarct could have TIMI 1 or 2 flow. A vessel with impaired flow is more likely to contain the culprit lesion for the patient's presentation than an equal or more severe lesion with normal TIMI 3 flow. A method of quantification using the concept of TIMI flow, TIMI frame count, has been developed in which the number of frames are counted in a cineangiogram (set at 30 frames/sec acquisition) from the first frame showing complete diameter contrast opacification (i.e., the first frame in which the column of contrast touches both sides of the artery) of the vessel to a predetermined landmark point of the vessel in question.[82] A correction factor of 1.7 is divided into the absolute TIMI frame count of the LAD to standardize it to the other major coronary vessels. A corrected TIMI frame count of < 20 frames/sec is associated with the lowest risk of in-house or out-of-hospital major adverse events. A corrected TIMI frame count of 20 to 40 frames/sec has a slightly greater risk of adverse events, and a count > 40 frames/sec has a poor outcome.[83]

COMPLICATIONS FOR INVASIVE PROCEDURES

Major complications, heart attack, stroke, and death, due to a diagnostic cardiac catheterization is a rare event consistently occurring in < 0.11% of procedures by reports from the Society for Cardiac Angiography and Interventions.[84] Although the risk of major complications is low, the "minor" complications can have equally serious outcomes.

Vascular access complications are the most common complication of a cardiac catheterization, but still occurring < 1% of the time. Complications range from hematoma, prolonged bleeding, ischemia, atrioventricular (AV) fistulas, retroperitoneal bleeding, infection, and pseudoaneurysms. Recently, closure devices, consisting of a suture or collagen plug delivered at the arteriotomy site, have been used to reduce bleeding complications. Although the minor bleeding rate was reduced, there was an increased trend for major complications (retroperitoneal bleeding,

large hematomas, need for transfusions) and infections.

Renal dysfunction is a worrisome complication after cardiac catheterization. It can be caused by contrast-induced nephropathy (CIN) or by cholesterol emboli. CIN occurs in 5% of procedures, however the risk is greatest is in those with advanced age, diabetes, volume depletion, underlying nephropathy, multiple myeloma, or those taking angiotensin-converting enzyme (ACE) inhibitors or nonsteroidal anti-inflammatory agents. Usually, contrast nephropathy occurs in the first 48 hours, as evidenced by a rise in creatinine. Less than 1% of those with CIN need chronic dialysis.[85] Prehydration[86] has been shown to have a beneficial impact on reducing the risk of CIN in those with an abnormal baseline creatinine. This includes 12 hours of hydration prior to and after the procedure. The use of N-acetylcysteine has recently been advocated,[87] as the data reveals improved outcomes after treatment. The modern management of patients with impaired renal function or at high risk for CIN include an early admission for prehydration, N-acetylcystine 600 mg twice daily the day before and the day of the procedure, and continuation of IV fluids for 12 hours after the procedure. Renal dysfunction due to cholesterol emboli carries a grave prognosis. Unlike CIN, the renal dysfunction continues to worsen over weeks to months after a procedure. Approximately half of the patients with cholesterol emboli renal failure progress to need chronic dialysis.

CONCLUSION

There is a growing trend for invasive assessments of coronary lesions in current practice. The need for adjunctive assessment of lesions is not limited to "indeterminate" lesions and allograft vasculopathy, but is also for defining the etiology of restenosis, successfulness of an intervention, and to accurately determine severity and lesion length. Correlation between the cardiac catheterization and nuclear laboratory techniques have been shown to be complementary. Although invasive techniques do carry some risk, the benefit of accurately evaluating the extent of disease present far outweighs the risk of the procedure.

Significant advances have been made in quantitative angiography, which now serves as a standard in many clinical investigations. Angioscopy is an exciting tool to directly visualize the lumen of a coronary artery and examine plaque and thrombus. Intravascular ultrasound assists in our understanding of coronary stenoses, providing clarification for lesions of indeterminate severity. Additionally, IVUS is a valuable tool following percutaneous intervention to assess the success of such treatments. In addition to the morphologic assessment of CAD, physiologic measurements are also obtainable by means of invasive techniques. Intracoronary Doppler flow measurements and the calculation of coronary flow reserve and fractional flow reserve have aided in the understanding microvascular circulation. These measurements correlate well with cinegraphic data.

In conclusion, cardiac catheterization and nuclear laboratory techniques are overall complementary. In many cases, either technique serves well to define the extent and severity of CAD. However, often the combination of the anatomic assessment performed in the cardiac catherization laboratory is complementary to the physiologic measurements obtained with nuclear cardiology techniques. Although invasive techniques do carry some risk, the benefits accurately evaluating the extent of disease and assisting in the delineation of physiologic significance of stenoses far outweigh the risks of these procedures.

REFERENCES

1. Mueller RL, Sanborn, TA. The history of interventional cardiology: Cardiac catheterization, angioplasty, and related interventions. *Am Heart J* 1995:129:146.
2. Principal investigators of CASS et al. The National Heart, Lung, and Blood Institute: As multi-center comparison of the effects of randomized medical and surgical treatment of mildly symptomatic patients with coronary artery disease, and a registry of consecutive patients undergoing coronary angiography. *Circulation* 1981;63:II.
3. Kennedy JW, Kaiser GC, Fischer LD, et al. Multivariate discriminant analysis of the clinical and angiographic predictors of operative mortality from the collaborative study in coronary artery surgery (CASS). *J Thorac Cardiovasc Surg* 1980;80:876.
4. Horn HR, Teichhola LE, Cohn PF, Herman MV, Gorlin R. Augmentation of left ventricular contraction pattern in coronary artery disease by an inotropic catecholamine: The epinephrine ventriculogram. *Circulation* 1974;49:1063.
5. Helfant RH, Pine R, Meister EG, et al. Nitroglycerin to unmask reversible asynergy: Correlation with post coronary bypass ventriculography. *Circulation* 1974;50:108.
6. Dyke SH, Cohn PF, Gorlin R, et al. Detection of residual myocardial function in coronary artery disease using postextrasystolic otentiation. *Circulation* 1974;50:694.
7. White C, Wright C, Doty D, et al. Does visual interpretation of the coronary arteriogram predict the physiologic importance of a coronary stenosis? *N Engl J Med* 1984;310:819.
8. Galbraith J, Murphy M, Desoyza N. Coronary angiogram interpretation: Interobserver variability. *JAMA* 1981;240:2053.
9. Grondin C, Dyrda I, Pasternac A, et al. Discrepancies between cineangiographic and post-mortem findings in patients with coronary artery disease and recent myocardial revascularization. *Circulation* 1974;49:703.
10. Arnett E, Isner J, Redwood C, et al. Coronary artery narrowing in coronary heart disease: Comparison of cineangiographic and necropsy findings. *Ann Intern Med* 1979;91:350.
11. Flemming RM, Kirkeeide RL, Smalling RW, Gould KL. Patterns in visual interpretation of coronary arteriograms as detected by quantitative coronary arteriography. *J Am Coll Cardiol* 1991;18:945.
12. Beauman GL, Vogel RA. Accuracy of individual and panel visual interpretations of coronary arteriograms: Implications for clinical decisions. *J Am Coll Cardiol* 1990;16:108.
13. Hermiller JB, Cusma JT, Spero LA, et al. Quantitative and qualitative coronary angiographic analysis: Review of methods, utility, and limitations. *Catheterization Cardiovasc Diagn* 1992;25:110.
14. Fischer L, Judkins M, Lesperance J, et al. Reproducibility of coronary arteriographic reading in the Coronary Artery Surgery Study (CASS). *Catheterization Cardiovasc Diagn* 1982;8:565.
15. Reiber JH, Van Eldik-Helleman P, Kooijman CD, et al. How critical is frame selection in quantitative coronary angiographic studies? *Eur Heart J* 1989;10:54.
16. Sanborn TA, Rygaard JA, Westbrook BM, et al. Intraoperative angioscopy of saphenous vein and coronary arteries. *J Thorac Cardiovasc Surg* 1986;91:339.

17. Waxman S, Saaower M, Mittleman MA, et al. Culprit lesion morphology in subtypes of unstable angina assessed by angioscopy. *Circulation* 1995;92:I353.

18. Waxman S, Mittleman MA, Zarich SW, et al. Angioscopic assessment of coronary lesions underlying thrombus. *Am J Cardiol* 1997;79:1106.

19. Ramee SR, White CJ, Collins TJ, et al. Percutaneous coronary angioscopy in patients with ischemic heart disease. *J Am Coll Cardiol* 1991;17:100.

20. Alfonso F, Hernandez R, Goicolea J, et al. Angiographic deterioration of the previously dilated coronary segment induced by angioscopic examination. *Am J Cardiol* 1994;74:604.

21. Kaplan BM, Safian RD, Grines CL, et al. Usefulness of adjunctive angioscopy and extraction atherectomy before stent implantation in high-risk aorto-coronary saphenous vein grafts. *Am J Cardiol* 1995;76:822.

22. Mintz GS, Nissen SE, Anderson WD, et al. ACC Clinical Expert Consensus Document on Standards for the acquisition, measurement and reporting of intravascular ultrasound studies: A report of the American College of Cardiology Task Force on Clinical Expert Consensus Documents (Committee to Develop a Clinical Expert Consensus Document on Standards for Acquisition, Measurement and Reporting of Intravascular Ultrasound Studies [IVUS]). *J Am Coll Cardiol* 2001;37:1478.

23. Metz JA, Yock PG, Fitzgerald PJ. Intravascular ultrasound: Basic interpretation. *Cardiol Clin* 1997;15:1.

24. Hodgson JM, Reddy KG, Suneja R, et al. Intracoronary ultrasound imaging: Correlation of plaque morphology with angiography, clinical syndrome and procedural results in patients undergoing coronary angioplasty. *J Am Coll Cardiol* 1993;21:35.

25. Rasheed Q, Dhawale PJ, Anderson J, et al. Intracoronary ultrasound-defined plaque compostition: Computer-aided plaque characterization and correlation with histologic samples obtained during directional coronary atherectomy. *Am Heart J* 1995;129:631.

26. Rickenbacher PR, Pinto FJ, Chenzbraun A, et al. Incidence and severity of transplant coronary artery disease early and up to 15 years after transplantation as detected by intravascular ultrasound. *J Am Coll Cardiol* 1995;25:171.

27. Yeung AC, Davis SF, Hauptman PJ, et al. Incidence and progression of transplant coronary artery disease over 1 year: Results of a multicenter trial with use of intravascular ultrasound. Multicenter Intravascular Ultrasound Transplant Study Group. *J Heart Lung Transplant* 1995;14:S215.

28. Canty JM Jr. Coronary pressure-function and steady-state pressure-flow relations during autoregulation in the unanesthetized dog. *Circ Res* 1988;63:821–836.

29. Smith TP Jr, Canty JM Jr. Modulation of coronary autoregulatory responses by nitric oxide: Evidence for flow-dependent resistance adjustments in conscious dogs. *Circ Res* 1993;73:232–240.

30. Lansman JB, Hallam TJ, Rink TJ. Single stretch-activated ion channels in vascular endothelial cells as mechanotransducers? *Nature* 1987;325:811–813.

31. Rouleau J, Boerboom LE, Surjadhana A, Hoffman JI. The role of autoregulation and tissue diastolic pressures in the transmural distribution of left ventricular blood flow in anesthetized dogs. *Circ Res* 1979;45:804–815.

32. Rajagopalan S, Dube S, Canty JM Jr. Regulation of coronary diameter by myogenic mechanisms in arterial microvessels greater than 100 microns in diameter. *Am J Physiol* 1995;268:H788–H793.

33. Weber KT, Janicki JS. The metabolic demand and oxygen supply of the heart: Physiologic and clinical considerations. *Am J Cardiol* 1979;44:722.

34. De Bruyne B, Bronzwaer JG, Heyndrickx GR, Paulus WJ. Comparative effects of ischemia and hypoxemia on left ventricular systolic and diastolic function in humans. *Circulation* 1993;88:461–471.

35. Braunwald E. Control of myocardial oxygen consumption: Physiologic and clinical considerations. *Am J Cardiol* 1971;27:416–432.

36. Bache RJ, Dymiek DJ. Local and regional regulation of coronary vascular tone. *Prog Cardiovasc Dis* 1981;24:191.

37. Kloke FJ. Coronary blood flow in man. *Prog Cardiovasc Dis* 1976;19:117.

38. Moncada S. Nitric oxide: Discovery and impact on clinical medicine. *J R Soc Med* 1999;92:164–169.

39. Ignarro LJ, Cirino G, Casini A, Napli C. Nitric oxide as a signaling molecule in the vascular system: An overview. *J Cardiovasc Pharmacol* 1999;34:879–886.

40. Murad F. Nitric oxide signaling: Would you believe that a simple free radical could be a second messenger, autacoid, paracrine substance, neurotransmitter, and hormone? *Rec Prog Horm Res* 1998;53:43–49.

41. Braunwald E, Zipes DP, Libby P, et al. *Heart Disease: A Textbook of Cardiovascular Medicine*, 6th ed. Philadelphia: WB Saunders, 2001.

42. Kinlay S, Selwyn AP, Delagrange D, et al. Biological mechanisms for the clinical success of lipid-lowering in coronary artery disease and the use of surrogate end-points. *Curr Opin Lipidol* 1996;7:389–397.

43. Anderson TJ, Meredith IT, Yeung AC, et al. The effect of cholesterol-lowering and antioxidant therapy on endothelium-dependent coronary vasomotion. *N Engl J Med* 1995;332:488–493.

44. Anderson TJ, Meredith IT, Charbonneau F, et al. Endothelium-dependent coronary vasomotion relates to the susceptibility of LDL to oxidation in humans. *Circulation* 1996;93:1647–1650.

45. Steinberg D: Lewis A. Conner Memorial Lecture: Oxidative modification of LDL and atherogenesis. *Circulation* 1997;95:1062–1071.

46. Williams SB, Goldfine AB, Timimi FK, et al. Acute hyperglycemia attenuates endothelium-dependent

vasodilatation in humans in vivo. *Circulation* 1998;97:1695–1701.

47. Miura H, Liu Y, Gutterman DD. Human coronary arteriolar dilation to bradykinin depends on membrane hyperpolarization: Contribution of nitric oxide and calcium activated potassium channels. *Circulation* 1999;99:3132–3138.

48. Quilley J, Fulton D, McGiff JC: Hyperpolarizing factors. *Biochem Pharmacol* 1997;54:1059–1070.

49. Doucette JW, Corl PD, Payne HM, et al. Validation of a Doppler guide wire for intravascular measurement of coronary artery flow velocity. *Circulation* 1992;85:1899.

50. Tadaoka S, Kigiyama M, Hiramatsu O, et al. Accuracy of 20 MHz Doppler catheter coronary artery velocimetry for measurement of coronary blood flow velocity. *Catheterization Cardiovasc Diagn* 1990;19:205.

51. Hatle L, Angelsen B. *Physics of Blood Flow: Doppler Ultrasound in Cardiology.* Philadelphia: Lea and Febiger, 1985.

52. McGinn AL, White CW, Wilson RF. Interstudy variability of coronary flow reserve. *Circulation* 1990;81:1319–1330.

53. Cobb FR, McHale PA, Rembert JC. Effects of acute cellular injury on coronary vascular reactivity I awake dogs. *Circulation* 1978;57:962–968.

54. Gould KL. Dynamic coronary stenosis. *Am J Cardiol* 1980;45:286–292.

55. Chauhan A, Mullins PA, Petch MC, Schofield PM. Is coronary flow reserve in response to papaverine really normal in syndrome X? *Circulation* 1994; 89:1998–2004.

56. Marcus ML, Mueller TM, Gascho JA, Kerber RE. Effects of cardiac hypertrophy secondary to hypertension on the coronary circulation. *Am J Cardiol* 1979;44:1023–1028.

57. Akasaka T, Yoshida K, Hozumi T, et al. Retinopathy identifies marked restriction of coronary flow reserve in patients with diabetes mellitus. *J Am Coll Cardiol* 1997;30:935–941.

58. Marcus ML, Doty DB, Hiratzka LF, et al. Decreased coronary reserve: A mechanism for angina pectoris in patients with aortic stenosis and normal coronary arteries. *N Engl J Med* 1982;307:1362–1366.

59. Marcus ML, Doty DB, Hirratzka LF, et al. Decreased coronary reserve a mechanism of angina pectoris in patients with aortic stenosis and normal coronary arteries. *N Engl J Med* 1982;37:1362–1366.

60. Houghton JL, Prisant LM, Carr AA, et al. Relationship of left ventricular mass to impairment of coronary vasodilator reserve in hypertensive heart disease. *Am Heart J* 1991;21:1107.

61. Cannon RO, Bonow RO, Bacharach SL, et al. Left ventricular dysfunction in patients with angina pectoris, normal epicardial coronary arteries, and abnormal vasodilator reserve. *Circulation* 1985;71:218–226.

62. Baumgart D, Haud M, Goerge G, et al. Improved assessment of coronary stenosis severity using the relative flow velocity reserve. *Circulation* 1998; 98(1):40–46.

63. Kern MJ, Puri S, Bach RG, et al. Abnormal coronary flow velocity reserve after coronary artery stenting in patients. Role of relative coronary flow reserve to assess potential mechanisms. *Circulation* 1999; 100:2491–2498.

64. Wieneke H, Haud M, Ge J, et al. Corrected coronary flow velocity reserve: A new concept for assessing coronary perfusion. *J Am Coll Cardiol* 2000; 35:1713–1720.

65. Meuwissen M, Chamuleau SA, Siebes M, et al. Role of variability in microvascular resistance on fractional flow reserve and coronary blood flow velocity reserve in intermediate coronary lesions. *Circulation* 2001;103:184–187.

66. Ofili EO, Labovitz AJ, Kern MJ. Coronary flow dynamics in normal and diseased arteries. *Am J Cardiol* 1993;71:3D–9D.

67. Donohue TJ, Kern MJ, Aguirre FV. Assessing the hemodynamic significance of coronary artery stenoses: Analysis of translesional pressure-flow velocity relations in patients. *J Am Coll Cardiol* 1993;22:449–458.

68. Miller DD, Donohue TJ, Wolford TL, et al. Myocardial ischemia/infarction/arteritis: Assessment of blood flow distal to coronary artery stenoses: Correlations between myocardial positron emission tomography and poststenotic intracoronary Doppler flow reserve. *Circulation* 1996;94:2447–2454.

69. Joye JD, Schulman DS, Lasorda D, et al. Intracoronary Doppler guide wire versus stress single-photon emission computed tomographic thallium-201 imaging in assessment of intermediate coronary stenoses. *J Am Coll Cardiol* 1994;24:940–947.

70. Heller LI, Cates C, Popma J, et al. Intracoronary Doppler assessment of moderate coronary artery disease: Comparison with 201Tl imaging and coronary angiography. FACTS Study Group. *Circulation* 1997;96:484–490.

71. Chamuleau SA, Rio RA, de Cock CC, et al. Prognostic value of coronary blood flow velocity and myocardial perfusion in intermediate coronary narrowings and multivessel disease. *J Am Coll Cardiol* 2002; 39:852–853.

72. Uren NG, Melin JA, De Bruyne B, et al. Relation between myocardial blood flow and the severity of coronary artery stenosis. *N Engl J Med* 1994; 330(25):1782–1788.

73. Pijls NHJ, Van Gelder B, Van der Voort P, et al. Fractional flow reserve: A useful index to evaluate the influence of an epicardial coronary stenosis on myocardial blood flow. *Circulation* 1995; 92:3183–3193.

74. Pijls NHJ, De Bruyne B, Peels K, et al. Measurement of fractional flow reserve to assess the functional severity of coronary artery stenoses. *N Engl J Med* 1996; 334:1703–1708.

75. Bech GJ, De Bruyne B, Bonnier HJ, et al. Long-term follow-up after deferral of percutaneous transluminal coronary angioplasty of intermediate stenosis on the basis of coronary pressure measurement. *J Am Coll Cardiol* 1998;31:841–847.

76. Pijls NHJ, De Bruyne B. Coronary pressure measurement and fractional flow reserve. *Heart* 1998;80:539–542.

77. De Bruyne B, Bartunek J, Sys SU, et al. Simultaneous coronary pressure and flow velocity measurements in humans: Feasibility, reproducibility, and hemodynamic dependence of coronary flow velocity reserve, hyperemic flow versus pressure slope index, and fractional flow reserve. *Circulation* 1996; 94(8):1842–1849.

78. De Bruyne B, Pijls NHJ, Heyndrickx GR, et al. Pressure derived fractional flow reserve to assess serial epicardial stenosis: Theoretical basis and animal validation. *Circulation* 2000;101:1840–1847.

79. Bartunek J, Pijls NHJ, Bech GJW, et al. Fractional flow reserve: who needs the pressure wire? *J Interventional Cardiol* 1999;12:425–430.

80. Pijls NHJ, Kern MJ, Yock PG, De Bruyne B. Practice and potential pitfalls of coronary pressure measurement. *Catheterization Cardiovasc Interventions* 2000;29:1–16.

81. The TIMI Study Group. The Thrombolysis in Myocardial Infarction (TIMI) trial. *N Engl J Med* 1985;31:932.

82. Gibson CM, Cannon CP, Daley WL, et al. TIMI frame count: A quantitative method of assessing coronary artery flow. *Circulation* 1996;93:879.

83. Gibson CM, Murphy SA, Rizzo MJ, et al. The relationship between the TIMI frame count and clinical outcomes after thrombolytic administration. *Circulation* 1999;99:1945.

84. Noto TJ, Johnson LW, Krone R, et al. Cardiac catheterization 1990: A report of the registry of the Society for Cardiac Angiography and Interventions. *Catheterization Cardiovasc Diagn* 1991;30:185.

85. Tommaso CL. Contrast-induced nephrotoxicity in patients undergoing cardiac catheterization. *Catheterization Cardiovasc Diagn* 1994;31:316.

86. Solomon R, Werner C, Mann D, et al. Effects of saline, mannitol, and furosemide on acute decreases in renal function induced by radiocontrast agents. *N Engl J Med* 1994;331:1416.

87. Tepel M, Van der Giet M, Schwarzfeld C, et al. Prevention of radiographic-contrast-agent–induced reductions in renal function by acetylcysteine. *N Engl J Med* 2000;343:180.

CHAPTER 19

Practical Guide to Risk Stratification Using Myocardial Perfusion Imaging

Rami Doukky
Robert C. Hendel

INTRODUCTION

In the past two decades, a great body of literature has established the use of nuclear imaging for risk stratification in patients with known or suspected coronary artery disease (CAD). The earlier studies have been reinforced, more recently, with the use of single photon emission computed tomography (SPECT) and electrocardiographic (ECG)-gated SPECT imaging. This chapter will review the use of stress radionuclide SPECT perfusion imaging for risk stratification of patients with chronic CAD, following myocardial infarction (MI), unstable angina. Risk stratification prior to major noncardiac surgery was discussed in Chapter 3.

RISK STRATIFICATION IN PATIENTS WITH CHRONIC CAD

Risk stratification is of crucial importance for the practice of contemporary medicine. Extending the paradigm of noninvasive cardiac testing beyond the detection of disease is especially important, as risk assessment permits patient management decisions to be formulated on an evidence-based approach. CAD patients who are identified as being at a high risk for subsequent cardiac events should receive aggressive management, possibly including cardiac catheterization for potential revascularization procedures that may improve their outcome. Conversely, the management focus in patients with low future event rate should be shifted toward risk factor modification and aggressive medical therapy, reserving invasive procedures for patients who fail medical management. A risk assessment, outcomes-based model strives for improved patient outcome and avoidance of complications from unnecessary procedures, and is cost-effective. In this section of the chapter, we will discuss the value of nuclear imaging as a powerful prognostic tool and its contribution to the management of patients with ischemic heart disease.

CAD is a disease with a wide spectrum of severity and extent with outcomes, such as nonfatal MI or cardiac death being related to the severity of disease. Clinical trials have shown that patients with severe CAD as left main coronary artery disease and multivessel disease, especially those with left ventricular (LV) dysfunction, can benefit from coronary artery bypass graft (CABG) surgery with significant reduction in their mortality rate.[1-5] Whereas patients with single-vessel disease or patients with two-vessel disease (without proximal left anterior descending [LAD] artery involvement) would have improved symptoms of angina following CABG and percutaneous transluminal coronary angioplasty (PTCA) without any effect on their mortality rate.[4,6,7] Assessing LV function is of extreme importance since impaired LV performance has a very negative prognostic value in all cardiac patients, especially in patients with CAD.[4,5]

Risk assessment based on clinical findings and resting ECG only is limited. Exercise testing can also help, especially when examining the patient's functional capacity. Exercise-induced ECG changes and risk indices, such as the Duke Treadmill Score, also have substantial prognostic value.[8] Unfortunately, using clinical data and the Duke Treadmill Score, most patients (55%) with suspected CAD would fall in an intermediate-risk group,[9] necessitating additional risk stratification.

Coronary angiography, considered the "gold standard" for the diagnosis of CAD, often does not provide information about the physiologic significance of atherosclerotic lesions, especially in borderline lesions (50–70% stenosis). More importantly, it does not provide a clear marker of risk of adverse events, especially in patients with moderate disease severity. Multiple studies have demonstrated that angiography is rarely an ideal method for risk stratification of CAD patients.

Risk Based on Nuclear Imaging Results

Normal SPECT Imaging Study The presence of a normal scintigraphic SPECT study at a high level of stress (≥ 85% of maximum pre-

dicted heart rate) or proper pharmacologic stress carries a very benign prognosis, with mortality rate less than 1% per year. Irrespective of patient's clinical risk, an abnormal perfusion study is associated with an increased incidence of nonfatal MI and/or cardiac death.[10,11] This finding has been reproduced in many studies.[12,13] Iskander and Iskandrian,[11] pooling the results of SPECT imaging from more than 12,000 patients in 14 studies, demonstrated that the event rate (death or MI) for patients with normal nuclear study is 0.6% per year, whereas abnormal study carries 7.4% per year event rate, a 12-fold increase, as shown in Figure 19-1.

One recent study has shown that technetium 99m (Tc-99m)-sestamibi has enhanced sensitivity in detecting reversible perfusion defects over Tc-99m-tetrofosmin.[14] However, this marginal difference in diagnostic performance did not translate into significant difference in prognostic predictive value.[15] In a more recent multicenter study, Shaw et al.[15] validated the excellent prognostic value of normal or near normal myocardial perfusion SPECT scan using Tc-99m-tetrofosmin with an annual mortality rate of 0.6%. Simi-

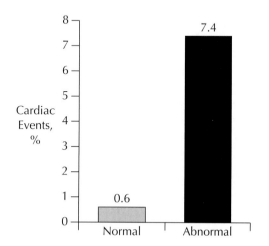

Figure 19-1. Differential risk of event rate in normal and abnormal myocardial perfusion imaging study. An abnormal SPECT study is associated with 12-fold increase in event rate compared to a normal study. (From Iskander et al.[11] with permission.)

larly, this excellent survival rate had been noted in male and female subsets of the population as well as in patients who underwent exercise or pharmacologic stress testing. In a meta-analysis of published literature on prognostic value of normal myocardial perfusion SPECT scan using various agents (thallium 201 [Tl-201] and Tc-99m-sestamibi), these investigators confirmed similar excellent survival rate regardless of the radiopharmaceutical agent used, ranging from 99.3% to 99.7%.[15]

In summary, the excellent prognostic value of a normal or near normal stress myocardial perfusion study has been confirmed in numerous studies using various radiopharmaceutical agents, stress modality (exercise vs. pharmacologic), or pharmacologic stress agent used (dipyridamole, adenosine, or dobutamine/atropine).[10–13,15–23] These findings have been noted in different subsets of patients regardless of gender,[15,24,25] race,[26] diabetic status,[27,28] or the presence of known CAD.[29]

Defining Risk in Patients with Abnormal SPECT Scan The value of myocardial perfusion scintigraphy comes from its ability to identify and quantify the degree of jeopardized myocardium during stress. The size of the perfusion abnormality provides powerful prognostic information and has been shown to directly relate to outcome.[16,30–33] Ladenheim et al.[32] have also shown that the magnitude of ischemia (severity and extent) correlates well with cardiac events, and this relationship is not linear but exponential (Figure 19-2). Vanzetto et al.[16] have shown correlation between event rate (death, nonfatal MI and revascularization) and extent of ischemia demonstrated by the number of ischemic segments on SPECT scan (Figure 19-3). Iskander and Iskandrian[11] have also shown that defect reversibility is an important predictor of type of cardiac events, as fixed perfusion defects are associated with cardiac death, whereas reversible perfusion defects are associated with nonfatal MI. This is a very important finding, since a re-

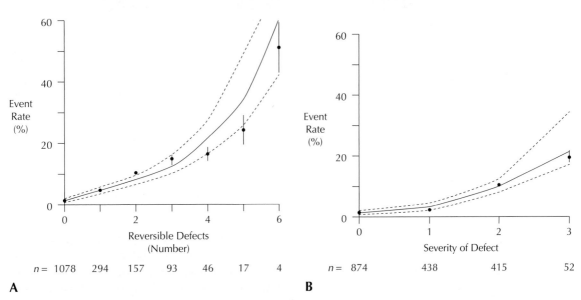

Figure 19-2. **A.** Correlation between cardiac event rate on the vertical axis and number of reversible segmental defects on the horizontal axis (six-segment model using planar imaging using thallium-201). **B.** Correlation between event rate (vertical axis) and ischemic severity on the horizontal axis (four-point scale: 0 = no defect, 1 = mild defect, 2 = moderate defect, 3 = severe defect). As ischemic extent or severity increases to moderate level, the event rate increases exponentially. (From Ladenheim et al.[32] with permission.)

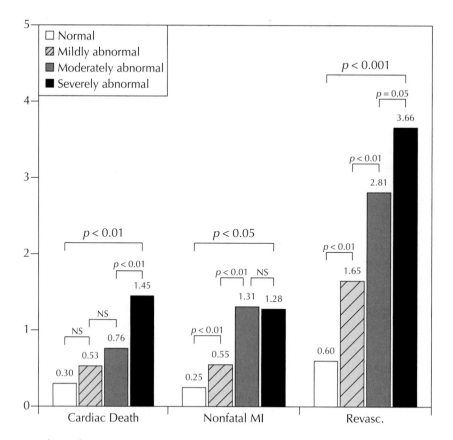

Figure 19-3. Correlation between event rates and the level of abnormality on thallium-201 SPECT myocardial perfusion imaging. Event rates of death, MI, and revascularization procedures increase with increasing level of abnormality of myocardial perfusion imaging. (From Vanzetto et al.[16] with permission.)

versible perfusion defect on SPECT imaging is the only available diagnostic tool that can independently predict the risk of nonfatal MI. Others have also demonstrated similar findings regarding long-term prognosis.[16,30,34] Therefore, stress perfusion studies should be reported documenting defect severity (mild, moderate, severe), size (small, moderate, large) and reversibility to provide essential risk stratification.[35]

In a fascinating study by Hachamovitch et al.,[33] these authors demonstrated a difference in the type of event predicted by a perfusion defect of varying severity/extent. A mildly abnormal study was associated with very low mortality rate (0.8%) but a slightly higher risk of nonfatal MI

(2.7%) compared to normal (0.5%), as shown in Figure 19-4. This interesting finding has important implications for patient management, as even the major CABG trials have not shown a reduction in nonfatal MI following bypass surgery when compared with medical therapy.[1-5] Further supporting the possible medical approach to patients with a mildly abnormal perfusion study are several recent primary and secondary prevention trials, which have shown conclusively that lipid-lowering agents (hydroxymethylglutaryl coenzyme A [HMG Co-A] inhibitors, "statins") are very effective in reducing event rate of death and MI by about one third.[36-39] The AVERT trial also suggests that aggressive lipid lowering is superior

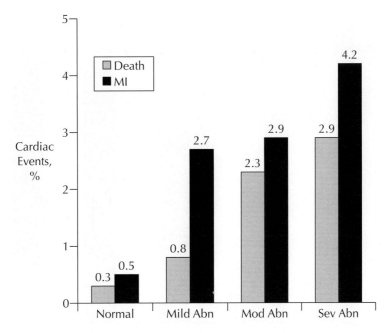

Figure 19-4. Cardiac events based on SPECT imaging results, differential stratification for risk of cardiac death and myocardial infarction. Patients with mildly abnormal SPECT scan have an increased rate of nonfatal MI but maintain very low risk of cardiac death. (From Hachamovitch et al.[33] with permission.)

to angioplasty in patients with mild to moderate CAD.[40] More recently, the Heart Outcomes Prevention Evaluation (HOPE) trial has shown that ramipril, an angiofensin-converting enzyme (ACE) inhibitor, reduces cardiovascular events including death and MI.[41] Based on these clinical trials, the Hachamovitch data suggests that patients with a mildly abnormal scintigraphic scan would benefit from secondary prevention measures, such as lipid lowering or ACE inhibitors, rather than revascularization procedures.

Incremental Prognostic Value of SPECT Imaging: Beyond Clinical, Electrocardiographic, and Angiographic Data

The prognostic value of the SPECT scan is not simply a substitute but a valuable addition to prognostic data that has been derived from clinical findings or from the results of stress testing.

Iskandarian et al.[42] and others[16,43–46] have shown the additive value of SPECT imaging to exercise stress testing and clinical data alone, especially if the number of perfusion defects is taken into account.[16] This incremental prognostic value has been confirmed using various stress modalities and radiopharmaceutical agents and protocols.[24,27,29,47–50] SPECT perfusion imaging is also more predictive of cardiac events than cardiac catheterization.[30,42] SPECT imaging, when added to stress and clinical data, has shown a higher incremental prognostic value than cardiac catheterization, which in fact failed to produce independent information,[42] as shown in Figure 19-5.

Even when SPECT data is compared with multivariate formulae incorporating several exercise and clinical parameters, it is more predictive of cardiac events. Hachamovitch et al.[9] compared the prognostic value of gated SPECT scan with the Duke Treadmill Score in predicting event

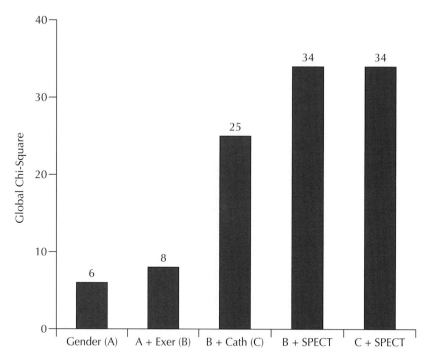

Figure 19-5. Incremental prognostic value of SPECT imaging for the prediction of nonfatal MI or death. SPECT data have incremental prognostic value to cardiac catheterization data, whereas cardiac catheterization does not provide additional prognostic value to SPECT. (From Iskandrian et al.[42] with permission.)

rate in 2,200 patients and revealed that gated SPECT was more predictive of event rate than the Duke Treadmill Score for each risk category (high, intermediate, and low). This is especially evident in the intermediate Duke risk group, as shown in Figure 19-6.

Value of ECG-Gated SPECT Imaging in the Evaluation of LV Function

The availability of Tc-99m based agents (i.e., Tc-99m sestamibi and Tc-99m tetrofosmin) has facilitated the widespread use ECG-gated acquisition of myocardial perfusion studies. Gated SPECT allows the evaluation of global and regional wall motion and an accurate evaluation of left ventricular ejection fraction (LVEF).[46,51] The evaluation of global and regional myocardial contractility not only increases the specificity of SPECT imaging[52–54] but also adds to its incremental prognostic value.[55,56] Sharir et al.[55] have

demonstrated an incremental prognostic value of LVEF when added to SPECT perfusion imaging data. In this study, LVEF ≤ 45% had very significant independent negative prognostic value in patients with severe perfusion defects and more so in patients with mild and moderate perfusion defects, as shown in Figure 19-7.

Value of Transient Ischemic Dilation (TID)

Transient ischemic dilation (TID) is the appearance of a larger LV cavity diameter on the post-stress images when compared with the resting study, which is most likely due to stress-induced subendocardial ischemia. This finding is predictive of extensive CAD and significantly increased cardiac events.[57–61] This finding appears to be independent of the perfusion imaging agent or the mode of stress. However, the value of TID in patients without perfusion defects is controversial.

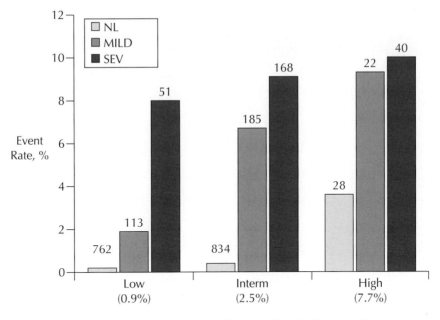

Figure 19-6.   Incremental prognostic value of SPECT to the Duke Treadmill Score. Note that most patients (55%) fell in an intermediate Duke risk group, and two thirds of those patients had normal SPECT scans with very low event rate. (From Hachamovitch et al.[9] with permission.)

Value of Increased Lung Uptake

This finding is a surrogate marker of stress-induced LV dysfunction, which results in pulmonary congestion. Increased lung uptake (lung–heart ratio [LHR]) has also been documented to predict patients at increased risk of severe disease and subsequent cardiac events, especially when noted in conjunction with Tl-201 scintigraphy.[62–64]

Cost-Efficacy of Nuclear Imaging

As SPECT imaging may identify those patients at high risk for subsequent cardiac event, perfusion imaging may be used to help guide further testing and revascularization procedures, functioning as a gatekeeper for more resource-intense techniques.[65] Nallamothu et al.[44] have demonstrated that SPECT imaging may help guide which patients undergo coronary angiography and thereby reduce "unnecessary" cardiac catheterizations. This obviously has important cost-effectiveness ramifications. In perhaps the most detailed analysis of the financial implications of perfusion imaging, Shaw et al.[66] evaluated 11,372 consecutive patients with stable angina gathered from several sites. In this cohort-matched study, they compared direct catheterization ("cath-all") with selective catheterization based on the results of SPECT imaging in patients with chronic stable angina. As a result, there was a substantial reduction (31–50%) in costs using SPECT with selective catheterization strategy. Event rate of death and nonfatal MI was identical in both cohorts. The only significant difference was in the rate of revascularization procedures, which was significantly reduced by nearly 50% in the SPECT cohort, as shown in Figure 19-8. Thus, available evidence supports the use of perfusion imaging for cost-effective risk stratification of patients with known or suspected CAD.

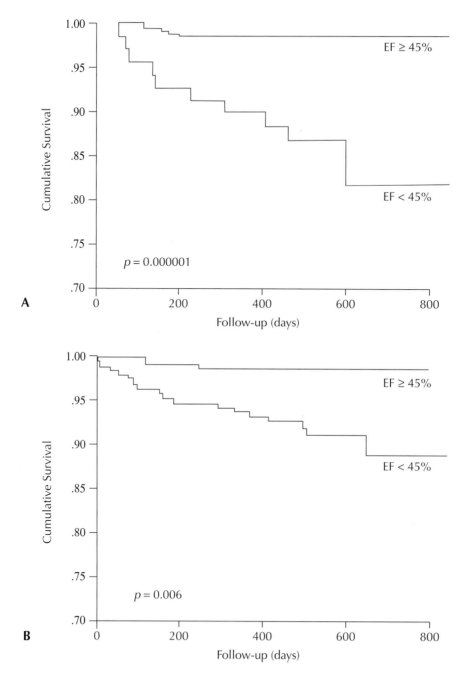

Figure 19-7. Incremental prognostic value for LVEF evaluation by gated SPECT. Cumulative survival in:
A. patients with mild/moderate perfusion abnormalities and, **B.** patients with severe perfusion abnormalities,
stratified into ejection fraction ≥ 45% and ejection fraction < 45%. (From Sharir et al.[55] with permission.)

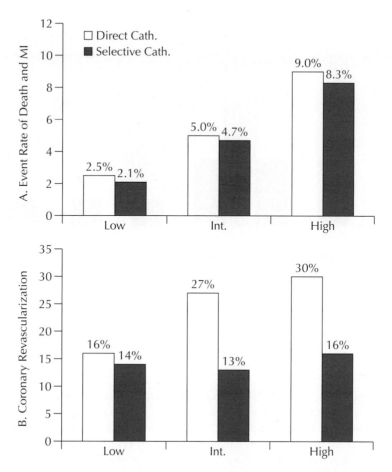

Figure 19-8. Direct catheterization approach versus selective catheterization based on the result of myocardial perfusion imaging study. Selective catheterization approach resulted in 50% reduction in revascularization procedures (PTCA, CABG) **(A).** but no significant difference in cardiac events of death or MI between the two groups **(B).** Selective catheterization approach was associated with 30 to 40% cost reduction compared to direct catheterization approach. (From Shaw et al.[66] with permission.) **(C)** See next page.

RISK STRATIFICATION FOLLOWING ST ELEVATION MYOCARDIAL INFARCTION

The need for risk stratification remains in patients who survive an acute MI, many of whom have an increased incidence of reinfarction or cardiac-related death. Postinfarction evaluation is often performed with submaximal exercise stress testing prior to hospital discharge, frequently followed by a symptom-limited test 6 to 12 weeks later.[67] Patients who demonstrate evidence of ischemia on submaximal exercise testing are usually referred for cardiac catheterization for further risk assessment and possible revascularization procedure, since these patients have increased risk for cardiac events.[67] However, SPECT imaging is more sensitive for the detection of the extent and severity of ischemia for the identification of patients at high risk.[16,32,68–71]

More than 15 years ago, Gibson et al.[72] compared the prognostic efficacy of exercise ECG,

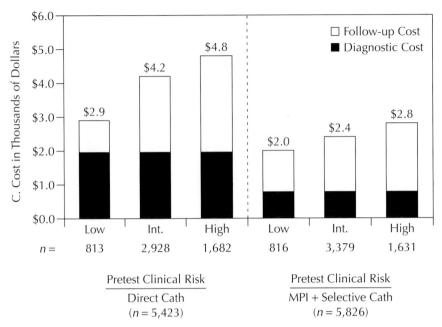

Figure 19-8. (continued)   (C). These findings were demonstrated in patients with all levels of pretest clinical risk (low, intermediate, or high). (From Shaw et al.[66] with permission.)

stress myocardial perfusion (using Tl-201) and cardiac catheterization performed prior to hospital discharge in patients with uncomplicated MI. High-risk characteristics in any of these tests was associated with high event rate (50%); however, only a negative stress myocardial perfusion study was predictive of low event rate (6%) versus 27% and 22% event rates, respectively, for negative submaximal exercise stress test and low-risk features on coronary angiogram. Myocardial perfusion imaging (MPI) can also assess the magnitude of jeopardized myocardium within the infarct zone. Ischemia within the infarct zone predicts increased risk of reinfarction and recurrent cardiac events.[68,73]

Pharmacologic stress MPI has been shown to be superior to the conventional submaximal exercise ECG stress testing as a risk stratification tool in this high-risk group of patients.[74,75] Additionally, stress testing with adenosine or dipyridamole may be performed safely as early as two to four days following an uncomplicated MI.[74,76,77] This approach can shorten hospital

stay, and more importantly, it has been shown to have an excellent prognostic value, as patients with low-risk myocardial perfusion scan (i.e., without evidence of reversible perfusion defect) have low risk for cardiac events.[74–77] Brown et al.[74] have demonstrated that early dipyridamole MPI following uncomplicated MI is not only safe, but also is superior to submaximal exercise stress imaging in identifying patients at increased risk. In the same study, these investigators have shown that event rate correlates well with the severity of the perfusion defects. Mahmarian et al.[77] have shown that large area of ischemia (> 10% of the left ventricle) on pharmacologic MPI using adenosine following noncomplicated MI is superior to coronary angiography findings in separating patients at increased risk for cardiac events from those at low risk, as shown in Figure 19-9. The value of MPI has been demonstrated in patients who did or did not receive thrombolytic therapy.[74,77] Patients who demonstrate evidence of peri-infarct ischemia or ischemia in a remote segment have an increased risk of cardiac

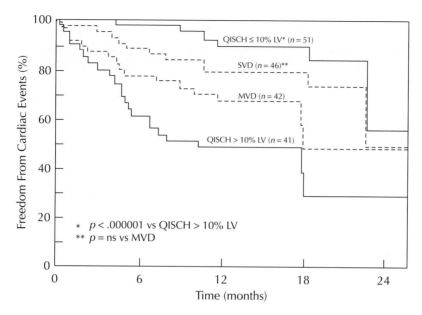

Figure 19-9. Early risk stratification of patients with uncomplicated MI with pharmacologic stress myocardial perfusion scintigraphy. Kaplan–Meier curves depicting freedom from cardiac events on the basis of quantified extent of ischemia (QISCH) and the extent of coronary artery disease. Quantified extent of ischemia separates low-risk from high-risk patients better than extent of coronary artery disease proven by coronary angiography. (SVD = single-vessel disease, MVD = multivessel disease.) (From Mahmarian et al.[77] with permission.)

events.[74–78] These high-risk patients may benefit from coronary revascularization.

In the era of thrombolytic therapy and percutaneous coronary intervention for acute MI, risk assessment with noninvasive testing remains an important component in patient care, despite the overall lower risk of this group of infarct survivors.[67] Clinical trials have shown that there is no role for "routine" PTCA of residual coronary lesion following successful thrombolytic therapy without any evidence of residual ischemia on stress testing.[79] Dakik et al.[69] revealed that the size of the perfusion defect on myocardial perfusion study and ejection fraction were the only significant predictors of cardiac events in patients after thrombolytic therapy, and these predictors had incremental prognostic value to clinical data. In fact, cardiac catheterization did not demonstrate further (incremental) prognostic value.

The LVEF remains one of the key predictors of cardiac events in post-MI patients.[69,77] There-

fore, the determination of LVEF using gated SPECT is often of vital importance for subsequent management decisions in these patients.[67,71]

RISK STRATIFICATION IN PATIENTS WITH UNSTABLE ANGINA AND NON– ST ELEVATION MI

Since the early 1990s, it has been shown that not all patients following a presentation of unstable angina or non-Q-wave MI require cardiac catheterization for optimal management. The Thrombosis in Myocardial Ischemia (TIMI)-IIIB trial showed that early conservative strategy in the management of unstable angina and non-Q-wave MI, followed by selective cardiac catheterization in patients with evidence of ischemia on noninvasive testing is associated with similar outcome to those patients who underwent an early invasive approach.[80] Subsequently, the Veterans Affairs Non-Q-Wave Infarction Strategies in Hospital (VANQWISH) study addressed the same issue and demonstrated increased event rate in patients who underwent an early invasive approach, likely due to increased complications related to revascularization.[81] These and other trials supported a conservative strategy following non-Q-wave MI or unstable angina, based on the lack of ischemia on noninvasive testing. However, these studies were completed prior to the common use of coronary stenting and glycoprotein IIb–IIIa inhibitors, which have been shown to have great impact on the outcome of coronary angioplasty and the outcome of patients with acute coronary syndromes.[82–84]

The TACTICS trial (TIMI-18)[85] recently demonstrated that an early invasive strategy using tirofiban and coronary stenting is superior to early conservative management and noninvasive testing. However, the TACTICS trial revealed that patients who benefit the most from early invasive approach are those with elevated troponin (I or T) level, and therefore those patients without troponin elevations upon admission are still likely candidates for a noninvasive risk assessment. Thus, there is a role for noninvasive testing for risk stratification in patients with low-risk unstable angina, as determined by a low TIMI risk score (The seven TIMI risk score predictor variables were age 65 years or older, at least three risk factors for CAD, prior coronary stenosis of ≥ 50%, ST-segment deviation on ECG at presentation, at least two anginal events in prior 24 hours, use of aspirin in prior 7 days, and elevated serum cardiac markers),[86] especially if they respond well to early medical management. Also, noninvasive risk stratification prior to cardiac catheterization should be considered in acute coronary syndrome patients with relative contraindication for coronary angiography, such as renal insufficiency.

Exercise or pharmacologic stress MPI can be used safely to assess risk for cardiac events (death or MI) in patients with unstable angina following the initial response to medical management.[87–89] Brown[87] has demonstrated in a follow-up study

(39 ± 11 months) that patients with unstable angina who underwent stress MPI using Tl-201 were effectively risk-stratified for long-term events, as a reversible perfusion defect was associated with a 26% event rate, versus a 3% incidence of MI or cardiac death for patients with no reversible perfusion defect. Similar results where shown by Stratmann et al.[89] using Tc-99m sestamibi SPECT perfusion imaging.

The data support the use myocardial perfusion scintigraphy for the risk stratification and management of patients with low-risk unstable angina or non-ST-segment elevation infarction. Patients who demonstrate evidence of ischemia on MPI have increased risk for cardiac events and should undergo cardiac catheterization and possible revascularization. Patients without evidence of ischemia can be treated medically and avoid invasive evaluation, as this group of patients has very low occurrence of ischemic cardiac events.

CONCLUSION

A wealth of literature supports the use of radionuclide MPI for risk stratification in patients with known or suspected CAD. Although an abnormal perfusion study predicts subsequent cardiac events such as MI or cardiac death, the ability of SPECT imaging to localize and define the extent/severity of disease adds additional prognostic value. Furthermore, specific applications of these nuclear cardiology techniques, such as postinfarction or in patients with unstable angina, have also successfully assessed risk of cardiovascular events. The prognostic applications of perfusion imaging are germane to all health care providers, as these methods may be used to guide subsequent tests and treatments. Thus, MPI has the potential to significantly impact on patient management decisions and the cost-effective utilization of health care dollars.

REFERENCES

1. Alderman EL, Bourassa MG, Cohen LS, et al. Ten-year follow-up for survival and myocardial infarction in the

randomized coronary artery surgery study (CASS). *Circulation* 1990;82:1629.

2. European Coronary Surgery Study Group: Long-term results of prospective randomized study of coronary artery bypass surgery in stable angina pectoris. *Lancet* 1982;2:1173.

3. The VA Coronary Artery Bypass Surgery Cooperative Study Group. Eighteen-year follow-up in the Veterans Affairs Cooperative of Coronary Artery Bypass Surgery for Stable Angina. *Circulation* 1992;86:121.

4. Yusuf S, Zucker D, Peduzzi P, et al. Effect of coronary artery bypass graft surgery on survival: Overview of 10-year results from randomized trials by Coronary Artery Bypass Graft Surgery Trialists Collaboration. *Lancet* 1994;344:563.

5. Pssamani E, Davis KB, Gillespi MJ, et al. A randomized trial of coronary artery bypass surgery (CASS): Survival in patients with a low ejection fraction. *N Engl J Med* 1985;312:1665.

6. Parisi AF, Folland ED, Hartigan P. A comparison of angioplasty with medical therapy in the treatment of single-vessel coronary artery disease. *N Engl J Med* 1992;326:10.

7. RITA-2 Trial Participants. Coronary angioplasty versus medical therapy for angina: The second Randomized International Treatment for Angina (RITA-2) trial. *Lancet* 1997;350:461.

8. Mark DB, Shaw l, Harrell FE Jr, et al. Exercise treadmill score for predicting prognosis in coronary artery disease. *Ann Intern Med* 1987;106:793.

9. Hachamovitch R, Berman DS, Kiat H, et al. Exercise myocardial perfusion SPECT in patients without known coronary artery disease: Incremental prognostic value and use in risk stratification. *Circulation* 1996;93:905.

10. Berman DS, Hachamovitch R, Kiat H, et al. Incremental value of prognostic testing in patients with known or suspected ischemic heart disease: A basis for optimal utilization of exercise technetium-99m sestamibi myocardial perfusion single-photon emission computed tomography. *J Am Coll Cardiol* 1995; 26:639.

11. Iskander S, Iskandrian A. Risk Assessment using single-photon emission computed tomographic technetium-99m sestamibi imaging. *J Am Coll Cardiol* 1998;32:57.

12. Brown KA, Altland E, Rowen M, et al. Prognostic value of normal technetium-99m-sestamibi cardiac imaging. *J Nucl Cardiol* 1994;35:554.

13. Heller GV, Brown KA. Prognosis of acute and chronic coronary artery disease by myocardial perfusion imaging. *Cardiol Clin* 1994;12:271.

14. Soman P, Taillefer R, DePuey EG, et al. Enhanced detection of reversible perfusion defects by Tc-99m sestamibi compared to Tc-99m tetrofosmin during vasodilator stress SPECT imaging in mild-to-moderate coronary artery disease. *J Am Coll Cardiol* 2001;37:458.

15. Shaw LJ, Hendel R, Borges-Neto S, Lauer MS, et al. Prognostic value of normal exercise and adenosine (99m) Tc-tetrofosmin SPECT imaging: Results from the multicenter registry of 4,728 patients. *J Nucl Med* 2003;44:134.

16. Vanzetto G, Ormezzano O, Fagret D, et al. Long-term additive prognostic value of thallium-201 myocardial perfusion imaging over clinical and exercise stress test in low to intermediate risk patients: Study in 1137 patients with 6-year follow up. *Circulation* 1999;100:1521.

17. Schinkel AF, Elhendy A, van Domburg RT, et al. Prognostic value of dobutamine–atropine stress (99m) Tc-tetrofosmin myocardial perfusion SPECT in patients with known or suspected coronary artery disease. *J Nucl Med* 2002;43:767.

18. Calnon DA, McGrath PD, Doss AL, et al. Prognostic value of dobutamine stress technetium-99m sestamibi single-photon emission computed tomography myocardial perfusion imaging: stratification of a high-risk population. *J Am Coll Cardiol* 2001;38:1511.

19. Soman P, Parsons A, Lahiri N, Lahiri A. The prognostic value of a normal Tc-99m sestamibi SPECT study in suspected coronary artery disease. *J Nucl Cardiol* 1999;6:252.

20. Groutars RG, Verzijlbergen JF, Muller AJ, et al. Prognostic value and quality of life in patients with normal rest thallium-201/stress technetium 99m-tetrofosmin dual-isotope myocardial SPECT. *J Nucl Cardiol* 2000;7:333.

21. Levine MG, Ahlberg AW, Mann A, et al. Comparison of exercise, dipyridamole, adenosine, and dobutamine stress with the use of Tc-99m tetrofosmin tomographic imaging. *J Nucl Cardiol* 1999;6:389.

22. Heller GV, Herman SD, Travin MI, et al. Independent prognostic value of intravenous dipyridamole with technetium-99m sestamibi tomographic imaging in predicting cardiac events and cardiac-related hospital admissions. *J Am Coll Cardiol* 1995;26:1202.

23. Elhendy A, Sozzi FB, Valkema R, et al. Dobutamine technetium-99m tetrofosmin SPECT imaging for the diagnosis of coronary artery disease in patients with limited exercise capacity. *J Nucl Cardiol* 2000;7:649.

24. Amanullah AM, Berman DS, Erel J, et al. Incremental prognostic value of adenosine myocardial perfusion single-photon emission computed tomography in women with suspected coronary artery disease. *Am J Cardiol* 1998;82:725.

25. Geleijnse ML, Elhendy A, van Domburg RT, et al. Prognostic significance of normal dobutamine–atropine stress sestamibi scintigraphy in women with chest pain. *Am J Cardiol* 1996;77:1057.

26. Akinboboye OO, Idris O, Onwuanyi A, et al. Incidence of major cardiovascular events in black patients with normal myocardial stress perfusion study results. *J Nucl Cardiol* 2001;8:541.

27. Kang X, Berman DS, Lewin HC, et al. Incremental prognostic value of myocardial perfusion single photon emission computed tomography in patients with diabetes mellitus. *Am Heart J* 1999;138:1025.

28. Schinkel AF, Elhendy A, van Domburg RT, et al. Prognostic value of dobutamine–atropine stress myocardial perfusion imaging in patients with diabetes. *Diabetes Care* 2002;25:1637.

29. Galassi AR, Azzarelli S, Tomaselli A, et al. Incremental prognostic value of technetium-99-tetrofosmin exercise myocardial perfusion imaging for predicting outcomes in patients with suspected or known coronary artery disease. *Am J Cardiol* 2001;88:101.

30. Marie PY, Danchin N, Durand JF, et al. Long-term prediction of major ischemic events by exercise thallium-201 single-photon emission computed tomography: Incremental prognostic value compared with clinical, exercise testing, catheterization and radionuclide angiographic data. *J Am Coll Cardiol* 1995;26:879.

31. Heller GV, Brown KA. Prognosis of acute and chronic coronary artery disease by myocardial perfusion imaging. *Cardiol Clin* 1994;12:271.

32. Ladenheim ML, Pollock BH, Rozanski A, et al. Extent and severity of myocardial hypoperfusion as predictors of prognosis in patients with suspected coronary artery disease. *J Am Coll Cardiol* 1986;7:464.

33. Hachamovitch R, Berman DS, Shaw LJ, et al. Incremental prognostic value of myocardial perfusion single photon emission computed tomography for the prediction of cardiac death: Differential stratification for risk of cardiac death and myocardial infarction. *Circulation* 1998;97:535.

34. Hendel RC, Whitfield SS, Villegas BJ, et al. Prediction of late cardiac events by dipyridamole thallium imaging in patients undergoing elective vascular surgery. *Am J Cardiol* 1992;70:1243.

35. Ritchie JL, Bateman TM, Bonow RO, et al. Guidelines for clinical use of cardiac radionuclide imaging. Report of the American College of Cardiology/American Heart Association Task Force on Assessment of Diagnostic and Therapeutic Cardiovascular Procedures (Committee on Radionuclide Imaging), developed in collaboration with the American Society of Nuclear Cardiology. *J Am Coll Cardiol* 1995;25:521.

36. Randomized trial of cholesterol lowering in 4444 patients with coronary heart disease: The Scandinavian Simvastatin Survival Study (4S). *Lancet* 1994;344:1383.

37. The Long-Term Intervention with Pravastatin in Ischemic Disease (LIPID) Study Group: Prevention of cardiovascular events and death with pravastatin in patients with coronary heart disease and a broad range of initial cholesterol levels. *N Engl J Med* 1998;339:1349.

38. Shepherd J, Cobbe SM, Ford I, et al. Prevention of coronary heart disease with pravastatin in men with hypercholesterolemia: West of Scotland Coronary Prevention Study Group. *N Engl J Med* 1995;333:1301.

39. Sacks FM, Pfeffer MA, Moye LA, et al. The effect of pravastatin on coronary events after myocardial infarction in patients with average cholesterol levels: Cholesterol and Recurrent Events (CARE) Trial investigators. *N Engl J Med* 1996;335:1001.

40. Pitt B, Waters D, Brown WV, van Boven AJ, et al. Aggressive lipid-lowering therapy compared with angioplasty in stable coronary artery disease. *N Engl J Med* 1999;341:70.

41. Yusuf S, Sleight P, Pogue J, Bosch J, et al. Effects of an angiotensin-converting enzyme inhibitor, ramipril, on cardiovascular events in high-risk patients: The Heart Outcomes Prevention Evaluation Study Investigators. *N Engl J Med* 2000;342:145.

42. Iskandrian AS, Chae SC, Heo J, et al. Independent and incremental prognostic value of exercise single-photon emission tomographic (SPECT) thallium imaging in coronary artery disease. *J Am Coll Cardiol* 1993;22:665.

43. Sharir T, Berman DS, Lewin HC, et al. Incremental prognostic value of rest-redistribution Tl-201 single-photon emission computed tomography. *Circulation* 1999;100:1964.

44. Nallamothu N, Ghods M, Heo J, Iskandrian AS. Comparison of thallium-201 single-photon emission computed tomography and electrocardiographic response during exercise in patients with normal rest electrocardiographic results. *J Am Coll Cardiol* 1995;25:830.

45. Pollock SG, Abbott RD, Boucher CA, et al. Independent and incremental prognostic value of tests performed in hierarchical order to evaluate patients with suspected coronary artery disease: Validation of models based on these tests. *Circulation* 1992;85:237.

46. Germano G, Berman D. On the accuracy and reproducibility of quantitative gated myocardial perfusion SPECT. *J Nucl Med* 1999;40:810.

47. Schinkel AF, Elhendy A, van Domburg RT, et al. Incremental value of exercise technetium-99m tetrofosmin myocardial perfusion single-photon emission computed tomography for the prediction of cardiac events. *Am J Cardiol* 2003;91:408.

48. Hachamovitch T, Berman DS, Kiat H, et al. Value of stress myocardial perfusion single photon emission computed tomography in patients with normal resting electrocardiograms: An evaluation of incremental prognostic value and cost-effectiveness. *Circulation* 2002;105:823.

49. Zerahn B, Jensen BV, Nielsen KD, Moller S. Increased prognostic value of combined myocardial perfusion imaging and exercise electrocardiography in patients with coronary artery disease. *J Nucl Cardiol* 2000;7:616.

50. Groutars RG, Verzijlbergen JF, Zwinderman AH, et al. Incremental prognostic value of myocardial SPECT with dual-isotope rest (201) TI/stress (99m) T-tetrofosmin. *Eur J Nucl Med Mol Imaging* 2002;29:46.

51. Germano G, Kavanagh PB, Kavanagh TJ, et al. Repeatability of automatic left ventricular cavity volume measurements from myocardial perfusion SPECT. *J Nucl Cardiol* 1998;5:477.

52. Depuey EG, Rozanski A. Using gated tecnetium-99m sestamibi SPECT to characterize fixed myocardial defects as infarct or artifact. *J Nucl Med* 1995;36:952.

53. Smanio PE, Watson DD, Segalla DL, et al. Value of gating of technetium-99m sestamibi single-photon emission computed tomography. *J Am Coll Cardiol* 1997;30:1687.

54. Taillefer R, Depuey EG, Udelson JE, et al. Comparative diagnostic accuracy of thallium-201 and technetium-99m sestamibi SPECT imaging (perfusion and ECG-gated SPECT) in detecting coronary artery disease in women. *J Am Col Cardiol* 1997;29:69.

55. Sharir T, Germano G, Kavanagh PB, et al. Incremental prognostic value of post-stress left ventricular ejection fraction and volume by gated myocardial perfusion single photon emission computed tomography. *Circulation* 1999;100:1035.

56. Sharir T, Germano G, Kang X, et al. Prediction of myocardial infarction versus cardiac death by gated myocardial perfusion SPECT: Risk stratification by the amount of stress-induced ischemia and the post-stress ejection fraction. *J Nucl Med* 2001;42:831.

57. Weiss AT, Berman DS, Lew AS, et al. Transient ischemic dilatation of the left ventricle on stress thallium-201 scintigraphy: A marker of severe and extensive coronary artery disease. *J Am Coll Cardiol* 1987;9:752.

58. Chouraqui P, Rodrigues EA, Berman DS, et al. Significance of dipyridamole-induced transient dilatation of the left ventricle during thallium-201 scintigraphy in suspected coronary artery disease. *Am J Cardiol* 1990;66:689.

59. McClellan JR, Travin MI, Herman SD, et al. Prognostic importance of scintigraphic left ventricular cavity dilatation during intravenous dipyridamole technetium-99m sestamibi myocardial tomographic imaging in predicting coronary events. *Am J Cardiol* 1997;79:600.

60. Mazzanti M, Germano G, Kiat H, et al. Identification of severe and extensive coronary artery disease by automatic measurement of transient ischemic dilatation of the left ventricle in dual-isotope myocardial perfusion SPECT. *J Am Coll Cardiol* 1996;27:1612.

61. Kinoshita N, Sugihara H, Adachi Y, et al. Assessment of transient left ventricular dilatation on rest and exercise on Tc-99m tetrofosmin myocardial SPECT. *Clin Nucl Med* 2002;27:34.

62. Boucher CA, Zir LM, Beller GA, et al. Increased lung uptake of thallium-201 during exercise myocardial imaging: Clinical, hemodynamic and angiographic implications in patients with coronary artery disease. *Am J Cardiol* 1980;46:189.

63. Gibson RS, Watson DD, Carabello BA, et al. Clinical implication of increased lung uptake of thallium-201 during exercise scintigraphy 2 weeks after myocardial infarction. *Am J Cardiol* 1982;49:1586.

64. Kaminek M, Myslivecek M, Skvarilova M, et al. Increased prognostic value of combined myocardial perfusion SPECT imaging and the quantification of lung TI-201 uptake. *Clin Nucl Med* 2002;27:255.

65. Brown KA. Cardiac risk defined by stress myocardial perfusion imaging: Impact on physician decision making and cost savings. *J Nucl Cardiol* 2002;9:124.

66. Shaw LJ, Hachamovitch R, Berman DS, et al. The economic consequences of available diagnostic and prognostic strategies for the evaluation of stable angina patients: an observational assessment of the value of precatheterization ischemia. *J Am Coll Cardiol* 1999;33:661.

67. Ryan TJ, Antman EM, Brooks NH, et al. 1999 update: ACC/AHA guidelines for the management of patients with acute myocardial infarction. A report of the American College of Cardiology/American Heart Association Task Force on Practice Guidelines (Committee on Management of Acute Myocardial Infarction). *J Am Coll Cardiol* 1999;34:890.

68. Brown KA, Weiss RM, Clements JP, et al. Usefulness of residual ischemic myocardium within prior infarct zone for identifying patients at high risk after acute myocardial infarction. *Am J Cardiol* 1987;60:15.

69. Dakik HA, Mahmarian JJ, Kimball KT, et al. Prognostic value of exercise 201 thallium tomography in patients treated with thrombolytic therapy during acute myocardial infarction. *Circulation* 1996;94:2735.

70. Zellweger MJ, Dubois EA, Lai S, et al. Risk stratification in patients with remote prior myocardial infarction using rest-stress myocardial perfusion SPECT: Prognostic value and impact on referral to early catheterization. *J Nucl Cardiol* 2002;9:23.

71. Kroll D, Farah W, McKendall GR, et al. Prognostic value of stress-gated Tc-99m sestamibi SPECT after acute myocardial infarction. *Am J Cardiol* 2001;87:381.

72. Gibson RS, Watson DD, Graddock GB, et al. Prediction of cardiac events after uncomplicated myocardial infarction: A prospective study comparing predischarge exercise thallium-201 scintigraphy and coronary angiography. *Circulation* 1983;68:321.

73. Wilson WW, Gibson RS, Nygaard TW, et al. Acute myocardial infarction associated with single vessel coronary disease: An analysis of clinical outcome and the prognostic importance of vessel patency and residual ischemic myocardium. *J Am Coll Cardiol* 1988;11:223.

74. Brown KA, Heller GV, Landin RS, et al. Early dipyridamole (99m) Tc-sestamibi single photon

emission computed tomographic imaging 2 to 4 days after acute myocardial infarction predicts in-hospital and postdischarge cardiac events: Comparison with submaximal exercise imaging. *Circulation* 1999;100:2060.

75. Gimple LW, Hutter AM, Guiney TE, et al. Prognostic utility of predischarge dipyridamole–thallium imaging compared to predischarge submaximal exercise electrocardiography and maximal exercise thallium imaging after uncomplicated acute myocardial infarction. *Am J Cardiol* 1989;64:1243.

76. Brown KA, O'Meara J, Chambers CE, et al. Ability of dipyridamole–thallium-201 imaging one to four days after acute myocardial infarction to predict in-hospital and late recurrent myocardial ischemic events. *Am J Cardiol* 1990;65:160.

77. Mahmarian JJ, Mahmarian AC, Marks GF, et al. Role of adenosine thallium-201 tomography for defining long-term risk in patients after acute myocardial infarction. *J Am Coll Cardiol* 1995;25:1333.

78. Leppo JA, O'Brien J, Rothendler JA, et al. Dipyridamole–thallium-201 scintigraphy in the prediction of future cardiac events after acute myocardial infarction. *N Engl J Med* 1984;310:1014.

79. Ellis SG, Mooney MR, George BS, et al. Randomized trial of late elective angioplasty versus conservative management for patients with residual stenoses after thrombolytic treatment of myocardial infarction: Treatment of Post-Thrombolytic Stenoses (TOPS) Study Group. *Circulation* 1992;86:1400.

80. Thrombolysis in Myocardial Ischemia TIMI-IIIB investigators. Effects of tissue plasminogen activator and a comparison of early invasive and conservative strategies in unstable angina and non-Q-wave myocardial infarction: Results of the TIMI IIIB Trial. Thrombolysis in Myocardial Ischemia. *Circulation* 1994;89:1545.

81. Boden WE, O'Rourke RA, Crawford MH, et al. Outcomes in patients with acute non-Q-wave myocardial infarction randomly assigned to an invasive as compared with a conservative management strategy: Veterans Affairs Non-Q-Wave Infarction Strategies in Hospital (VANQWISH) Trial Investigators. *N Engl J Med* 1998;338:1785.

82. The CAPTURE Investigators. Randomized placebo-controlled trial of abciximab before and during coronary intervention in refractory unstable angina: The CAPTURE study. *Lancet* 1997;349:1429.

83. The Platelet Receptor Inhibition in Ischemic Syndrome Management in Patients Limited by Unstable Signs and Symptoms (PRISM-plus) Study Investigators. Inhibition of the platelet glycoprotein IIb/IIIa receptor with tirofiban in unstable angina and non-Q-wave myocardial infarction. *N Engl J Med* 1998;338:1488.

84. The PURSUIT Trial Investigators. Inhibition of platelet glycoprotein IIb/IIIa with eptifibatide in patients with acute coronary syndromes. *N Engl J Med* 1998;339:436.

85. TACTICS—Thrombolysis in Myocardial Infarction (TIMI)-18 Investigators: Comparison of Early Invasive and Conservative Strategies in Patients with Unstable Coronary Syndromes Treated with the Glycoprotein IIb/IIIa Inhibitor Tirofiban. *N Engl J Med* 2001;344:1879.

86. The TIMI Risk Score for Unstable Angina/Non-ST Elevation MI. A method for prognostication and therapeutic decision making. *JAMA* 2000;284:835.

87. Brown KA. Prognostic value of thallium-201 myocardial perfusion imaging in patients with unstable angina who respond to medical treatment. *J Am Coll Cardiol* 1991;17:1053.

88. Freeman MR, Chishom RJ, Armstrong PW. Usefulness of exercise electrocardiography and thallium scintigraphy in unstable angina pectoris in predicting the extent and severity of coronary artery disease. *Am J Cardiol* 1988;62:1164.

89. Stratmann HG, Younis LT, Wittry MD, et al. Exercise technetium-99m myocardial tomography for the risk stratification of men with medically treated unstable angina pectoris. *Am J Cardiol* 1995;76:236.

CHAPTER 20

Selection for Referral for Cardiac Catheterization

William E. Boden

APPROACH TO EARLY MANAGEMENT: INITIAL ORIENTATION

Guidelines have been published for the management of patients with unstable angina.[1,2] Patients at low risk with new-onset exertion angina or minor exacerbation of chest pain during exercise, which is promptly relieved by nitroglycerin, can be safely managed as outpatients, assuming close follow-up and rapid investigation. Patients with prolonged pain and a ruled-out diagnosis of myocardial infarction (MI) are observed in the emergency room or in a chest pain unit, where clinical status, electrocardiogram (ECG), cardiac enzymes, and, wherever possible, troponin T or troponin I plasma levels are monitored. Blood tests are obtained at admission and repeated 8 to 12 hours after the onset of chest pain to rule out myocardial damage. Patients with a more definite diagnosis and one or more features of high risk, including repetitive pain, hemodynamic compro-

mise, ST-segment shift, or elevation in cardiac enzymes or troponin T or I levels, are best monitored in a coronary care unit (CCU) setting and are generally regarded as candidates for early diagnostic coronary angiography, followed by myocardial revascularization with coronary artery bypass graft (CABG) surgery or percutaneous coronary intervention (PCI). Management of patients with an intermediate risk is directed by the physician's judgment, often dictated by local facilities and pattern of practice.

USE OF NONINVASIVE AND INVASIVE TESTING IN RISK STRATIFICATION

The management of acute coronary syndromes has been largely predicated on the performance of routine, diagnostic coronary angiography to define abnormal coronary anatomy. Such an approach seeks to identify the so-called culprit stenosis, or stenoses, for which the goal is to perform myocardial revascularization with either coronary bypass surgery or PCI. Presumably, the purpose of performing early coronary angiography and myocardial revascularization is to improve both short-term and long-term clinical outcomes. Unquestionably, this management approach is associated with improved symptoms and quality of life short term, but it remains unclear whether such a strategy favorably alters clinical outcomes such as death or recurrent nonfatal MI.

Prior to undertaking an invasive evaluation, it seems most appropriate to achieve control of symptoms and objective findings of myocardial ischemia in patients who present to the hospital with unstable angina. In the majority of patients, bed rest and intensification of antithrombotic (IV heparin and aspirin), anti-ischemic (IV nitroglycerin plus calcium channel blocker and/or beta blocker), and/or platelet glycoprotein IIb/IIIa receptor antagonist therapy will be effective pharmacotherapy.

In patients who have persistent or refractory symptoms of angina, or recurrent ECG findings of myocardial ischemia, despite maximal medical therapy, or if patients demonstrate hemodynamic instability, use of intra-aortic balloon counterpulsation may be extremely effective, until cardiac catheterization and myocardial revascularization can be safely performed.

If coronary angiography cannot be deferred as an elective procedure because the patient exhibits persistent or recurrent ischemia despite intensification of medical therapy, prompt coronary angiography must be undertaken, followed by myocardial revascularization, if possible. Clearly, the risk of undertaking PCI or CABG surgery is higher in such patients, compared to the morbidity associated with performing such revascularization procedures on stable elective coronary artery disease (CAD) patients. Nevertheless, myocardial revascularization may be the most appropriate strategy to undertake in patients with unstable angina whose myocardium is at risk for infarction and should be reserved for those patients who do not adequately respond to medical therapy.

The approach to the "stabilized" unstable angina patient is somewhat more controversial. One approach would be to subject *all* unstable angina patients to diagnostic coronary angiography, irrespective of their initial response to medical therapy in the CCU. The rationale for this approach is that the acute coronary syndrome was likely presaged by accelerated coronary atherosclerosis, and the "stabilization" achieved with medical therapy is likely only to be temporary, and is not likely to affect the underlying coronary stenosis or stenoses.

However, studies have indicated that most coronary lesions that presage plaque rupture in unstable angina are minor (< 50% stenosis), and that high-grade CAD is not invariably the angiographic finding in patients who present with acute coronary syndromes.[1,2] Thus, it remains unproven that *all* patients with unstable angina should undergo *routine* coronary angiography prior to hospital discharge. Such a decision must be individualized, taking into account several factors (patient's age, physical activity level, ECG findings of ischemia, other medical conditions, etc.) that may influence diagnostic and therapeutic decision making.

An alternative strategy may be employed. According to this approach, intensive medical therapy (antithrombotic, antiplatelet, and anti-ischemic), as previously described, should be initiated as soon as the patient has been admitted to a monitored care facility. If the patient stabilizes on maximal medical therapy in the CCU or telemetry unit, these intravenous medications can be changed to equivalent oral therapy. If the patient does not develop spontaneous angina or ECG findings of recurrent ischemia as his or her physical activity is advanced, urgent coronary angiography can be deferred, and myocardial perfusion imaging (MPI) with sestamibi or thallium can be performed.

If the patient exhibits objective findings of a "high-risk" scan (multiple perfusion defects, an extensive anteroseptal perfusion defect, increased lung uptake, increased left ventricular [LV] cavity dilatation [increased cardiac blood pool]), he or she should undergo prompt diagnostic coronary angiography followed by myocardial revascularization, as outlined above. On the other hand, if the patient exhibits a normal or low-risk myocardial perfusion scan, it would be appropriate to continue antithrombotic and anti-ischemic therapy, and to follow the patient's clinical course closely post-discharge.

MEDICAL MANAGEMENT VERSUS CORONARY INTERVENTION

In an effort to define better therapeutic modalities, intervention therapy has been compared with medical therapy. The two main trials that have compared bypass surgery with medical therapy, the National Cooperative Study[3] and the Veterans Administration Cooperative Study,[4] have shown similar survival rates with the two therapeutic modalities. In the former study, mortality at 1 year was 8% in surgical patients and 50% in medical patients. In the latter, the rates of MI after 2 years were 11.7% and 12.2%, respectively. Rates of crossover to surgery were 19% at 1 year in the National Cooperative Study and 34% at 2 years in the Veterans Administration Study. Importantly, subsets of patients in the Veterans Administration Study benefited in the long term from surgery. Thus, the 5-year survival rate in patients with three-vessel disease was 89% with surgery, compared with 75% with medical treatment ($p = 0.02$), and the mortality in patients with an ejection fraction between 30% and 49% was reduced from 27 to 14%.

With the development of percutaneous procedures for myocardial revascularization, trials have been reoriented to conservative strategy. The TIMI-IIIB Trial was the prototype of these trials.[5] By study design, patients in the early invasive strategy arm had coronary angiography within 24 to 48 hours after randomization, followed by coronary angioplasty or bypass surgery in the presence of suitable anatomy. These procedures were performed in the conservative strategy arm with failure of medical therapy, defined by recurrent chest pain with ST-T changes, a 20-minute period of ischemic ST-segment shifts on a 24-hour Holter monitor, a predischarge positive stress thallium exercise test before completion of stage 2 of the Bruce protocol, rehospitalization for unstable angina, or angina class III or IV with a positive exercise test during follow-up. A total of 1,473 patients with unstable angina or non-Q-wave MI were randomized. The primary end point included death, MI, or positive treadmill test at 6 weeks; it occurred in 18.1% of patients assigned to the conservative strategy and in 16% of patients assigned to invasive strategy ($p = $ NS). Death or MI occurred in 7.8% and 7.2% of patients at 6 weeks ($p = $ NS) and in 12.2% and 10.8% at 1 year ($p = $ NS). A large proportion of patients (64%) assigned to medical treatment crossed over to invasive treatment because of recurrent angina or an early positive test for ischemia. Also, the average length of initial hospital stay, the incidence of rehospitalization within 6 weeks, and the number of days of rehospitalization were all decreased with invasive treatment. Another important subset of acute coronary syndromes includes patients with non-Q-wave myocardial infarction (MI). It is generally agreed that patients recovering from acute non-Q-wave MI sustain less myocardial necrosis and have a lower in-hospital mortality, whereas most (but not all) studies indicate that such patients have the same or higher long-term mortality than do patients recovering from acute Q-wave MI. Moreover, the majority of published studies indicate that both early and late ischemic complications (reinfarction, postinfarction angina) are consistently higher in non-Q-wave MI patients compared to Q-wave MI patients, presumably due to the large degree of residually ischemic, jeopardized myocardium that remains at risk within the perfusion zone of the infarct-related coronary artery.

Accordingly, the management of acute non-Q-wave MI patients has become increasingly aggressive during the last decade, although the hypothesis (that an invasive approach would be superior to a conservative approach) has never been adequately tested prospectively in a large group of such patients with this type of acute coronary syndrome.

Most data in the management of non-Q-wave MI have been retrospectively acquired, and certain clinical variables have emerged as powerful predictors of adverse 1-year outcome. These include recurrent infarct extension (reinfarction), postinfarction angina associated with transient electrocardiographic changes (early recurrent ischemia), followed by persistent ST-segment depression on serial post–non-Q-wave MI ECGs, congestive heart failure (CHF), and left ventricular hypertrophy (LVH).

Such data support a balanced diagnostic approach to identify high-risk subsets of post–non-Q-wave MI management. Approximately 30 to 35% of non-Q-wave MI patients comprise this high-risk subset, defined as those with reinfarction, postinfarction angina, CHF, or persistent ST-segment depression. Invasive testing and interventional maneuvers should be reserved for patients considered at high risk according to the presence of two or more of the above covariates of risk. Alternatively, the remaining asymptomatic or low-risk patients appear to be appropriate candidates for conservative management, which would include a functional assessment of risk (stress test, preferably with sestamibi or thallium) followed by diagnostic coronary angiography only for clinical need or for objective evidence of inducible ischemia.

Acute coronary syndromes (ACSs) represent a spectrum of disease, including unstable angina, non–ST elevation MI, and ST elevation MI. In patients with cardiovascular disease, ACS represents the most common diagnosis for hospital admission, accounting for nearly 1.5 million hospital admissions in 1999. Similarly, although improvements in medical therapy have resulted in a dramatic decline in mortality from acute MI over the last four decades, MI remains the most common cause of in-hospital death in industrialized nations.

The approach to managing patients with ACSs has evolved dramatically over the past decade and, in many respects, represents a rapidly moving target in light of recent advances in pharmacotherapy and catheter-based revascularization. A number of recently published studies, including the TACTICS Trial[6], the ADMIRAL Trial[7], the TARGET Trial[8], and the GUSTO V study[9], provide novel information about the relative merits of pharmacologic therapy and invasive intervention. A common theme from these studies is that there is a growing consensus among cardiologists that *combination* therapy with these two modalities may actually provide the best clinical outcomes in ACS patients.

ST ELEVATION MYOCARDIAL INFARCTION

ST elevation myocardial infarction (STEMI) is a medical emergency that is most often caused by occlusive coronary thrombus. Approximately 33% of patients with STEMI die, one half of them within the first hour of symptom onset. Mortality can be significantly reduced by rapid transport to the hospital, institution of prompt pharmacologic or mechanical reperfusion, treatment of ventricular arrhythmias, and recognition and treatment of hemodynamic complications.

Perhaps the most important advance that has occurred in STEMI therapy over the last 10 years has been general acceptance of the "open-artery hypothesis." This hypothesis, derived from the results of numerous clinical trials, states that early restoration of antegrade blood flow in the infarct-related artery results in beneficial salvage of ischemic myocardium and significantly reduces both patient morbidity and mortality. Rapid restoration of brisk antegrade flow in the culprit vessel of patients with evolving acute myocardial infarction (AMI) has been incontrovertibly shown to decrease infarct size and to improve survival. Acceptance of this hypothesis has resulted in the widespread testing of reperfusion modalities to open the occluded infarct vessel, including both pharmacologic and mechanical techniques, used alone or in combination.

Pharmacologic reperfusion with intravenous thrombolytic therapy became widely used initially in the 1980s. Based on the results of the GISSI-1[10], ISIS-2[11], ASSET[12], ISIS-3[13], GUSTO-1[14], LATE[15], and the EMERAS Trials[16], thrombolytic therapy has been shown to result in an estimated average reduction of early mortality of 20 to 30%. The obvious benefits of thrombolytic therapy include its widespread availability in all centers, its ease of administration, and the fact that its efficacy is not operator dependent. Furthermore, the clinical benefits of thrombolytic reperfusion have been undeniably documented in multiple rigorous scientific trials with large numbers of patients.[17]

Since its introduction, however, deficiencies in the use of intravenous thrombolysis have clearly emerged. First, despite widespread availability, a majority of patients (70–75%) have not been considered eligible for receiving thrombolytic therapy, including patients with cerebrovascular disease, hemorrhagic diatheses, active bleeding, recent surgery, severe hypertension, or recent cardiopulmonary resuscitation. Second, regardless of the dose or combination of thrombolytic agents given, use of this technique results in a maximal 80% incidence of infarct-vessel patency and a maximal 55 to 60% incidence of optimal TIMI-III flow. Third, despite rapid administration of thrombolytic agents in the emergency department, there is a median lag time of approximately 45 minutes prior to pharmacologic reperfusion and there are indistinct parameters to measure the return of optimal infarct-vessel blood flow. Finally, use of these agents is associated with a significant 0.5 to 1.5% incidence of intracranial bleeding and a 15 to 30% incidence of recurrent ischemic events.

As an alternative to intravenous thrombolysis, mechanical reperfusion of the infarct vessel in the catheterization laboratory emerged in the 1990s. Several early studies demonstrated clear superiority of mechanical over pharmacolgic reperfusion, including the PAMI[18], Mayo Clinic[19] and Zwolle[20] studies. These potential benefits included use in patients who were thrombolytic in-

eligible, a higher (85 to 95%) incidence of infarct-vessel patency and TIMI-III flow, a reduced incidence of recurrent ischemia/reinfarction and intracranial bleeding, and shorter hospital stays. In addition, a recent meta-analysis of 10 randomized trials conducted in 2,606 AMI patients has shown a significant reduction in mortality in patients treated with mechanical versus pharamacologic reperfusion.[21]

Like thrombolytic therapy, however, substantial deficiencies of mechanical reperfusion have emerged. First, widespread use of mechanical reperfusion is limited by the small number of hospitals that are capable of performing the procedure. Currently, only 20% of U.S. hospitals have suitable catheterization facilities, on-site surgical backup, and appropriately trained personnel, which are needed for safe, immediate catheterization and percutaneous intervention.[22,23] As a result, there is a significant time delay for a majority of AMI patients presenting to community hospitals necessitated by the need for rapid transport to a tertiary centers and the mobilization of appropriate catheterization resources. Second, like thrombolytic therapy, percutaneous revascularization is still associated with a significant incidence of recurrent ischemia and reinfarction. Finally; despite the short-term benefits of percutaneous revascularization, the impact of mechanical reperfusion on long-term clinical outcomes has not been rigorously tested and remains less certain.

The ongoing debate over the relative superiority of PCI versus thrombolytic therapy has been further complicated by recent improvements in fibrinolytic agents, adjunctive antiplatelet/antithrombin pharmacology, and the refinement of mechanical techniques. The advent of newer recombinant DNA technologies has created a new generation of "bolus thrombolytics" that have enhanced fibrin sensitivity and facilitated greater ease of use.[9,24] Although additional testing is needed, use of these newer fibrinolytic agents in AMI has been associated with earlier and superior coronary infarct-artery patency in some preliminary trials. In addition, use of these newer agents in reduced doses (i.e., half-dose thrombolytics) may potentially reduce the prothrombotic effects indigenous to intravenous thrombolysis and may also reduce serious bleeding complications.

Equally important to improvements in fibrinolytic agents have been recent advances in antiplatelet and antithrombin pharmacology. Over the last several years, glycoprotein platelet [GP] IIb/IIIa receptor blockers have emerged as potent platelet inhibitors which have been shown to provide significant benefit in all classes of patients with ACSs. Preliminary studies, including the TAMI-8[25], the IMPACT-AMI[26], the PARADIGM[27], the TIMI 14A[28], and SPEED Trials[29], have shown that combined use of IIb/IIIa agents with thrombolytics is safe and efficacious in AMI patients, with theoretic potentiation of fibrinolysis by platelet disaggregation that engenders more stable reperfusion. In addition, better anticoagulants, including low-molecular-weight heparins, direct thrombin inhibitors, and agents that block higher in the anticoagulation cascade, have emerged and are in various states of testing. The potential use of these agents may theoretically provide for more comprehensive clot lysis with more rapid, complete, and sustained myocardial perfusion.

Improvements in pharmacologic reperfusion have been paralleled by simultaneous refinement of mechanical revascularization techniques. Over the last several years, intracoronary stenting in the AMI patient has been shown to be superior to balloon angioplasty with less recurrent ischemia and reduced late infarct-vessel restenosis. Mechanical thrombectomy devices and distal embolization protection devices are two additional modalities that are currently being tested and that may have a role in the treatment of the AMI patient.

Perhaps more important than refinement in pharmacologic and mechanical therapy has been the recent documentation that the *combination* of these two approaches may be particularly beneficial and synergistic. Despite theoretic considerations that optimal reperfusion would be achieved with pharmcologic treatment of thrombus and mechanical stabilization of underlying atheroma, early attempts to combine these therapies in the AMI setting were disappointing. Previous reports, including the TIMI-IIA[30], the TAMI-1,[23] and the European Cooperative Group[31] trials, demonstrated that PCI performed immediately after the administration of thrombolytic therapy did not provide any benefit over performing mechanical reperfusion at a later time or as part of a conservative strategy in which intervention was utilized only if indicated by noninvasive testing. In some of these studies, the combined use of thrombolysis followed by immediate intervention was associated with a higher incidence of adverse clinical events. More recent studies, however, have documented the safe use of combined pharmacologic–mechanical therapy.[33,34] In particular, the concept of "facilitated percutaneous intervention" has emerged and involves so-called "triple therapy" employing reduced-dose thrombolytics, GP IIb/IIIa inhibitors, and immediate catheterization with percutaneous intervention as indicated. Preliminary reports have suggested that this approach may be the most efficacious revascularization technique to date.

As an important step in recognizing the potential benefits of combined therapy in STEMI, Montalescot and co-workers have reported the results of the ADMIRAL Trial. In AMI patients randomized either to abciximab plus stenting or placebo plus stenting, the authors report a significant 59% reduction at 30 days and a 54% reduction at 6 months in the abciximab versus the placebo group for the triple composite primary end point of death, reinfarction, or urgent target vessel revascularization (TVR). For the "hard" end points of death, reinfarction, or a composite of death or reinfarction, there were important trends (but no significant between-group differences) in the abciximab plus primary stenting group at 30 days or 6 months, indicating that the benefits of GP IIb/IIIa inhibition were driven largely by the reductions in TVR. Nevertheless, the results of ADMIRAL indicate that the improved clinical outcomes were related to enhanced TIMI-III flow rates and coronary patency, as well as improved LV function, suggesting an important role for "facilitated PCI" in this group of patients.

The results of the ADMIRAL Trial differ somewhat from the recently reported CADILLAC Trial,[35] which also investigated the potential benefits of stenting plus GP IIb/IIIa receptor inhibition with abciximab in AMI patients. Although the CADILLAC investigators documented individual benefit of either primary stenting or abciximab use, there appeared to be no incremental value of adjunctive abciximab use in stented patients, other than a significant decrease in the incidence of subacute thrombosis. One potential explanation for the disparity between these two studies involves the upstream use of abciximab in ADMIRAL study. In particular, over 25% of ADMIRAL patients received the drug prior to cardiac catheterization. As a possible consequence of this upstream treatment, the incidence of baseline TIMI-III flow in the infarct vessel was significantly higher for the stent plus abciximab patients versus the stent alone patients in the ADMIRAL trial, with no significant differences between these two patients groups in the CADILLAC Trial. This suggests a possible benefit for upstream use of GP IIb/IIIa agents in the AMI population in the earlier establishment of optimal infarct-vessel flow prior to intervention, and further emphasizes the complementary importance of combined pharmacotherapy and mechanical reperfusion in this setting.

UNSTABLE ANGINA AND NON-ST-SEGMENT ELEVATION MYOCARDIAL INFARCTION (NSTEMI)

Unstable angina (UA) and non-ST-segment elevation myocardial infarction (NSTEMI) are two components of the ACSs. These syndromes are currently considered to be conditions with similar pathogenesis and clinical presentations that differ only in severity.[2] The most common cause is thrombus formation secondary to plaque disruption.[1] The presence of markers of cardiac necrosis, such as the I and T subunits of the troponin complex (TnI, TnT) or the MB isoenzyme of creatine kinase (CK-MB), establishes a diagnosis of NSTEMI.[2] Most patients with NSTEMI do not evolve a Q wave and are subsequently diagnosed as having non-Q-wave MI (NQMI).

In the management of patients with ACS, particularly those with NSTEMI, a fundamental question underlies the debate regarding invasive versus conservative strategies. The American College of Cardiology/American Heart Association Task Force on Practice Guidelines has published recommendations regarding diagnosis and treatment of patients with known or suspected UA/NSTEMI.[2] The acute ischemia pathway presented in these guidelines encompasses both an early invasive strategy and an early conservative strategy. However, the continued technical evolution of stents, and widespread availability and success of catheter-based revascularization has prompted many clinicians to question the need for noninvasive risk stratification of any kind as we enter the third millennium.

It is essential to consider a balanced approach to managing patients with non-ST-segment elevation ACS: an aggressive ("early invasive") approach for patients with increased risk as manifested by persistent pain or ECG or enzymatic changes; and an "ischemia-guided" strategy for patients who do not manifest these signs of increased risk. A "conservative strategy" is defined as including intensive antiplatelet, antithrombotic, and anti-ischemic therapy combined with careful clinical assessment and provocative testing (e.g., myocardial perfusion imaging with use of treadmill exercise or pharmacologic vasodilator stress testing). In these patients, selective catheterization and, if necessary, revascularization are performed only if spontaneous angina occurs or there is objective evidence of stress-induced myocardial ischemia. Randomized clinical trials focused on the various treatment approaches will be reviewed.

STUDIES COMPARING INVASIVE VERSUS CONSERVATIVE STRATEGIES IN UA/NSTEMI

TIMI-IIIB (Enrollment 1989–1992)

No significant differences in outcome between the invasive and conservative strategies for treating patients with unstable angina and non-Q-wave MI were shown in the Thrombolysis in Myocardial Infarction (TIMI-IIIB) trial, which was published in 1994.[5] This trial included 1,473 patients who were considered to have unstable angina or non-Q-wave MI. Study subjects were randomized using a 2 × 2 factorial design to compare the following:

- Tissue plasminogen activator (TPA) versus placebo as initial therapy
- An early invasive strategy (cardiac catheterization, LV angiography, and coronary arteriography 18 to 48 hours after randomization) versus an early conservative strategy (catheterization and angiography only after failure of initial therapy)

The composite end point for the comparison of the two strategies of death, MI, or an unsatisfactory exercise stress test at 6 weeks occurred in 18.1% of patients assigned to the early strategy and 16.2% of those assigned to the invasive strategy (Table 20-1). Although the early invasive strategy indicated more rapid relief of angina than the conservative approach, by 6 weeks, anginal status was similar between patients, as was the major clinical outcome of death or MI.

VANQWISH (Enrollment 1993–1995)

In the Veterans Affairs Non-Q-Wave Infarction Strategies in Hospital (VANQWISH) trial,[36] which was also conducted during the early 1990s, an unexpected difference was found in outcomes between the two approaches. The study compared early and late clinical outcomes (death or recurrent MI) in 462 patients randomly assigned to the early invasive strategy, with 458 patients who received the early conservative treatment. As shown in Figure 20-1, patients treated with the routine, early invasive strategy (heart catheterization followed by myocardial revascularization) had significantly worse clinical outcomes during the first year of follow-up than those treated with a conservative strategy (intervention guided by rigorous ischemia management, noninvasive stress testing, and medical therapy). VANQWISH is the largest trial of its kind to test the efficacy of long-term management strategies in patients recovering from non-Q-wave MI. The number of patients who had one of the components of the primary end point was significantly higher in the invasive-

Table 20-1

Invasive Versus Conservative Strategies in Patients with Non-ST-Segment Elevation MI: Outcomes at 6 Weeks in the TIMI-IIIB Trial

	Invasive Strategy (n = 740) n (%)	Conservative Strategy (n = 733) n (%)	P
Death	18 (2.4)	18 (2.5)	NS
MI	38 (5.1)	42 (5.7)	NS
Positive 6-week ETT	64 (8.6)	73 (10.0)	NS
Combined	120 (16.2)	133 (18.1)	NS

MI = myocardial infarction; ETT = exercise tolerance test
Modified from The TIMI-IIIB Investigators[5] with permission.

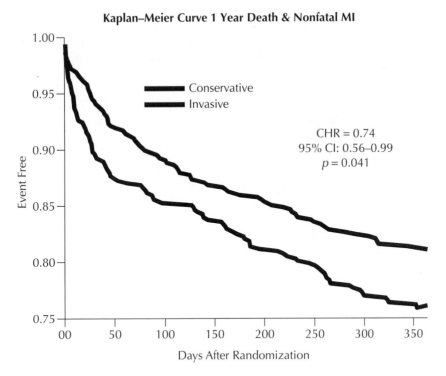

Kaplan–Meier Curve 1 Year Death & Nonfatal MI

CHR = 0.74
95% CI: 0.56–0.99
$p = 0.041$

Figure 20-1. From the VANQWISH trial, Kaplan–Meier analysis of the probability of event-free survival according to strategy group during 1 year of follow-up. Events included in the analysis were death and nonfatal MI (the composite end point). The Cox proportional hazards ratio for the conservative versus the invasive strategy was 0.74 (95% confidence interval, 0.56–0.99; $p = 0.041$). (Reprinted from Boden et al.[36] with permission.)

strategy group at hospital discharge (36 vs. 15 events, $p = 0.004$), at 1 month (48 vs. 26 events, $p = 0.012$), and at 1 year (111 vs. 85 events, $p = 0.05$).

An overlooked feature of the VANQWISH trial is that patients who remained in the conservative treatment arm and did not cross over to cardiac catheterization in the 44 months of follow-up (52% of this arm) had a remarkably low cardiac event rate; two patients (1%) died, and three patients (1%) experienced a clinical event at 30-day follow-up. This low rate of events occurred in patients with high clinical comorbidity and an almost 80% incidence of triple-vessel and left main coronary disease.

An interaction analysis to determine whether any subset of patients benefited with the invasive

strategy revealed no evidence of an interaction that supported improved outcomes in the patients with the invasive strategy.[36] In contrast, the ischemia-guided strategy benefited 4 of 10 prespecified subsets of patients (patients who underwent thrombolysis, those with no prior infarction, those with no ST-segment depression, and those ≥ 60 years).

Whether the results of TIMI-IIIB and VANQWISH are really relevant to the contemporary practice or management of patients with NSTEMI remains unclear. Both trials were conducted prior to a number of important advances that have occurred during the past 2 to 3 years, including the advent of stents and the newer catheter-based techniques. The use of glycoprotein IIb/IIIa receptor antagonists has expanded rapidly, based on a number of secondary prevention trials.[37-40] The benefits of low-molecular-weight heparins, particularly enoxaparin, have been convincingly demonstrated.[41-43] Evidence from the Organisation to Assess Strategies for Ischemic Syndromes (OASIS-2) trial revealed that hirudin (lepirudin), a direct thrombin inhibitor, may have benefit.[44] The Clopidogrel versus Aspirin in Patients at Risk of Ischemic Events (CAPRIE)[45] and the Clopidogrel in Unstable angina to prevent Recurrent ischemic Events (CURE)[46] trials showed that clopidogrel, a thienopyridine derivative similar to ticlopidine, to be an important adjunctive treatment in the management of patients with acute coronary syndromes.

However, the TIMI-IIIB[5] and VANQWISH[36] trials are relevant to risk stratification, because they reveal that both high- and low-risk subsets can be identified. In the VANQWISH trial, only 9% of patients were excluded during the first 48 to 72 hours for symptoms of refractory angina, persistent ischemia, heart failure, or significant ventricular tachyarrhythmia or fibrillation. As discussed, the 30-day event rate of death and MI was remarkably low (1%) with the conservative strategy, despite the high prevalence of clinical comorbidity and angiographic morbidity.

FRISC II (Enrollment 1996 to 1998)

The Fragmin and Fast Revascularisation during Instability in Coronary Artery Disease (FRISC II) invasive trial[47] showed for the first time, in a subset of patients with unstable angina and non-Q-wave infarction, a significant event rate reduction favoring the invasive over the noninvasive strategy at 6 months (Figure 20-2). In the trial, 2,457 patients in 58 Scandinavian hospitals were assigned an early invasive (1,222 patients) or noninvasive treatment strategy (1,235 patients) with placebo-controlled long-term low-molecular-weight heparin (dalteparin) for 3 months. In the invasive group, 96% of patients received angiography within 7 days; of those, 71% underwent revascularization within 10 days. For the noninvasive group, 10% received angiography within 7 days;

of those, 9% went on to undergo revascularization procedures. At 6 months, the rate of death, MI, or both, was 9.4% in the invasive group (113 of 1,207 patients) and 12.1% in the noninvasive group (148 of 1,226 patients) (risk ratio, 0.78; 95% CI, 0.62 to 0.98; $p = 0.031$).

The results favoring the invasive strategy were not uniformly shown among patient subsets in FRISC II, however. In a substudy examining the influence of troponin levels in study patients, plasma samples for central analyses of troponin T levels were available in 2,230 patients; of those, 42% had troponin-negative levels (< 0.1 ug/L).[48] The 6-month rate of death or MI was 8.3% in patients assigned to an invasive strategy versus 10.3% in those assigned to a conservative strategy. Although there was a trend toward improvement with the invasive strategy, the difference between groups was not statistically significant.

Similarly, in the evaluation of patients who had ST segment deviations on the admission electrocardiogram (ECG) in FRISC II, 418 patients had no demonstrable ST-T wave changes (Table 20-2).[49] The relative risk of an unfavorable outcome—death or MI at 6 months—was actually slightly higher for patients in the invasive group. No significant benefit was shown with the invasive strategy in patients who had isolated T wave inversion only. The early invasive strategy was not shown to be beneficial in fully 52% of patients who had either no ECG changes or T wave inversion only. The true benefit of early invasive treatment, when evaluated by ECG, was derived from the subset of patients with ST-segment depression MI.

In summary, patients who were troponin negative and those who had no ST-T wave changes or only isolated T wave inversions (> 50% of all patients) did not benefit from an invasive strategy. There are only observational data and registry data available to show a reduction of death or MI, or refractory ischemia, in NSTEMI patients who underwent PCI within 24 hours of presentation. Thus, much remains to be proven with regard to the overall benefit of applying an early aggressive invasive strategy in such patients.

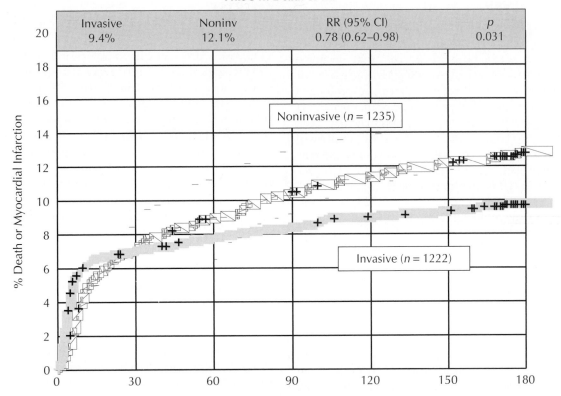

Figure 20-2. From the FRISC II study, probability of death or myocardial infarction in the invasive and noninvasive groups. (Reprinted from FRISC II Investigators[47] with permission.) Copyright by The Lancet Ltd, 2001.

Table 20-2

Subset Analysis of Primary End Point by Admission Electrocardiogram in the FRISC-II Trial

| ST-T Changes | n | Primary End Point % | | Inv. vs. Noninv. |
		Noninvasive	Invasive	RR (CI 95%)
No ST-T change	418	9.0	9.6	1.07 (0.59–1.95)
Inverted T only	866	8.5	7.7	0.90 (0.57–1.41)
ST depression	1100	14.9	10.3	0.69 (0.50–0.95)
All patients	2457	12.0	9.2	0.77 (0.61–0.97)

Reprinted from Diderholm et al.[49] with permission.

TACTICS-TIMI 18 (Enrollment 1997–1999)

The Treat Angina with Aggrastat and Determine Cost of Therapy with an Invasive or Conservative Strategy (TACTICS-TIMI 18) trial included 2,220 patients with UA/NSTEM.[6] Inclusion criteria were an accelerating pattern and prolonged or recurrent anginal pain at rest or minimal effort within the previous 24 hours, plus ischemia, ECG changes, elevated cardiac markers, or a history of prior CAD. Study subjects were immediately treated with aspirin, heparin, and the glycoprotein IIb/IIIa inhibitor tirofiban (admininstered for 48 to 108 hours). Patients were then randomized to one of the following two groups:

1. Catheterization and subsequent PCI/ CABG within 4 to 48 hours
2. Conservative strategy with catheterization performed only if there was objective evidence of recurrent ischemia or a positive exercise stress test

At 6 months, the primary outcome (death, MI, and rehospitalization for ACS) occurred in 15.9% of the invasive-strategy group and 19.4% of the conservative-strategy group (odds ratio, 0.78; $p = 0.025$). The rate of death or MI was also significantly lower in the invasive-strategy group (7.3% vs. 9.5%; odds ratio, 0.74; $p < 0.05$).

Subgroup analysis according to TnT status on admission revealed that the difference between the two strategies was largely due to a reduction in the primary outcome among TnT-positive patients. In this subgroup, the invasive strategy was associated with a primary outcome rate of 14.3% compared with 24.2% for the conservative strategy (odds ratio, 0.52; $p < 0.001$). The two strategies were comparable in their effects on the primary outcome in TnT-negative patients. Patients with an intermediate or high TIMI UA risk score also benefited from an invasive over a conservative strategy. In patients with a low TIMI UA score, the two strategies were comparable.

PROPOSED CLASSIFICATION OF RISK

High-Risk Patients

High-risk ACS patients who clearly warrant catheterization and early revascularization include those with rest angina with ST-segment depression and/or elevated serum concentrations of cardiac markers of ischemic injury (CK-MB, troponin, myoglobin). Those who have rest angina with hemodynamic instability, heart failure, or an ejection fraction < 40%, and those with rest angina and prior revascularization (PCI or CABG) should be sent to the catheterization laboratory and undergo revascularization as indicated.

Intermediate-Risk Patients

Patients at an intermediate level of risk for future cardiac events appear to benefit from catheterization and early revascularization. This subset includes patients with Canadian Cardiovascular Society (CCS) class III or IV angina within the past 2 weeks, those with diabetes mellitus, and those who have deep T wave inversions in more than five leads with chest discomfort or pain.

Low-Risk Patients

Patients with atypical or recurring symptoms that could be UA (CCS class I or II) are not likely to benefit from catheterization or early revascularization. These include patients with normal or nonspecific ECG changes, T wave inversion without ST-segment depression, and biochemical markers that are negative for CK-MB or troponin levels.

CONCLUSIONS

Risk stratification makes as much sense in 2001–2002 as it did 30 years ago because non-ST-segment elevation ACS is heterogeneous, with a spectrum of risk ranging from low to high. The approach of watchful waiting with medical therapy and no PCI, though advocated

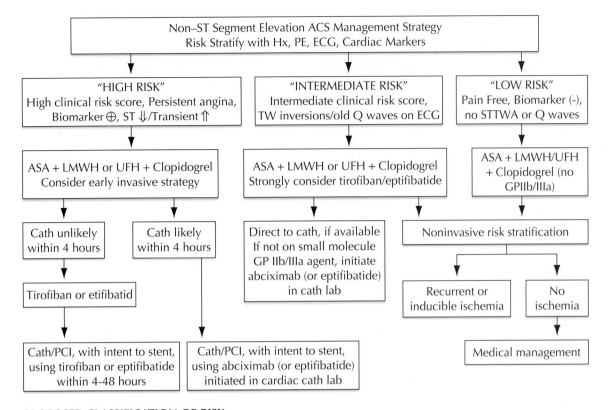

PROPOSED CLASSIFICATION OF RISK

High-Risk Patients   High-risk ACS patients who clearly warrant catheterization and early revascularization include those with rest angina with ST-segment depression and/or elevated serum concentrations of cardiac markers of ischemic injury (CK-MB, troponin, myoglobin). Those who have rest angina with hemodynamic instability, heart failure, or an ejection fraction < 40%, and those with rest angina and prior revascularization (PCI or CABG) should be sent to the catheterization laboratory and undergo revascularization as indicated.

Intermediate-Risk Patients   Patients at an intermediate level of risk for future cardiac events appear to benefit from catheterization and early revascularization. This subset includes patients with Canadian Cardiovascular Society (CCS) class III or IV angina within the past 2 weeks, those with diabetes mellitus, and those who have deep T wave inversions in more than five leads with chest discomfort or pain.

Low-Risk Patients   Patients with atypical or recurring symptoms that could be UA (CCS class I or II) are not likely to benefit from catheterization or early revascularization. These include patients with normal or nonspecific ECG changes, T-wave inversion without ST-segment depression, and biochemical markers that are negative for CK-MB or troponin levels.

Figure 20-3.

in the United Kingdom and other parts of Europe, has little basis for support. Conversely, a routine invasive approach with acute revascularization for all patients may not be clinically effective or cost-effective, and may result in unnecessary complications such as restenosis, need for revascularization, and risk of stroke (the VAN-QWISH trial demonstrated that 52% of non-Q-wave MI patients randomized to the ischemia-guided strategy had a very low 30-day event rate of 1%). The balanced approach reserves catheterization and revascularization for high-risk patients; as defined in this article, this subgroup comprises 25 to 50% of all patients. Stress myocardial perfusion imaging, preferably symptom-limited exercise-induced imaging, at 2 to 3 days in patients who are otherwise stable at the time of transfer to the CCU will clearly delineate high- and intermediate-risk subgroups.

Aggressive pharmacologic therapy is indicated in all patients, with use of aspirin, with or without clopidogrel; GP IIb/IIIa receptor antagonists; low-molecular-weight heparin, especially enoxaparin; intravenous nitroglycerin; beta-blockers; HMG Co-A reductase inhibitors (statins); and ACE inhibitors, as indicated.

Tailoring therapy to the level of risk is essential for optimizing efficacy and cost-effectiveness. Cardiac catheterization is an important diagnostic modality in delineating abnormal coronary anatomy and to configuring appropriate myocardial revascularization in intermediate- and high-risk subjects with symptomatic coronary heart disease. Its role in low-risk patients is not established and, unless there are compelling reasons to do otherwise, should be avoided in this setting.

REFERENCES

1. Braunwald E. Unstable angina: An etiologic approach to management. *Circulation*. 1998;98:2219–2222.
2. Braunwald E, Antman EM, Beasley JW, Califf RM, Cheitlin MD, Hochman JS, Jones RH, Kereiakes D, Kupersmith J, Levin TN, Pepine CJ, Schaeffer JW, Smith EE, 3rd, Steward DE, Theroux P, Alpert JS, Eagle KA, Faxon DP, Fuster V, Gardner TJ, Gregoratos G, Russell RO, Smith SC, Jr. ACC/AHA guidelines for the management of patients with unstable angina and non-ST-segment elevation myocardial infarction. A report of the American College of Cardiology/American Heart Association Task Force on Practice Guidelines (Committee on the Management of Patients With Unstable Angina). *J Am Coll Cardiol*. 2000;36:970–1062.
3. Unstable angina pectoris: national cooperative study group to compare surgical and medical therapy. III. Results in patients with S-T segment elevation during pain. *Am J Cardiol*. 1980;45:819–824.
4. Luchi RJ, Scott SM, Deupree RH. Comparison of medical and surgical treatment for unstable angina pectoris. Results of a Veterans Administration Cooperative Study. *N Engl J Med*. 1987;316:977–984.
5. Effects of tissue plasminogen activator and a comparison of early invasive and conservative strategies in unstable angina and non-Q-wave myocardial infarction. Results of the TIMI IIIB Trial. Thrombolysis in Myocardial Ischemia. *Circulation*. 1994;89:1545–1556.
6. Cannon CP, Weintraub WS, Demopoulos LA, Vicari R, Frey MJ, Lakkis N, Neumann FJ, Robertson DH, DeLucca PT, DiBattiste PM, Gibson CM, Braunwald E. Comparison of early invasive and conservative strategies in patients with unstable coronary syndromes treated with the glycoprotein IIb/IIIa inhibitor tirofiban. *N Engl J Med*. 2001;344:1879–1887.
7. Montalescot G, Barragan P, Wittenberg O, Ecollan P, Elhadad S, Villain P, Boulenc JM, Morice MC, Maillard L, Pansieri M, Choussat R, Pinton P. Platelet glycoprotein IIb/IIIa inhibition with coronary stenting for acute myocardial infarction. *N Engl J Med*. 2001;344:1895–1903.
8. Topol EJ, Moliterno DJ, Herrmann HC, Powers ER, Grines CL, Cohen DJ, Cohen EA, Bertrand M, Neumann FJ, Stone GW, DiBattiste PM, Demopoulos L. Comparison of two platelet glycoprotein IIb/IIIa inhibitors, tirofiban and abciximab, for the prevention of ischemic events with percutaneous coronary revascularization. *N Engl J Med*. 2001;344:1888–1894.
9. Topol EJ. Reperfusion therapy for acute myocardial infarction with fibrinolytic therapy or combination reduced fibrinolytic therapy and platelet glycoprotein IIb/IIIa inhibition: the GUSTO V randomised trial. *Lancet*. 2001;357:1905–1914.
10. Effectiveness of intravenous thrombolytic treatment in acute myocardial infarction. Gruppo Italiano per lo Studio della Streptochinasi nell'Infarto Miocardico (GISSI). *Lancet*. 1986;1:397–402.
11. Randomised trial of intravenous streptokinase, oral aspirin, both, or neither among 17,187 cases of suspected acute myocardial infarction: ISIS-2. ISIS-2 (Second International Study of Infarct Survival) Collaborative Group. *Lancet*. 1988;2:349–360.
12. Wilcox RG, von der Lippe G, Olsson CG, Jensen G, Skene AM, Hampton JR. Trial of tissue plasminogen activator for mortality reduction in acute myocardial

infarction. Anglo-Scandinavian Study of Early Thrombolysis (ASSET). *Lancet.* 1988;2:525–530.

13. ISIS-3: A randomised comparison of streptokinase vs tissue plasminogen activator vs anistreplase and of aspirin plus heparin vs aspirin alone among 41,299 cases of suspected acute myocardial infarction. ISIS-3 (Third International Study of Infarct Survival) Collaborative Group. *Lancet.* 1992;339:753–770.

14. The effects of tissue plasminogen activator, streptokinase, or both on coronary-artery patency, ventricular function, and survival after acute myocardial infarction. The GUSTO Angiographic Investigators. *N Engl J Med.* 1993;329:1615–1622.

15. Late Assessment of Thrombolytic Efficacy (LATE) study with alteplase 6–24 hours after onset of acute myocardial infarction. *Lancet.* 1993;342:759–766.

16. Randomised trial of late thrombolysis in patients with suspected acute myocardial infarction. EMERAS (Estudio Multicentrico Estreptoquinasa Republicas de America del Sur) Collaborative Group. *Lancet.* 1993;342:767–772.

17. Keeley EC, Boura JA, Grines CL. Primary angioplasty versus intravenous thrombolytic therapy for acute myocardial infarction: a quantitative review of 23 randomised trials. *Lancet.* 2003;361:13–20.

18. Stone GW, Grines CL, Browne KF, Marco J, Rothbaum D, O'Keefe JH, Hartzler GO, Overlie P, Donohue B, Chelliah N, Vlietstra R, Puchrowicz-Ochocki S, O'Neill WW. Outcome of different reperfusion strategies in patients with former contraindications to thrombolytic therapy: a comparison of primary angioplasty and tissue plasminogen activator. Primary Angioplasty in Myocardial Infarction (PAMI) Investigators. *Cathet Cardiovasc Diagn.* 1996;39:333–339.

19. O'Murchu B, Gersh BJ, Reeder GS, Bailey KR, Holmes DR, Jr. Late outcome after percutaneous transluminal coronary angioplasty during acute myocardial infarction. *Am J Cardiol.* 1993;72:634–639.

20. Zijlstra F, de Boer MJ, Hoorntje JC, Reiffers S, Reiber JH, Suryapranata H. A comparison of immediate coronary angioplasty with intravenous streptokinase in acute myocardial infarction. *N Engl J Med.* 1993;328:680–684.

21. Vaitkus PT. Percutaneous transluminal coronary angioplasty versus thrombolysis in acute myocardial infarction: a meta-analysis. *Clin Cardiol.* 1995;18:35–38.

22. Ryan TJ, Anderson JL, Antman EM, Braniff BA, Brooks NH, Califf RM, Hillis LD, Hiratzka LF, Rapaport E, Riegel BJ, Russell RO, Smith EE, Jr., Weaver WD. ACC/AHA guidelines for the management of patients with acute myocardial infarction. A report of the American College of Cardiology/American Heart Association Task Force on Practice Guidelines (Committee on Management of Acute Myocardial Infarction). *J Am Coll Cardiol.* 1996;28:1328–1428.

23. Grines CL, Browne KF, Marco J, Rothbaum D, Stone GW, O'Keefe I, Overlie P, Donohue B, Chelliah N, Timmis GC, et al. A comparison of immediate angioplasty with thrombolytic therapy for acute myocardial infarction. The Primary Angioplasty in Myocardial Infarction Study Group. *N Engl J Med.* 1993;328:673–679.

24. Efficacy and safety of tenecteplase in combination with enoxaparin, abciximab, or unfractionated heparin: the ASSENT-3 randomised trial in acute myocardial infarction. *Lancet.* 2001;358:605–613.

25. Kleiman NS, Ohman EM, Califf RM, George BS, Kereiakes D, Aguirre FV, Weisman H, Schaible T, Topol EJ. Profound inhibition of platelet aggregation with monoclonal antibody 7E3 Fab after thrombolytic therapy. Results of the Thrombolysis and Angioplasty in Myocardial Infarction (TAMI) 8 Pilot Study. *J Am Coll Cardiol.* 1993;22:381–389.

26. Ohman EM, Kleiman NS, Gacioch G, Worley SJ, Navetta FI, Talley JD, Anderson HV, Ellis SG, Cohen MD, Spriggs D, Miller M, Kereiakes D, Yakubov S, Kitt MM, Sigmon KN, Califf RM, Krucoff MW, Topol EJ. Combined accelerated tissue-plasminogen activator and platelet glycoprotein IIb/IIIa integrin receptor blockade with Integrilin in acute myocardial infarction. Results of a randomized, placebo-controlled, dose-ranging trial. IMPACT-AMI Investigators. *Circulation.* 1997;95:846–854.

27. Combining thrombolysis with the platelet glycoprotein IIb/IIIa inhibitor lamifiban: results of the Platelet Aggregation Receptor Antagonist Dose Investigation and Reperfusion Gain in Myocardial Infarction (PARADIGM) trial. *J Am Coll Cardiol.* 1998;32:2003–2010.

28. Antman EM, Giugliano RP, Gibson CM, McCabe CH, Coussement P, Kleiman NS, Vahanian A, Adgey AA, Menown I, Rupprecht HJ, Van der Wieken R, Ducas J, Scherer J, Anderson K, Van de Werf F, Braunwald E. Abciximab facilitates the rate and extent of thrombolysis: results of the thrombolysis in myocardial infarction (TIMI) 14 trial. The TIMI 14 Investigators. *Circulation.* 1999;99:2720–2732.

29. Trial of abciximab with and without low-dose reteplase for acute myocardial infarction. Strategies for Patency Enhancement in the Emergency Department (SPEED) Group. *Circulation.* 2000;101:2788–2794.

30. Comparison of invasive and conservative strategies after treatment with intravenous tissue plasminogen activator in acute myocardial infarction. Results of the thrombolysis in myocardial infarction (TIMI) phase II trial. The TIMI Study Group. *N Engl J Med.* 1989;320:618–627.

31. Topol EJ, Califf RM, George BS, Kereiakes DJ, Abbottsmith CW, Candela RJ, Lee KL, Pitt B, Stack RS, O'Neill WW. A randomized trial of immediate versus delayed elective angioplasty after intravenous

tissue plasminogen activator in acute myocardial infarction. *N Engl J Med.* 1987;317:581–588.

32. de Bono DP. The European Cooperative Study Group trial of intravenous recombinant tissue-type plasminogen activator (rt-PA) and conservative therapy versus rt-PA and immediate coronary angioplasty. *J Am Coll Cardiol.* 1988;12:20A–23A.

33. Zijlstra F, Beukema WP, van't Hof AW, Liem A, Reiffers S, Hoorntje JC, Suryapranata H, de Boer MJ. Randomized comparison of primary coronary angioplasty with thrombolytic therapy in low risk patients with acute myocardial infarction. *J Am Coll Cardiol.* 1997;29:908–912.

34. Herrmann HC, Molitemo DJ, Ohman EM, Stebbins AL, Bode C, Betriu A, Forycki F, Miklin JS, Bachinsky WB, Lincoff AM, Califf RM, Topol EJ. Facilitation of early percutaneous coronary intervention after reteplase with or without abciximab in acute myocardial infarction: results from the SPEED (GUSTO-4 Pilot) Trial. *J Am Coll Cardiol.* 2000;36:1489–1496.

35. Stone GW, Grines CL, Cox DA, Garcia E, Tcheng JE, Griffin JJ, Guagliumi G, Stuckey T, Turco M, Carroll JD, Rutherford BD, Lansky AJ. Comparison of angioplasty with stenting, with or without abciximab, in acute myocardial infarction. *N Engl J Med.* 2002;346:957–966.

36. Boden WE, O'Rourke RA, Crawford MH, Blaustein AS, Deedwania PC, Zoble RG, Wexler LF, Kleiger RE, Pepine CJ, Ferry DR, Chow BK, Lavori PW. Outcomes in patients with acute non-Q-wave myocardial infarction randomly assigned to an invasive as compared with a conservative management strategy. Veterans Affairs Non-Q-Wave Infarction Strategies in Hospital (VANQWISH) Trial Investigators. *N Engl J Med.* 1998;338:1785–1792.

37. A comparison of aspirin plus tirofiban with aspirin plus heparin for unstable angina. Platelet Receptor Inhibition in Ischemic Syndrome Management (PRISM) Study Investigators. *N Engl J Med.* 1998;338:1498–1505.

38. Inhibition of the platelet glycoprotein IIb/IIIa receptor with tirofiban in unstable angina and non-Q-wave myocardial infarction. Platelet Receptor Inhibition in Ischemic Syndrome Management in Patients Limited by Unstable Signs and Symptoms (PRISM-PLUS) Study Investigators. *N Engl J Med.* 1998;338:1488–1497.

39. Inhibition of platelet glycoprotein IIb/IIIa with eptifibatide in patients with acute coronary syndromes. The PURSUIT Trial Investigators. Platelet Glycoprotein IIb/IIIa in Unstable Angina: Receptor Suppression Using Integrilin Therapy. *N Engl J Med.* 1998;339:436–443.

40. Effects of platelet glycoprotein IIb/IIIa blockade with tirofiban on adverse cardiac events in patients with unstable angina or acute myocardial infarction undergoing coronary angioplasty. The RESTORE Investigators. Randomized Efficacy Study of Tirofiban for Outcomes and REstenosis. *Circulation.* 1997;96:1445–1453.

41. Cohen M, Demers C, Gurfinkel EP, Turpie AG, Fromell GJ, Goodman S, Langer A, Califf RM, Fox KA, Premmereur J, Bigonzi F. A comparison of low-molecular-weight heparin with unfractionated heparin for unstable coronary artery disease. Efficacy and Safety of Subcutaneous Enoxaparin in Non-Q-Wave Coronary Events Study Group. *N Engl J Med.* 1997;337:447–452.

42. Antman EM, McCabe CH, Gurfinkel EP, Turpie AG, Bernink PI, Salein D, Bayes De Luna A, Fox K, Lablanche JM, Radley D, Premmereur J, Braunwald E. Enoxaparin prevents death and cardiac ischemic events in unstable angina/non-Q-wave myocardial infarction. Results of the thrombolysis in myocardial infarction (TIMI) 11B trial. *Circulation.* 1999;100:1593–1601.

43. Long-term low-molecular-mass heparin in unstable coronary-artery disease: FRISC II prospective randomised multicentre study. FRagmin and Fast Revascularisation during InStability in Coronary artery disease. Investigators. *Lancet.* 1999;354:701–707.

44. Effects of recombinant hirudin (lepirudin) compared with heparin on death, myocardial infarction, refractory angina, and revascularisation procedures in patients with acute myocardial ischaemia without ST elevation: a randomised trial. Organisation to Assess Strategies for Ischemic Syndromes (OASIS-2) Investigators. *Lancet.* 1999;353:429–438.

45. A randomised, blinded, trial of clopidogrel versus aspirin in patients at risk of ischaemic events (CAPRIE). CAPRIE Steering Committee. *Lancet.* 1996;348:1329–1339.

46. Yusuf S. Clopidogrel in unstable angina to prevent recurrent ischemic events (CURE). *Presented at the 50th Annual Scientific Session of the American College of Cardiology; March 19, 2001; Orlando, Florida.*

47. Invasive compared with non-invasive treatment in unstable coronary-artery disease: FRISC II prospective randomised multicentre study. FRagmin and Fast Revascularisation during InStability in Coronary artery disease Investigators. *Lancet.* 1999;354:708–715.

48. Lagerqvist B, Diderholm E, Lindahl B. An early invasive treatment strategy reduces cardiac events regardless of troponin levels in unstable coronary artery (UCAD) with and without troponin-elevation: A FRISC II substudy. *Circulation.* 1999;100 (Suppl I):I–497 (abstract).

49. Diderholm E, Andren B, Frostfeldt G. ST depression in ECG at entry identifies patients who may benefit most from early revascularisation in unstable coronary artery disease: A FRISC II substudy. *Circulation.* 1999;100 (Suppl I):I–497 (abstract).

CHAPTER 21

Introduction to the Physics of Myocardial Perfusion SPECT Imaging

James A. Case
S. James Cullom
Timothy M. Bateman

HISTORY AND INTRODUCTION

The origin of nuclear imaging can be traced back to the late 1800s when physicists began investigating the fundamental properties of matter. In 1896, Henri Becquerel announced the discovery of a strange new property of matter, radioactivity, for which he shared the Nobel prize in physics with Marie and Pierre Curie in 1903[1] (Figure 21-1). This award could have just as easily been for medicine because of the tremendous impact it would have on the care of patients for the next century.* Soon after, radioactivity was being investigated as a treatment for certain ailments. In 1905, the first uses of natural radioactivity in

medicine were made in attempts to treat thyroid cancer using radium. The first uses of radionuclides for medical imaging were in the late 1930s with ^{131}I to study the thyroid, using a single detector to measure the total uptake by the thyroid. By the late 1940s, the increased availability of radioisotopes allowed researchers to develop clinical procedures for diagnostic imaging. However, routine use of radionuclides for imaging patients began with the introduction of the rectilinear scanner. This scanner used a focusing collimator to identify structures at a particular depth in the patient, and to blur structures in front of and behind the specified depth. By scanning the patient with this device, a crude three-dimensional image could be made of the activity in the patient.

The first electronic gamma camera with multiple photomultiplier tubes was developed in 1957 by Hal Anger.[2] This camera employed a lead collimator in front of a scintillating crystal to effec-

---

*Ironically, the marriage between physics and medicine was already underway in the Nobel Prize in 1903 for medicine. That year, the Nobel Laureate for Medicine was awarded to Dr. Niels Finsen for his work on treating lupus vulgaris using concentrated "light therapy".

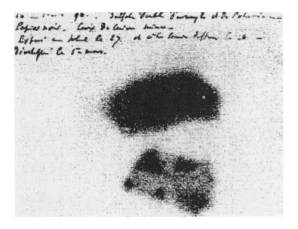

Figure 21-1. From Henri Becquerel's Nobel lecture. Displayed is the first image created by radioactivity. Dr. Becquerel report to the guests at the Nobel lecture, "We were thus faced with a spontaneous phenomenon of a new order. Shown here is the first print, which revealed the spontaneity of the radiation emitted by the uranium salt. The rays passed through both the black paper which enveloped the plate, and a thin sheet of copper in the shape of a cross." (Reprinted from Becquerel[1] with permission.)

tively "focus" the gamma-rays and create an image.* Similar to a "pin-hole" camera, the Anger camera could produce planar images of radionuclide distributions. Myocardial perfusion imaging began in 1973 when H. William Straus introduced the first protocol for imaging the heart at stress and at rest using a planar Anger camera.[3] This technique revolutionized the imaging of coronary disease, however it suffered from many of the same limitations of the geometry as conventional planar x-ray imaging. Planar imaging acquires a single projection of the three-dimensional activity in the patient onto a planar detector. These difficulties result in ambiguity as to where the photons originate along the line of sight.

*Unlike visible light that has photon energies in the 1-eV range, high energy of x-rays and gamma rays (50,000–1,000,000 eV) cannot be focused using lenses. Though some investigators are studying collimatorless gamma ray imaging, no practical solution has been found.

Because of the computerized nature of the Anger camera, it became clear that the Anger camera could be adapted to acquire data in a true three-dimensional mode. Ronald Jaszczak and John Keyes in 1976 independently reported the invention of a system for acquiring 3D nuclear images.[4,5] This technique, single photon emission computed tomography (SPECT), estimates the 3D activity distribution by acquiring a large number of projections at different angles around the patient and then mathematically determines a source distribution that could have produced those projections. This is accomplished by mounting gamma cameras (one, two, or three camera heads) on a rotating gantry and imaging at evenly spaced projection angles. By using a model for the formation of the 2D projection images, a reconstruction of the original 3D distribution is calculated (this is referred to as computed tomography [CT]).

RADIOACTIVE DECAY

SPECT imaging relies on the production of high-energy photons that can be imaged using a specialized camera. This is accomplished by using naturally occurring or artificially created atoms that decay and emit photons. In general, radioactive decay can be classified into four broad types of processes: (1) alpha particles (ionized helium nuclei); (2) beta particles (high energy electrons or positrons); (3) gamma rays (photons produce via a relaxation of the nuclei from a higher energy state to a lower energy state); and (4) electron capture (x-rays are produced from an electron being captured by the nucleus of an atom). The last two of these processes are the most common source of radiation in SPECT (see Figure 21-2A and B).

Radioactive decay can be described in terms of the "half-life" of a radionuclide. A half-life is defined as the time for half of a radioactive sample to undergo the radioactive transition. For example, technetium 99m (Tc-99m) has a natural half-life of 6.03 hours. If one begins with 10 mCi of Tc-99m, 6.03 hours later only 5 mCi will remain, and after 12.06 hours only 2.5 mCi will

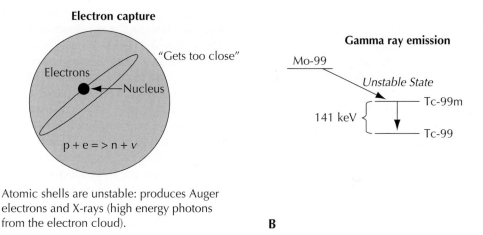

Electron capture

Electrons

Nucleus

"Gets too close"

$p + e => n + v$

A   Atomic shells are unstable: produces Auger electrons and X-rays (high energy photons from the electron cloud).

Gamma ray emission

Mo-99

Unstable State

Tc-99m

141 keV

Tc-99

B

Figure 21-2.   The two primary nuclear mechanisms for creating high energy photons in nuclear medicine are electron capture (**A**) and the relaxation of an internal energy state of a nuclei (**B**).

remain, and so forth. In addition to natural decay, the radionuclide can be excreted through biological processes. Therefore, the lifetime of a radionuclide in the body (the biological half-life) is less than the natural half-life.

Thallium-201 (Tl-201) decays via an electron capture process. This occurs when a proton in the nucleus is converted to a neutron by capturing an orbital electron. This process reduces the atomic number of the atom by one, changing the Tl-201 atom into Mercury-201 (Hg-201). This change in the charge of the nucleus tips off a cascade in the lower atomic electron shells (Auger electron emission), which radiate x-rays. For Tl-201, this is a "dirty" process, in which numerous energy photons are produced, the bulk of which are around 70 keV, but higher-energy gamma photons can be found at 137 keV and 167 keV.

In contrast, Tc-99m is a monochromatic emitter that is a result of beta decay. Tc-99m has been described as the "perfect" imaging isotope because of its 6.03-hour half-life and the single 141-keV photon that it emits (Figure 21-2B). The 140-keV photon is nearly optimal for imaging using the Anger camera and the 6.03 hour half-life for imaging during a single day and short enough to minimize patient dose. Unfor-

tunately, these favorable imaging characteristics are not matched with favorable biokinetics. Complex chemistry is needed for attaching the technetium atoms onto molecules that can be used for physiological imaging.

ISOTOPES IN MYOCARDIAL PERFUSION STUDIES

The isotopes Tl-201 and Tc-99m have proven themselves to be very useful in cardiac SPECT for perfusion studies. Tc-99m has a primary gamma ray at 141 keV and a half-life of 6.03 hours. Tl-201 has several x-rays in the energy range of 70 to 80 keV, two low-abundance gamma rays at 135 keV and 167 keV, and a half-life of 73 hours. Tl-201 biological kinetics make it a very useful agent for imaging cardiac viability, because it is a potassium analog, allowing it to passively penetrate the cell membrane.[6,7]

Using Tc-99m for perfusion studies is done by chelating the technetium atom to a molecule that will be absorbed by the myocardium. Two of the most commonly used radiopharmaceuticals are Tc-99m-methoxyisobutyl isonitrile (sestamibi) and Tc-99m 1,2-bis[bis (2-ethoxyethyl)phophino] ethane (tetrofosmin). These agents interact with the cells in the heart by reacting to changes in the metabolism caused by ischemia or hypoxia.[7] During stress, metabolism changes the polarization of the cell membrane, driving the agent into the cells. These radiopharmaceuticals have been demonstrated to have good target-to-background characteristics, and because of its short half-life, higher activity levels than Tl-201 can be used within acceptable radiation exposure to the patient. Unfortunately, these agents are readily absorbed by the liver and bowel. Because these organs are close to the heart, scattered photons from these organs can contaminate the image of the heart.

Several groups have advocated using both Tl-201– and Tc-99m–based agents in the same protocol (dual-isotope SPECT imaging).[8] In cardiac SPECT, the redistribution study is performed first by injecting the patient with Tl-201. The patient is then imaged 15 minutes later. Following the resting study the patient is stressed and injected with 20 to 30 mCi of a Tc-99m tracer at peak stress. Thirty minutes to an hour later the patient is imaged. Because the Tc-99m photopeak energy is significantly higher than the main photo-peak energy of Tl-201, there is little contamination of the Tc-99m stress image by the Tl-201. It has the advantage of reducing the total time in which the patient is required for the study. The acquisition of a simultaneous dual-isotope protocol has also been explored. Though initial investigation of this technique was not encouraging,[9] recent studies indicate that scatter contamination of the Tc-99m photons into the Tl-201 window can be mitigated and reasonable accuracy may be possible.[10,11]

Imaging System: Anger Camera

Modern SPECT has relied almost exclusively on the Anger camera for the acquisition of images. The Anger camera has changed little in its fundamental workings since it was invented in the 1950s. This is because the Anger camera combines nearly 100% photon collection efficiency with relatively low-cost materials.

The Anger camera uses lead collimators for "focusing" the gamma rays by excluding photon that are not traveling in the direction of the holes in the collimator. Behind the collimator is the sensitive part of the camera consisting of a NaI(Tl) scintillator crystal and an array of photomultiplier tubes. This camera has a good energy resolution in the range typically used in nuclear medicine and a high quantum efficiency (nearly 100%) for photons absorbed in the crystal.[12] The crystals also have a high atomic number (Z), necessary for efficient photon collection.

When high-energy photons are absorbed in the scintillation crystal, a pulse of optical light is generated. This pulse is detected by an array of photomultipliers which generate an electronic pulse. Electronic circuits convert the pulses generated into an x-y location of the interaction in the crystal and the integral of the electrical pulse received in all photomultiplier tubes (referred to as the z-coordinate) which is used to determine the incident energy of a photon (see Figure 21-3). A typical Anger camera has an energy resolution of 10% FWHM at 141 keV.

Determination of the interaction point on the crystal is not sufficient to determine the direction from which the photon originated. Typically, a collimator is used to allow only those photons traveling in particular direction to enter the camera. The

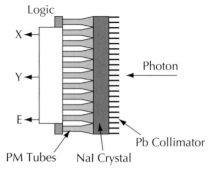

Figure 21-3. Components of the Anger camera determine the incident energy of the photon. The x-y and z coordinates are digitized and stored by computer.

collimator is a lead sheet that has been perforated with an array of narrow holes. These holes have a length roughly 50 times the diameter of the hole, allowing photons traveling within 1 degree of the axis of the hole to penetrate the collimator (i.e., 1 in 20,000 photons). Because of the low efficiency of transmission through the collimator, the number of counts in SPECT images is low. Parallel hole collimators allow only photons that are traveling nearly perpendicular to the camera face to penetrate the collimator (see Figure 21-4A). Another type of collimator is the fan-beam collimator. This collimator allows radiation emitted from a line source at a specific focal distance to penetrate the collimator (see Figure 21-4B).

Reconstruction of Images

In SPECT, multiple images of the patient are taken at different rotation angles to obtain three-dimensional information about the activity distribution within the patient. A three-dimensional picture of the patient can be "reconstructed" from the projection data using a mathematical model. This is accomplished by modeling the system that created the projection images as a system of simultaneous linear equations and then inverting that matrix to reveal the source distri-

bution. As simple as that sounds, finding the projector matrix that describes the physics of a SPECT camera and then inverting that matrix (typically of order $10,000 \times 10,000$ or larger) to obtain an inverse is very difficult. In reality, approximations must be made to reconstruct 3D volumes of activity distributions. The most common of these techniques are filtered backprojection, which is an analytical approximation to the image reconstruction problem and iterative reconstruction, a stepwise approach to reconstructing the images.

Filtered Backprojection (FBP)

The physics of the image formation process is modeled mathematically by a projector matrix. A simple model for this process is the Radon transform, which integrates all of the activity along the line of sight onto the detector. The inverse Radon transform can be solved (creating 3D reconstructions) using an algorithm called filtered backprojection. This method "inverts" the Radon transform by convolving the projection data with a ramp filter in the frequency domain. This has the effect of eliminating the "rays" that project outward from each point in the image and creating an accurate 3D representation of the source dis-

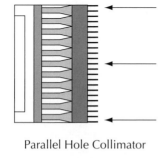

A   Parallel Hole Collimator

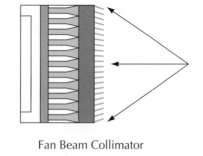

B   Fan Beam Collimator

Figure 21-4. Gamma rays are "focused" by excluding those photons that are not traveling along a preferred trajectory. **A.** In parallel collimation, the collimator allows only those photons that are traveling perpendicular to the surface of the detector to be recorded. **B.** In fan beam collimation, only those photons traveling along rays originating from a line are accepted.

tribution (see Figure 21-5). (For a review of filtered backprojection, see Herman [1980][13]).

The Radon transform has been used extensively in CT with extremely high precision. However, FBP is not easily adapted to projector models that are not the Radon transform, as is the case with SPECT. In the case of cardiac SPECT, the activity measured at a particular detector is not the sum of the activity along the line of site of the detector. Photon scatter, camera blurring, attenuation, and partial volume effects all combine to increase the complexity of the projector. Techniques that model the true imaging properties of SPECT are required to correct for the myriad of "real-world" imaging artifacts.

Iterative Image Reconstruction

Iterative algorithms are often used for reconstructions because the physics of the photon transport problem can be included into the algorithm. Thus, reconstructions that accurately compensate for nonuniform attenuation, scatter, collimator response, and the like can be devised

without having to explicitly determine an inverse to the projector matrix (which can be nearly impossible in most real-world examples). Iterative SPECT image reconstruction begins with an initial estimate of the activity distribution (typically a uniform estimate). Then, at each step of the iteration sequence, an update of the present estimate is calculated according to some strategy for improving the estimate (see Figure 21-6). The most common strategy for performing iterative reconstruction is the Maximum Likelihood–Expectation Maximization algorithm.[14,15] One of the limitations of iterative algorithms is that the computation time can be 20 to 30 times longer than FBP techniques. Recent advances in the mathematics of iterative reconstruction have created techniques that improve reconstruction times often 5- to 10-fold and clinically acceptable.[16] However, work is ongoing to improve the speed and reliability of these accelerated reconstruction techniques.

IMAGE ARTIFACTS

Attenuation Artifacts

Attenuation artifacts are considered to be one of the most troubling and significant limitations to myocardial perfusion SPECT imaging.[17–19] These artifacts can appear as false perfusion defects that, on follow-up, have no corresponding lesion. This has a significant impact on the accuracy of nuclear cardiology interpretations. Diaphragmatic attenuation in males and breast attenuation in females are commonly identified attenuation artifacts. In particular, the diaphragm can suppress counts from the inferior wall of the heart, leading to poor specificity in the right coronary artery (RCA) territory. In females, breast attenuation often affects the anterior as well as septal and lateral walls of the left ventricle, suppressing the count from the left anterior descending (LAD) and left circumflex (LCX) artery territories.

One technique that has been employed to account for difference in male and female attenuation is the use of a library of normal and abnormal perfusion patterns to differentiate

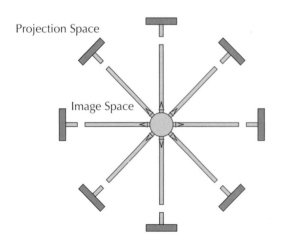

Figure 21-5. The Radon transform assumes the counts received at the detector are the sum of all source along a line of sight. The Radon is reconstructed using filter backprojection. That process filtered the projection data using a ramp filter and backprojects the filtered data into the iamge space.

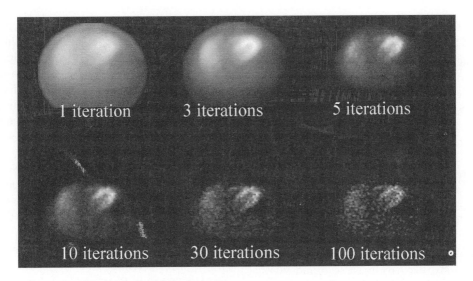

Figure 21-6. Iterative reconstruction accomplishes the same task as the ramp filter in FBP. At each step, artifacts of the backprojection process are removed iteratively, successively improving the image quality. At high iteration numbers, the noise tends to dominate the image.

between normal or abnormal perfusion patterns. Eisner et al.[20] demonstrated that most attenuation artifacts can be described by either a male or female normal database.

Electrocardiographic (ECG) gating of myocardial perfusion SPECT studies has been shown to be valuable in discriminating fixed perfusion defects from attenuation artifacts in patients without prior myocardial infarction.[21,22] In segments in which there is concern about the presence of fixed defects, adequate thickening and contraction can be attributed to attenuation. However, ECG gating is not helpful in assessing patterns in which attenuation may be superimposed on true perfusion defects due to ischemia.

Other adjunctive methods have been utilized to identify attenuation artifacts, including the use of external breast markers and breast positioning protocols to identify and standardize breast position, recording breast (bra) size, breast density, patient body habitus, and the use of prone and left-decubitus planar imaging for diaphragmatic attenuation assessment.[23,24] Although the value of these methods has been demonstrated, they lack standardization and significantly hamper laboratory efficiency and operation.

The potential clinical ramifications of a fully implemented attenuation correction approach are substantial. Enhanced visual and quantitative analyses through improved count density distribution that approach homogeneity in the presence of normal perfusion should be possible with attenuation correction. One might also expect higher sensitivity for detection of disease including mild–moderate single-vessel and multivessel disease with relative balanced flow reduction, higher specificity due to reduced artifacts from attenuation and improved delineation of myocardial viability in terms of accuracy of assessment of tracer uptake in dysfunctional areas. It is likely that with recent improvements designed to overcome "first-generation" hardware/software systems for attenuation correction that these long awaited investigations will soon appear in the literature. The American Society of Nuclear Cardiology and the Society of Nuclear Medicine publish a joint position statement endorsing the use of attenuation correction and should be considered.[25]

Photopeak Scatter and Nonstationary Spatial Resolution

Attenuation correction is not "everything correction." In addition to attenuation, other physical limitations continue to challenge physicians and physicists. Photon scatter, partial volume effects, and depth-dependent spatial resolution are factors that are important to correct for physical limitations of SPECT.[26] Compton scattered photons detected in the photopeak form a greater proportion of the emission image with Tl-201 than for Tc-99m agents because of the lower energy of the Tl-201 photons.

A major source of diagnostic uncertainty in SPECT is the contamination of the photopeak data by photons that have been scattered by the electrons in the object. This can affect the image in several ways. First, the scattered photons can reduce the contrast of the image because they tend to "blur" the image. This increases the background that is in the images and reduces the relative differences between the features in the image. The second effect is the blurring of an object into neighboring objects. This can have a significant effect on the diagnostic quality of the image. It has been demonstrated[27] that activity in the liver can have a significant influence on the estimated activity in the inferior wall of the heart. Furthermore, King et al.[28] demonstrated in a Monte Carlo investigation that the liver can cause negative artifacts in activity estimates of the myocardium. It was demonstrated that both scatter correction and attenuation correction were needed to improve cardiac images; otherwise, the "cold" attenuation and scatter artifacts observed in the inferior wall might be exchanged for "hot" scatter artifacts due to the liver uptake.

Scatter correction is important for Tc-99m–based agents because of the affinity these agents have for subdiaphragmatic structures. Extracardiac activity adjacent to the myocardium can cause overcorrection of the inferior wall causing artifactual decrease in anterior wall intensity.[27] The clinical literature on attenuation correction consistently reports some small but significant complications to image interpretation from extracardiac scatter. Several methods have recently been investigated to correct for scatter. These methods use scatter information collected in a separate window for subtraction of a fraction of this from the photopeak image, intrinsically model scatter in the reconstruction algorithm, and use of filtering methods that compensate for spatial and contrast resolution.[29–32]

The problem of liver uptake is significantly less in Tl-201 studies than with Tc-99m tracers due to the lower liver uptake of Tl-201. However, because of the low-energy resolution of the Anger camera (14% Full Width at Half-Maximum [FWHM] at 73 keV) and the angle-energy dependence of Compton scattering, many scattered photons remain in the energy window of the photopeak. For example, for Tl-201, a FWHM = 7.5% energy window centered at 73 keV will include photons scattered up to 65 degrees. Thus, the image from the photopeak data will include scattered photons traveling in different directions than the primary, unscattered radiation, degrading the spatial resolution of the image.

Quality Control Issues

Though some artifacts, such as attenuation and scatter, are unavoidable and must be dealt with through correction or training, many image artifacts can be prevented through proper image acquisition and quality control procedures. The International Committee for the Accreditation of Nuclear Laboratories (ICANL) recommends that certain procedures be in place to receive accreditation. Each laboratory should put in place procedures consistent with ICANL guidelines for ensuring that quality data are acquired according to those standards.[33]

In addition to quality control programs to ensure camera performance, processes should be in place to ensure that quality data are acquired on all patient studies. Many image artifacts can be traced to poor data acquisition techniques such as patient motion.[34] Technologists must review data immediately after acquisition to ensure that it is suitable for interpretation.

Uniformity Detector uniformity is one of the most common quality control problems that can arise in a gamma camera. Because of the intricate electronics in the gamma camera, the photomultiplier tubes can shift out of tune, leading to problems in the uniformity of the performance of the detector. Unchecked, these problems can lead to poor performance of the system and image artifacts being introduced into the acquired images.

Daily quality control floods should be checked to ensure system performance. Overall integral uniformity should not exceed 7%.[35]

Users must check uniformity daily, weekly, and after any work is performed on the camera. Daily floods (3–5 million counts) should be acquired on every instrument. According to NEMA and ICANL standards, all detectors should have a differential uniformity (without smoothing) of 7% or better (Figure 21-7). Weekly high-count floods (30 million counts) are also recommended for detecting more subtle deviations in camera performance (see Figure 21-7).

Center of Rotation Center of rotation (COR) errors are not as common in fixed dual-detector gantry design; however, they are very common in single-head detector systems. COR errors can lead to "swirl-like" image artifacts being introduced in images. Though most COR artifact can be recognized after the reconstruction, it is often difficult to salvage an acquisition that has a COR problem. COR should be checked on all systems on at least a weekly basis (or according to manufacturer's recommendations) and after any camera maintenance.

Count Density One of the most correctable problems in a nuclear image is insufficient counts. Because count density is directly proportional to imaging time, virtually every patient can be imaged with adequate counts if the acquisition time is extended to a proper amount. To date there has been very little work to establish what are sufficient counts necessary for imaging.[36-38] In addition, more counts will be need for performing gated imaging versus traditional nongated techniques.[39]

In 1999, the American Society of Nuclear Cardiology and the American College of Cardiology released imaging guidelines to help guide protocol utilization in nuclear laboratories to ensure that adequate counts is acquired in the majority of nuclear cardiology images. Adherence to these guidelines is essential for achieving sufficient count in routine nuclear cardiology.

CONCLUSION

An understanding of physics is an essential component of performing high-quality nuclear cardiology. From image interpretation to laboratory management, the clinician will be called upon to understand these physical principles in daily routine. Basic physics, statistics, mathematics, and radiation physics all play a vital role in daily service. Understanding the fundamental principles of these disciplines can help the physician make sound judgments in daily practice.

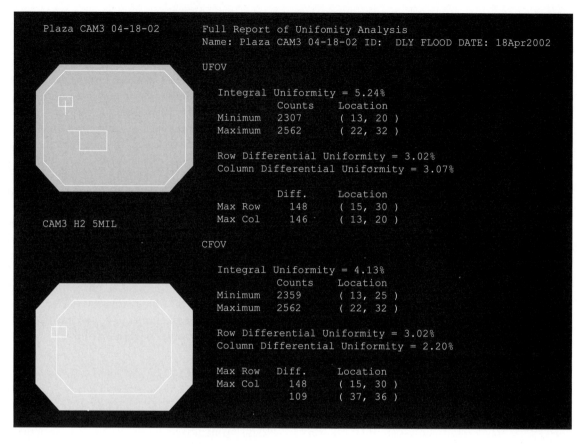

Figure 21-7. An example of a high-quality uniformity study. Both useful field of view (UFOV) and center field of view (CFOV) uniformity are below 6% but UFOV is above 5%. Close inspection of the flood should be done to ensure that the cause of the UFOV uniformity will not impact study image quality.

REFERENCES

1. Becquerel AH. On radioactivity, a new property of matter, Noble Lectures, Physics, 1901–1921.
2. Anger HO. A new instrument for mapping gamma ray emitters. *Biol Med Quarterly Rep* 1957; UCRL-3653:38.
3. Strauss, HW, Zaret, BL, Hurley, PJ, et. al., A scintiphotographic method for measuring left ventricular ejection fraction in man without cardiac catheterization, *Am J Cardiol,* 1971;28,:575.
4. Jaszczak RJ, Murphy PH, Huard D, Burdine JA, Radionuclide emission computed tomography of the head with Tc-99m and a scintillation camera. *J Nucl Med Inst Phys* 1977;18(4):373–375
5. Keyes WI. The fan-beam gamma camera. *Phys Med Biol* 1975;20:489–491.
6. Istandrian AE, and Veran, MS, Nuclear Cardiac Imaging, New York, Oxford Press, 2003;51–73.
7. Beller GA. *Clinical Nuclear Cardiology.* Philadelphia: WB Saunders, 1995.
8. Berman DS, Kiat H, Friedman JD, Wang FP, Van Train K. Separate acquisition rest thallium-201/technetium-99m sestimibi dual-isotope myocardial perfusion single photon emission computed tomography: A clinical validation study. *J Am Coll Cardiol* 1993;22:1455–1464.
9. Kiat H, Germano G, Friedman J, et al. Comparative feasibility of separate or simultaneous rest thallium-201/stress technetium-99m sestamibi dual-isotope myocardial perfusion SPECT. *J Nucl Med* 1994;35(4);542–548.
10. Bateman TM, Case JA, Moutray KL, et al. Clinical evaluation of a novel dual-simultaneous SPECT

myocardial perfusion protocol: Blinded comparison to dual-sequential images. *J Am Coll Cardiol* 1999;33:418A.

11. Case JA, Bateman TM, Moutray KL, et al. Critical evaluation of a simultaneous acquisition dual Tl-201/sestamibi imaging protocol in patients with known CAD. *J Nucl Cardiol* 1999;6:S115.

12. Sorenson JA, and Phelps ME. Physics in Nuclear Medicine, Second Edition. Chapter 15. WB Saunders Company, 1987.

13. Herman GT. Image reconstruction from projections: The fundamentals of computed tomography. New York: Academic Press, 1980.

14. Shepp LA, Vardi Y. Maximum likelihood reconstruction for emission tomography. *IEEE Trans Med Imaging* 1982; MI-1(2):113–122.

15. Lange K, Carson R. EM reconstruction algorithms for emission and transmission tomography. *J Comput Assist Tomogr* 1984;8(2):306–316.

16. Hudson MH, Larkin RS. Accelerated image reconstruction using ordered subsets of projection data. *IEEE Trans Med Imaging* 1994;13(4):601–609.

17. DePuey EG, Garcia EV. Optimal specificity of thallium-201 SPECT through recognition of imaging artifacts. *J Nucl Med* 1989;30:441–449.

18. DePuey EG. How to detect and avoid myocardial perfusion SPECT artifacts. *J Nucl Med* 1994;35(4):699–702.

19. Hendel RC, Corbett JR, Cullom SJ, et al. The value and practice of attenuation correction for myocardial perfusion SPECT imaging: A joint position statement from the American Society of Nuclear Cardiology and the Society of Nuclear Medicine. *J Nucl Med* 2002;9(1):135–143.

20. Eisner RL, Tamas MJ, Cloninger K, et al. Normal SPECT thallium-201 bull's eye display: Gender differences. *J Nucl Med* 1988;29(12):1901–1909.

21. DePuey EG, Rozanski AR. Using gated technetium-99m-sestamibi SPECT to characterize fixed defects as infarct or artifact. *J Nucl Med* 1995;36:952–955.

22. Smanio PE, Watson DD, Segalla DL, et al. Value of gating of technetium-99m sestamibi single-photon emission computed tomographic imaging. *J Am Coll Cardiol* 1997;30(7):1687–1692.

23. Esquerre JP, Coca FJ, Martinez SJ, Guiraud RF. Prone decubitus: A solution to inferior wall attenuation in thallium-201 myocardial tomography. *J Nucl Med* 1989;30(3):398–401.

24. Kiat H, Van Train KF, Friedman JD, et al. Quantitative stress-redistribution thallium-201 SPECT using prone imaging: Methodologic development and validation. *J Nucl Med* 1992;33(8):1509–1515.

25. Hendel RC, Corbett JR, Cullom SJ, et al. The value and practice of attenuation correction for myocardial perfusion SPECT imaging: A joint position statement

from the American Society of Nuclear Cardiology and the Society of Nuclear Medicine. *J Nucl Cardiol* 2002;9(1):135–143.

26. Hutton BF. Cardiac single-photon emission tomography: Is attenuation correction enough? *Eur J Nucl Med* 1997;24(7):713–715.

27. Heller EN, DeMan P, Liu YH, et al. Extracardiac activity complicates quantitative cardiac SPECT imaging using a simultaneous transmission–emission approach. *J Nucl Med* 1997;38(12):1882–1890.

28. King MA, Weishi X, deVries DJ, A Monte Carlo investigation of artifacts caused by liver uptake in single photon emission computed tomography perfusion imaging with technetium 99m-labeled agents. *J Nucl Cardiol* 1996;3(1):18–29.

29. Liu L, Cullom SJ, White ML. A modified wiener filter method for nonstationary resolution recovery with scatter and iterative attenuation correction for cardiac SPECT. *J Nucl Med* 1996;37(5):210P.

30. Jaszczak RJ, Greer KL, Floyd CE, et al. Improved SPECT quantification using compensation for scattered photons. *J Nucl Med* 1984;25:893–900.

31. Bowsher JE, Floyd CE Jr. Treatment of Compton scattering in maximum-likelihood, expectation-maximization reconstructions of SPECT images. *J Nucl Med* 1991;32(6):1291–1293.

32. Ogawa K, Harata Y, Ichihara T, et al. A practical method for position-dependent Compton-scatter correction in single photon emission CT. *IEEE Trans Med Imaging* 1991;MI-10(3):408–412.

33. Intersocietial Commision for the Accreditation of Nuclear Laboratories. *ICANL Essentials and Standards*, 2000.

34. Moutray K, Williams M, Bateman T, et al. Management of a wide-area network: Study of patient motion as a proxy for technologist performance. *J Nucl Cardiol* 2000;7:S5.

35. NEMA. *Performance Measurements of Scintillation Cameras*, NU-1, 2001.

36. Garcia EV, Bacharach SL, Mahmarian JJ, et al. Imaging guidelines for nuclear cardiology procedures. Part 1. *J Nucl Cardiol* 1996;3:G1–46.

37. O'Conner MK, Bothun E, Gibbons RJ. Influence of patient height and weight and type of stress on myocardial count density during SPECT imaging with Tl-201 and Tc-99m-sestamibi. *J Nucl Cardiol* 1998;5:304–312.

38. Case JA, Cullom SJ, Bateman TM, et al. Count density and filter requirements for accurate LVEF measurements from gated Tl-201 SPECT. *J Nucl Med* 1997;38:27P.

39. Germano G, Kiat H, Kavanagh P, et al. Automatic quantification of ejection fraction from gated myocardial perfusion SPECT. *J Nucl Med* 1995;36:2138–2148.

CHAPTER 22

Basics of ECG-Gated SPECT Imaging

Vanessa Go
Robert C. Hendel

INTRODUCTION

One of the most important recent developments in single photon emission computed tomography (SPECT) myocardial perfusion imaging (MPI) is the ability to acquire these studies in conjunction with electrocardiogram (ECG) gating. Initially developed in the late 1980s, it has now evolved into a standard for MPI in the United States. The American Society of Nuclear Cardiology in its position paper from March 1999 recommends the routine incorporation of ECG gating during SPECT cardiac perfusion scintigraphy.[1,2] By allowing simultaneous assessment of perfusion and function in a single-injection, single-acquisition sequence, it adds to the quality control of myocardial perfusion SPECT, improves its diagnostic accuracy and prognostic value and expands its clinical applications in a practical and user-friendly manner.

New developments in radiopharmaceuticals, as well as in imaging hardware and computer technology, have contributed significantly to the development of gated SPECT. The technetium-99m (Tc-99m)-based perfusion tracers, because of their higher count rates and stable myocardial distribution with time, permit evaluation of regional myocardial wall motion and wall thickening throughout the cardiac cycle. The development of automatic algorithms to quantitatively measure left ventricular (LV) volume and ejection fraction (EF), and even regional myocardial wall motion and thickening from gated SPECT rapidly and accurately with minimal operator interaction, has contributed to its widespread use.

TECHNICAL CONSIDERATIONS

Hardware Requirements

Gated SPECT images can be acquired using single- or multiple-detector cameras. More recently, dual-headed cameras in the 90-degree configuration have been preferred, as images can be ac-

303

quired in half the time required using a single-headed system without sacrificing image quality. The majority of gated SPECT imaging is performed with high-resolution parallel hole collimators for Tc-99m studies, while all-purpose collimators are used for thallium 201 (Tl-201) studies. A 180-degree imaging arc (45-degree right anterior oblique to 45-degree left posterior oblique projections), with a circular orbit is most commonly used, although noncircular (body contour) orbits can also be used. The most common detector rotation mode is the "step and shoot" acquisition method, in which the detector records events while stationary at each projection, but not while it is moving from one projection to the next. A "continuous" acquisition or a "pseudocontinuous" or "modified step and shoot" acquisition, wherein the data are collected even as the detector moves between projections, is often provided by some manufacturers, and is thought to be desirable in gated studies, as they provide a modest increase in counts with only a slight loss of spatial resolution. The standard image matrix size for gated and nongated SPECT imaging is 64×64 pixels, in conjunction with pixel sizes of 5 to 7 mm. This size offers adequate image resolution for interpretation and quantitation of both Tl-201 and Tc-99m tomograms. Computers with adequate processing speed and internal hard disk space are needed to process and store large amounts of scintigraphic data. Acquisition computers are usually separate from processing computers to allow for efficient laboratory operations. In addition, unsophisticated, relatively inexpensive, three-lead gating devices are provided by manufacturers to supply the trigger to the acquisition computer.[3]

Gated SPECT Acquisition and Processing

In a gated acquisition, a three-lead ECG provides the R-wave trigger to the acquisition computer, with two successive R-wave peaks on the ECG defining a cardiac cycle. Counts from each phase of the cardiac cycle are binned to a corresponding temporal "frame" within the computer. Perfusion projection images are obtained from summation of the individual frames (Figure 22-1). There is a trade-off between the temporal resolution of gated Tc-99m sestamibi images and the count density of the individual frames. Gating of myocardial perfusion is usually performed at eight frames per R-R interval per projection to maintain the count density using a single-headed camera, although 16 and 32 frames per cycle are also possible. With a multiheaded SPECT system, more frames can be acquired with no increase in acquisition time, as these systems can obtain higher count density images.

Most manufacturers provide either of two modes of gated SPECT acquisition, either "fixed" or "variable" to define the R-R interval.[4] In the fixed acquisition mode, the R-R interval is estimated by the acquisition computer prior to the study, based on the previously observed 10 to 20 heartbeats, and remains fixed throughout the study. In the variable acquisition mode, the heart rate is continuously monitored throughout

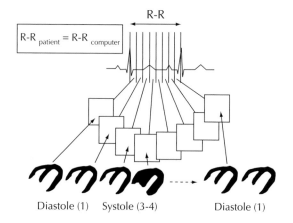

Diastole (1)   Systole (3-4)   Diastole (1)

Figure 22-1. Principle of ECG-gated SPECT acquisition. Separate temporal frames corresponding to different phases of the cardiac cycle are acquired for each angular projection. Perfusion images are obtained from summation of the individual frames. (From Cullom et al.[10] with permission).

the study and the acquisition computer alters the duration of temporal frames as needed to bin all counts equally into eight intervals per each previously detected R-R interval. In the fixed and variable modes, the data typically cannot be reformatted after the acquisition is complete. Another alternative to this is the list mode, which is a technique commonly used in radionuclide angiography.[6] This technique allows counts to be reformatted into temporal frames after the acquisition is complete. In this mode, the computer records the spatial coordinates of each detected count as well as a timing marker that identifies at what time the count was detected. After the acquisition, gated SPECT frames are generated by selecting a mean R-R interval and beat rejection criteria followed by appropriate binning of data. Some computers allow analysis of R-R intervals in the form of a histogram to derive mean heart rate and variability parameters as a guide to reformatting of data. The advantage of list mode acquisition is its flexibility, and can be used to aid in the identification of potential gating artifacts in fixed and variable mode acquisitions. A major disadvantage is that it requires storage of massive amounts of data, and as a result, is almost never used in clinical practice.[3]

Variations in heart rate due to a variety of factors (sinus arrhythmia, other arrhythmias, patient anxiety or motion, poor ECG lead contact, etc.) can result in temporal "blurring," that is, mixing of counts from adjacent frames. To limit acquired data to those heartbeats that are representative of the patient's average heartbeat and to minimize temporal blurring, a beat rejection window is set by specifying the acceptable deviation of R-R interval from the expected value. A 20% (± 10) window has historically been applied, although in patients with highly variable heart rates, up to a 100% (± 50) acceptance window can be set. Some camera manufacturers provide an extra frame in which counts from all rejected beats are accumulated. The counts within the extra frame can be added to the gated data after the acquisition is complete in order to generate a summed SPECT data set for interpretation of the static perfusion images. If a beat is rejected, the response to counts from the next R-R interval may be affected. On most commercial systems, a premature ventricular contraction (PVC) mode may be set that programs the computer to skip one or more cardiac beats before the R-R gating is reestablished. This is done to avoid mixing counts from the two successive cardiac cycles.[3]

As inferred from these quality control measures for gated acquisitions, the detection of an adequate R-wave signal is essential to the successful collection of image data synchronized to heart rate. In patients with severe arrhythmias, wherein the triggering mechanism is incapable of properly identifying the R wave, it has been demonstrated that EF fluctuations, perfusion differences, and, in particular, wall thickening discordance may occur.[6] Thus, in cases of extreme variation in heart rate or rhythm, an ungated SPECT study is preferred.

A variety of single-day and 2-day protocols may be used in conjunction with gated SPECT. As long as counts are adequate, either Tl-201 or Tc-99m perfusion tracers may be used. Either or both the acquisitions composing the stress/rest or rest/stress protocol can be gated, although the most commonly utilized is the high-dose technetium stress study because of its superior count density. Although the common practice is to gate only the poststress image, a small study by Johnson et al.[7] reports that in 36% of patients with reversible perfusion defects, the poststress LVEF was > 5% lower than at rest. This implies that global and regional LV function obtained from poststress gated acquisitions are not representative of basal LV function in patients with stress-induced ischemia, and that perhaps both rest and stress images should be gated routinely, as long as count density is adequate.

Injected doses of radiopharmaceuticals and injection-to-imaging intervals are the same as in nongated SPECT imaging. Acquisition times, energy windows, and poststress imaging delay are similar as well.[8] As in nongated studies, the supine position is most often used, although the prone position may be indicated for patients with suspected diaphragmatic attenuation.

Quality control measures need to be instituted after acquisition of images as well. Specially designed software can detect gating errors caused by variations in the cardiac cycle during the middle of an acquisition by means of superimposed graphs displaying accepted counts as a function of the projection number. If there are no gating errors, all eight projection curves should superimpose nearly perfectly.[9] In addition, simple visual inspection of the cinematic playback of data will also detect chaotic rhythms such as atrial fibrillation, which manifest as "flickering" of the display from one projection to the next.

Several types of artifacts are unique to gated SPECT imaging. If the R-R duration is less than the expected duration, but within the window of acceptance, the later frames of the gated SPECT study may contain a reduced number of counts. The computer will attempt to normalize the counts in all frames to the counts in the first temporal frame. If there are very few counts in that frame, the normalization step requires that they be multiplied by a very large factor, and this will have the effect of amplifying the noise in that frame to a level that will cause severe corruption of the gated SPECT data. "Flashing" artifacts will then be seen on cinematic display of the projected images. The same artifacts will be propagated into the tomographic images by filtered backprojection reconstruction, resulting in "streaking". Another type of artifact is radial blurring in the gated tomographic images, which may be caused by a marked and persistent R-R interval variability. This may limit definition of the systolic frame, affecting end-systolic volume and LVEF measurements.[10]

Quantitative Analysis of Gated SPECT Data

Functional Quantitation Overall ventricular function (end-diastolic and end-systolic LV cavity volumes and LVEF), as well as regional cardiac function (myocardial wall motion and thickening) can calculated separately using different automated programs requiring minimal operator input. There are multiple approaches to calculating ventricular function using different ventricular modeling assumptions as to the means by which endocardial locations are offset from midmyocardial points. All approaches assume the myocardial center to correspond to the location of the brightest midmyocardial count, and the different models approach this using either a geometric or count-based schema, or a hybrid of both. The Dodge–Sandler formula,[11] widely used in radiographic contrast angiography, has been applied to gated SPECT data. End-diastolic (ED) volumes from outlines drawn manually or automatically are obtained using area–length calculations, and LVEF is computed from the differences between end-diastolic volume and end-systolic volume. The Dodge–Sandler method utilizes only the midventricular vertical long-axis (VLA) tomogram, and as such, embodies the most restrictive assumptions about cardiac shape.[12] Biplane Simpson's method,[12,13] commonly used in echocardiography[14] and magnetic resonance imaging (MRI),[15] utilizes paired biplane midventricular tomographic sections. The method assumes that each short-axis slice is an ellipsoidal solid. Volumes are then computed by summing elliptical slices from apex to base.

More recently, fully three-dimensional approaches have been developed and validated to calculate LV volume and EF. The most widespread of these approaches is Gaussian count profile fitting to generate midmyocardial location estimates to detect epicardial and endocardial surface points.[16] Another approach to quantitating LV function is the count-based model, which uses observed changes secondary to partial volume effect in myocardial perfusion counts between end-diastole and end-systole to measure the percentage of myocardial thickening.[17] The advantage of three-dimensional approaches over slice-based methods is that they provide a better assessment of regional function. Regional function can be quantitated as well by measuring wall motion (i.e., endocardial excursion from end-diastole to end-systole) or wall thickening (i.e., brightening of the myocardium from end-diastole to end-systole) or a combination of both.[18] All these approaches are fully or semi-automated, but retain the possibility of manual intervention or correction (Figure 22-2).

Perfusion Quantitation

Historically, perfusion analysis is performed separately from functional analysis. However, because functional quantitation uses perfusion images to identify myocardial boundaries, both are intimately related. Currently, most systems are inte-

grated and use the same coordinates to quantify perfusion, motion, and thickening.[19] Traditionally, the patient's circumferential profile is displayed in a two-dimensional profile referred to as a *polar map*. Relative counts, defect extent, severity, and reversibility maps all can be generated. Most commercial systems also provide three-dimensional perfusion maps with defect and reversibility maps, which can be freely manipulated and reoriented by the reader using a computer "mouse" or trackball. To determine if an individual patient's study is normal or abnormal, the patient's sampled values must be compared to a set of profiles that are taken to be normal. Normality is usually determined from a

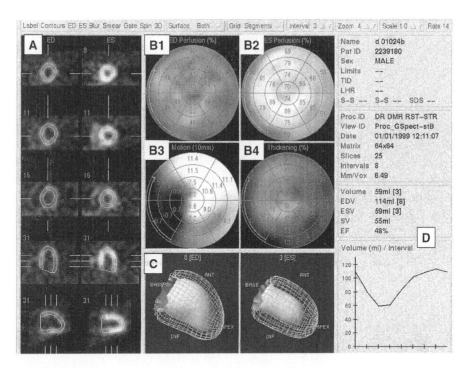

Figure 22-2. Quantification of ejection fraction, regional myocardial wall motion, and thickening from gated myocardial perfusion SPECT (QPS™) **A.** Myocardial contours displaying endocardial and epicardial surfaces overlying the end-diastolic (ED) and end-systolic (ES) frames, three short-axis images, a midcavity horizontal, and a midcavity vertical long axis. **B.** Quantitative polar plots measuring regional myocardial wall perfusion (B1, B2), motion (B3) and wall thickening (B4) from gated SPECT. **C.** Three-dimensional display of the endocardial (solid) and epicardial (grid) left ventricular surfaces calculated by the automatic algorithm. **D.** Endocardial time–volume curve and calculated LVEF from end-systolic and end-diastolic volumes. (*See also Color Insert*).

population of patients defined as having a low Bayesian likelihood of coronary artery disease (CAD) correlated with visual readings from a panel of experts.[8]

Validation of LVEF and Regional Function Quantitation by Gated SPECT

The two most widely distributed software packages for LV function analysis from gated myocardial perfusion scans are QGS (Cedars-Sinai, Los Angeles, CA) and the Emory Cardiac Toolbox or ECTb (Emory University, Atlanta, GA). The QGS methodology uses Gaussian fit to determine endocardial and epicardial offsets, while the ECTb is a count-based method. While both programs have, in general, compared favorably to other modalities for determining LVEF and volumes (Tables 22-1 and 22-2), it is important to note that the choice of gold standard as well as rigorousness in comparing different methodologies in these validation studies vary. Some modalities, including two-dimensional echocardiography, radionuclide ventriculography, and first-pass radionuclide angiography have their own inherent inaccuracies. Also, it is important to note that not all reports provided the statistical analysis of the variability around the correlation line, such as the standard error of estimates (SEE), which indicates the likelihood that the EF measured by the new technique will be within a certain range of the EF measured by the gold standard. If there is a large range, this usually indicates that a study is not as reliable. A small study done in canines by Vallejo et al.,[20] which showed that the automated QGS program consistently overestimated LVEF and LV volumes when compared to MRI, highlights the confounding effects that perfusion defects, background activity, time after injection, and the injected dose may have on the accuracy of such a determination. Furthermore, since this was a canine study, it is postulated that perhaps in smaller hearts, the limited spatial resolution of SPECT makes endocardial border recognition problematic and that perhaps a count-based method

would be more appropriate. A larger human study by the same author, comparing gated SPECT with first-pass radionuclide angiography (FPRNA), showed a better correlation in studies with low extracardiac activity, higher counts, and larger hearts.[21] This emphasizes the critical importance of quality control and optimizing image acquisition, as well as meticulousness on the part of the reader to recognize the presence of such variables. A comparison between both programs showed that QGS consistently provided significantly lower volumes and EFs compared to the ECTb algorithm for both CAD and low-likelihood patients, but that both methods showed close correlation with each other ($r = 0.91 - 0.94$).[22] If both programs are used in one institution, it would be important to take these differences into consideration and establish normal limits for each set of algorithms (Table 22-3).

In addition, an automated algorithm was also developed to measure regional function by measuring the motion of the three-dimensional endocardial surface using a modification of the centerline method, as well as wall thickening using both geometry (Gaussian fit) and partial volume (counts). This was tested against expert visual assessments of regional wall motion and regional wall thickening and was shown to have significant correlation.[18] This was validated in another study comparing semiquantitative assessments of regional wall motion and regional wall thickening by gated SPECT and MRI, which showed a high degree of agreement (kappa > 0.70, $p < .001$).[23]

CLINICAL APPLICATIONS
Artifact Identification

Gated SPECT initially found its clinical role in the enhanced ability to identify artifacts. Soft tissue attenuation artifacts often appear as fixed defects and are difficult to differentiate from infarct, thereby reducing the test specificity of SPECT MPI. Gated acquisitions may help differentiate scar from artifact as fixed defects with decreased function likely represent a myocardial infarction (MI), while attenuation artifacts will

Table 22-1

Validation of Quantitative Measurements of LVEF by Different Software Programs for Gated Myocardial Perfusion SPECT

Authors	Year	Software	Gold Standard	# of Patients	Correlation Coefficient	Isotope
Ioannidis et al.[61]	2002	QGS	MRI	164	0.89	
Baba et al.[62]	2002	QGS	Contrast ventriculography	20	0.80	Tl-201
Itti et al.[63]	2001	QGS	Equilibrium radionuclide angiography (ERNA)	50	0.88–0.92	Tl-201
Vourvouri et al.[64]	2001	QGS	2D echocardiography	32	0.83	
Higuchi et al.[65]	2001	QGS	Gated blood pool (GBP)		0.90	Tc-99 sestamibi
Germano et al.[16]	1995	QGS	First-pass radionuclide ventriculography	65	0.90	Tc-99 sestamibi
Faber et al.[19]	1999	ECTb	MRI	10	0.88	Tc-99 sestamibi
			First-pass radionuclide ventriculography	79	0.82	
Vallejo et al.[20]	2000	QGS	MRI	16 (canine)	0.51	Tc-99 sestamibi
Tadamura et al.[23]	1999	QGS	MRI	20	0.92	Tl-201
					0.94	Tc-99 sestamibi
Yoshioka et al.[66]	1999	QGS	First-pass RNA ventriculography	21	0.91	Tc-99 tetrofosmin
					0.87	
Vallejo et al.[21]	2000	QGS	FPRNA	400	0.66	
Nichols et al.[67]	1998	SPECT EF[a]	LV angiography	58	0.86	Tc-99 sestamibi
Nichols et al.[68]	1997	SPECT EF	FPRNA	22	0.90	Tc-99 sestamibi
Atsma et al.[69]	2000	QGS	Contrast ventriculography	74	0.84	Tc-99 tetrofosmin
Wright et al.[70]	2000	QGS	Radionuclide ventriculography	70	0.70–0.71	Tl-201 (low dose)
Bax et al.[71]	2000	QGS	MRI	22	0.90	Tc-99 tetrofosmin
Bavelaar-Croon et al.[72]	2000	QGS	MRI	21	0.85	
Cwajg et al.[73]	2000		2D ECHO	109	≥ 0.68	Tl-201 Tc-99
Nichols et al.[74]	2000	SPECT EF QGS ECTb	2D ECHO	33	0.92 overall 0.82 SPECT EF 0.75 QGS 0.72 ECTb	
He et al.[75]	1999		FPRNA	63	0.84–0.85	Tc-99 sestamibi Tl-201
Vaduganathan et al.[76]	1999		MRI	25	0.93	Tc-99

(continued)

Table 22-1 (continued)

Validation of Quantitative Measurements of LVEF by Different Software Programs for Gated Myocardial Perfusion SPECT

Authors	Year	Software	Gold Standard	# of Patients	Correlation Coefficient	Isotope
Tadamura et al.[23]	1999	QGS	MRI	16	0.89	Tc-99 sestamibi BMIPP[b]
Inubushi et al.[77]	1999	QGS	FPRNA	44	0.919	Tc-99 sestamibi
Nichols et al.[12]	1996		Equilibrium GBP FPRNA	75 65	0.87 0.87	Tc-99 sestamibi
Nakajima et al.[58]	2001	QGS ECT 4D-MSPECT pFAST[c]	RNA GBP	30	0.82 QGS 0.78 ECTb 0.69 4DM 0.84 pFAST	Tc-99 sestamibi
Everaert et al.[78]	1997	QGS Stanford	ERNA	40	0.89 QGS 0.93 SU	Tc-99 tetrofosmin
Chua et al.[79]	2000	QGS	ERNA	62	0.94	Tc-99
Abe et al.[80]	2000	QGS	Contrast ventriculography	229	0.78	Tc-99 tetrofosmin
Manrique et al.[81]	2000	QGS	ERNA	55	0.71–0.94	Tl-201
Williams and Taillon[82]	1996	U Chicago (Image inversion)	FPRNA Contrast ventriculography	38 54	0.83 0.93	Tc-99 sestamibi

[a] St. Luke's Roosevelt.

[b] Beta-methyl-p-iodophenyl-pentadecanoic acid.

[c] Perfusion and function analysis for gated SPECT.

have a fixed defect with normal or relatively normal wall motion. By incorporating regional wall motion data in the interpretation of perfusion imaging, DePuey and Rozanski[24] demonstrated that false-positive perfusion studies could be reduced from 14 to 3%. In women, the false-positive rate of stress ECGs is relatively high and the incidence of breast soft tissue attenuation artifact is a consideration; ECG gating was shown to further enhance the diagnostic specificity of Tc-99m

Table 22-2

Assessment of Left Ventricular Ejection Fraction by Five Methods: Range and Lower Normal Limits

Method	Gated SPECT (QGS)	Echocardiography	MRI	Angiography	GBP
Mean LVEF ± SD	63% ± 10%	60% ± 5%	65% ± 5%	67% ± 8%	55% ± 7%
Normal (lower limit)	44%	48%	57%	51%	43%

Reprinted from Rozanski et al.[83] with permission.

Table 22-3

Comparison of Two Software Programs for Quantitation of LV Function and Volumes in Normal or Low-Risk Subjects

	QGS	ECTb
EF (%)	62 ± 9	67 ± 8
EDV (mL)	84 ± 26	105 ± 33
ESV (mL)	33 ± 17	35 ± 17

Reprinted from Nichols et al.[22] with permission.

perfusion imaging from 84 to 94%.[25] Subsequently, Smanio et al.[26] demonstrated that the addition of gated SPECT for the assessment of regional systolic function reduces the degree of uncertainty in the interpretation of Tc-99m sestamibi perfusion studies. The number of "borderline normal" or "borderline abnormal" inter-

pretations were significantly reduced. In patients with low likelihood of CAD, the normalcy rate increased from 74 to 93% (Figure 22-3). In patients with a high likelihood for CAD, the trend was also toward a higher number of unequivocally abnormal interpretations.

Coronary Artery Disease Detection

In addition to improving diagnostic specificity, the capability to obtain functional information through gating may also enhance the detection of CAD, particularly multivessel disease. While proven in various studies that SPECT MPI reliably detects CAD, the question of underestimating ischemia in the case of multivessel disease or left main disease because of balanced global hypoperfusion comes into question. Several reports have estimated that only 13 to 50% of patients with three-vessel CAD or left main disease actually have perfusion abnormalities in multiple ter-

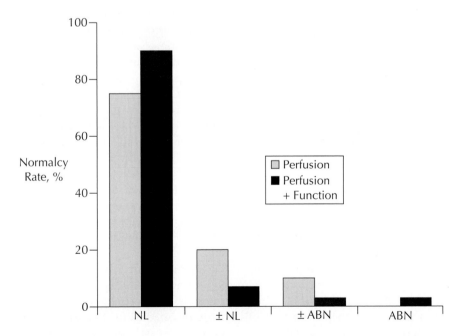

Figure 22-3. In patients with low likelihood of CAD, normalcy rate increased from 74% to 93%, and borderline readings decreased from 32% to 10% when the functional data from gating is incorporated into study interpretation. (Modified from DePuey and Rozanski[24] with permission.)

ritories,[27–29] thus potentially leading clinicians to underestimate risk or mispredict prognosis. Several studies have clearly demonstrated the incremental value of utilizing both functional and perfusion data in detecting multivessel disease or high-grade stenoses over perfusion data alone, although there is some conflicting data on sensitivity and specificity. Sharir et al.[30] examined a population of 99 patients who underwent dual-isotope resting Tl-201/exercise gated Tc-99m sestamibi SPECT with normal resting perfusion. Multivariate regression analysis showed that both extensive perfusion abnormalities and the presence of wall motion abnormalities in multiple territories were independent predictors of severe multivessel CAD, but that the addition of wall motion variables to perfusion data resulted in a significant increase in the global chi-square for predicting severe proximal left anterior descending (LAD) as well as multivessel CAD. For perfusion alone, sensitivity was 49%, while combined perfusion and wall motion abnormality yielded a sensitivity of 82%. Furthermore, the use of rest and stress LVEF may assist in the detection of multivessel coronary disease, as demonstrated in a study by Yamagishi et al.[31] wherein the combination of perfusion data and worsening of the LVEF significantly increased sensitivity in detecting multivessel CAD over Tl-201 perfusion defects or rest LVEF and postexercise LVEF alone (43.3% vs. 26.9%, 25.4%, and 25.4%, respectively). Of note, while sensitivity increased, there was also a significant decrease in specificity, although this remained acceptable at approximately 90%. Another study sought to correlate degree of angiographic stenosis with the presence of regional wall motion abnormalities (RWMAs) on exercise stress/rest–gated technetium-99m SPECT studies.[32] Reversible RWMAs were found to be highly specific for angiographic stenoses > 70%, both overall and for specific vascular territories (94–100%). Furthermore, when patients were stratified according to severity of angiographic stenoses (50–79% and 80–99%), the presence of reversible RWMA distinguished a higher angiographic severity with positive predic-

tive values between 77% and 88% for specific vascular territories. Notably, these improvements in specificity were at the expense of sensitivity, which were much less compared to perfusion alone (53% for reversible RWMA vs. 89% for perfusion alone).

Prognosis and Risk Stratification

As is the case with perfusion imaging in general, gated SPECT imaging has also found an important role in the risk assessment of patients with known or suspected CAD. This is not surprising, given the well-recognized prognostic role of LV function with regard to long-term survival, as has been shown using a variety of techniques for LV functional assessment. Among a large series of 1,690 consecutive patients who underwent dual-isotope–gated SPECT imaging, those whose EFs were < 45% were associated with reduced survival, irrespective of the perfusion defect size or severity. Additionally, those patients with normal end-systolic volumes of < 70 mL or an EF of > 45% had a very low cardiac mortality rate, despite severe perfusion abnormalities[33] (Figure 22-4). This group also examined the relative value of perfusion and function in the risk stratification in 2,686 patients into low-, intermediate-, and high-risk categories for cardiac death and MI.[34] LVEF was most predictive of death, and the amount of ischemia (summed difference score on perfusion imaging) was the best predictor of nonfatal MI. Functional information was found to be of incremental value in the prediction of cardiac death beyond the perfusion imaging parameters. Interestingly, the presence of ischemia did not influence prognosis in patients with LVEF < 30%, due to the already high mortality rate.

LV function has long been a key determinant for survival following an acute MI. Recently, a study of 128 postinfarct survivors confirmed the value of gated SPECT imaging for risk stratification in post-MI patients, as an LVEF of < 40% with this method was found to increase the risk of subsequent cardiac event by almost three-

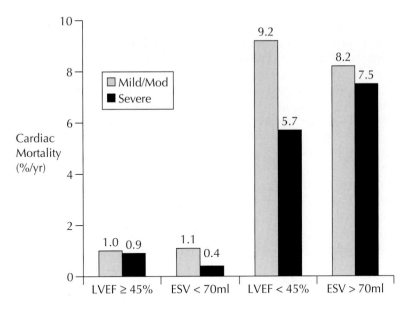

Figure 22-4. Annual cardiac death rates stratified by LV volume and ejection fraction. Patients with an LVEF of ≥ 45% or ESV < 70 mL have a low mortality rate regardless of severity of perfusion defects. Similar findings are noted for patients with a low ejection fraction (< 45%). (Modified from Yamagishi et al.[31] with permission.)

fold.[35] Interestingly, the presence of a fixed or reversible defect had no independent predictive value in this study, although the latter finding may be a result of the censoring of high-risk patients who underwent early revascularization.

Ischemic Cardiomyopathy and Viability Determination

Among patients with a dilated cardiomyopathy, the distinction between an ischemic and nonischemic etiology has clinical relevance and may greatly affect management decisions. Danias et al.[36] demonstrated that ischemic and nonischemic cardiomyopathy can be reliably distinguished from each other noninvasively with the use of gated SPECT imaging. Not only do patients with ischemic cardiomyopathy have greater summed stress scores than nonischemic cardiomyopathies, but the amount of regional variability in function is also an important parameter in distinguishing between these broad categories.

In patients with CAD and LV dysfunction, the issue of myocardial viability is often highly relevant in the decision-making process regarding revascularization. Several modalities have been studied and used for the assessment of viability, including Tl-201 stress-redistribution, rest-redistribution, or reinjection scintigraphy with both Tl-201 or Tc-99 sestamibi,[37–44] low-dose dobutamine echocardiography,[45] contrast-enhanced MRI, and F-18 fluorodeoxyglucose positron-emission tomography (FDG-PET).[46–48] Although FDG-PET is widely considered the gold standard, with sensitivities ranging from 71 to 100%, a recent meta-analysis by Bax et al.[49] showed no clear advantage of one technique over another. The principal limitation of FDG-PET is the fairly high cost of the equipment, thus limiting its availability in all medical centers. Other modalities are usually utilized to determine viability before employing PET. The addition of functional information provided by ECG gating is thought to have an incremental value for the prediction of viability over perfusion studies alone. In a small study by Levine and colleagues,[50] perfusion and wall motion combined significantly improved sensitivity and accuracy for the prediction of viability, as defined by a ≥ 20% improvement in perfusion and/or function when compared with perfusion imaging alone (95% vs. 86% sensitivity, 91% vs. 85% accuracy). Specificity remained the same at 55%. In another trial, gated SPECT Tc-99m tetrofosmin assessment of wall thickening (rather than wall motion), combined with perfusion data, increased the sensitivity for assessment of viability using FDG-PET imaging as the gold standard, from 79 to 85%, but decreased specificity from 79 to 56%.[51] Other investigators have demonstrated that the assessment of wall thickening on gated SPECT may have its potential impact on improved specificity with regard to postrevascularization recovery of regional function, depending on tracer activity on perfusion. When segments with > 50% tetrofosmin activity have detectable wall thickening, there is a higher likelihood of functional improvement when compared with segments with no contractile function; however, in segments with < 50% tracer activity, there was no significant difference.[52] While these particular studies demonstrate an advantage of combined function and perfusion assessment, the actual sensitivities and specificities are not significantly different from the weighted mean sensitivities and specificities of the meta-analysis,[49] keeping in mind that most of these studies are small and have varied study designs.

Low-dose dobutamine has been used successfully to demonstrate contractile reserve for many imaging modalities including echocardiography,[45] radionuclide angiography,[53] MRI,[54] and most recently with gated SPECT imaging.[55–57] Overall, viability measurements based on contractile reserve have higher specificity than perfusion imaging; this finding has been confirmed for gated SPECT imaging as well. In a study by Leoncini et al.,[55] the use of low-dose dobutamine-gated SPECT significantly improved the specificity and overall accuracy for predicting functional recovery

after coronary revascularization. The visual assessment of regional function following low-dose dobutamine was especially useful for hypokinetic segments in which specificity for postrevascularization functional improvement increased to 94%, as compared with 23% for perfusion imaging. However, the sensitivity for prediction of improvement in akinetic regions was inferior with dobutamine-gated SPECT compared with quantitative perfusion imaging (Figure 22-5). This study suggests a combined approach, using data from both contractile reserve and quantitative tracer activity.[55] In the same series, they also assessed global LV function with low-dose dobutamine infusion as a predictor of postrevascularization functional improvement. An increase in the LVEF of > 5 EF units was found to be a good predictor of improvement in EF post-revascularization.[56] Again, it is important to note that the main limitation of these, as well as other studies looking at functional recovery, is the small population size.

Other Diagnostic Applications

Aside from its well-studied applications in determining systolic function, attempts have been made to expand the clinical applications of ECG-gated SPECT imaging. Echocardiography has been the most commonly utilized method for assessing diastolic function. Radionuclide techniques, specifically equilibrium radionuclide angiography, have more recently been applied as well. Several diastolic parameters have been used, including peak filling rate (PFR), which measures the most rapid change in ventricular counts in early to mid-diastole, the time to peak filling (the time interval from the nadir of LV counts to the moment of the PFR), and the filling fraction (percentage of filling that has occurred at one third, one half, and two thirds of diastole). A small study has applied ECG-gated SPECT to assess the same diastolic parameters (specifically PFR), and found a close correlation between PFR generated by equilibrium radionuclide angiography (ERNA) and gated SPECT using a higher frame rate of 32 frames per cardiac cycle

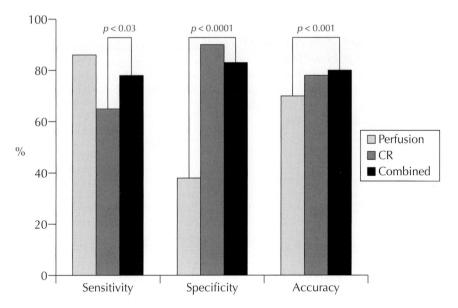

Figure 22-5. Prediction of functional recovery with nitrate-enhanced Tc-99m sestamibi dobutamine-gated imaging. For all asynergic segments, using a combination of tracer activity and contractile reserve (black bars—combined) improved specificity and overall accuracy significantly when compared to perfusion quantification alone (stippled—perfusion). Sensitivity was not altered significantly with the combined approach, but was higher than using contractile reserve alone (hatched bars—CR). (From Stollfuss et al.[52] with permission.)

(the most commonly used frame rate is 8 frames per cycle).[58] In another study, the diastolic parameters of a small group of patients with systemic sclerosis were examined using gated SPECT, and again a closer correlation and higher accuracy was found when using 16 frames per cycle.[59] Both these studies utilized three-detector SPECT systems. These findings are consistent with the concept that accurate assessment of diastolic function by radionuclide techniques require a high temporal resolution and reliability of the diastolic filling phase of the time–activity curve. In addition, the fidelity of the diastolic filling phase of the time–activity curve is also affected by the traditional problems associated with gating based on R-R interval, such as arrhythmias or PVCs, and thus alternative acquisition modes (such as list mode acquisition) or "bad beat rejection" filters have to be applied. These technical considerations have currently limited the usefulness of gated SPECT for assessment of diastolic function.

Another potential novel application of gated SPECT is the assessment of right ventricular size and wall motion. An unsuspected pulmonary embolism was diagnosed when unexplained right ventricular (RV) dilatation and hypokinesis was detected on gated SPECT imaging.[60] More studies are definitely warranted for this application, but routine examination of RV size and motion when interpreting studies may provide additional clinical information.

CONCLUSION

In conclusion, gated SPECT imaging provides a wealth of additional information that is useful not only to the reader interpreting MPI studies but also to the referring clinician. Although the major benefit of perfusion imaging has been its ability to improve artifact recognition, the use of functional information also improves the detection of severe and extensive coronary disease, provides independent and incremental prognostic information, and aids in the evaluation of myocardial viability. Numerous other applications have also been described, and unique values of this technique will undoubtedly continue to evolve.

REFERENCES

1. Bateman TM, Berman DS, Heller GV, et al. American Society of Nuclear Cardiology position statement on electrocardiographic gating of myocardial perfusion SPECT scintigrams. *J Nucl Cardiol* 1999;6:470.
2. Anonymous. Imaging guidelines for nuclear cardiology procedures, part 2: American Society of Nuclear Cardiology. *J Nucl Cardiol* 1999;6:G47.
3. Germano G, Nichols K, Cullom SJ. Gated perfusion SPECT: Technical considerations. In: DePuey EG, Garcia EV, Berman DS, eds. *Cardiac SPECT Imaging*, 2nd ed. Philadelphia: Lippincott Williams and Wilkins, 2001:103.
4. Bacharach SL, Bonow RO, Green MV. Comparison of fixed and variable temporal resolution methods for creating gated cardiac blood-pool image sequences. *J Nucl Med* 1994;35:38.
5. Port S. First-pass radionuclide angiography. In: Marcus ML, Braunwald E, eds. *Marcus Cardiac Imaging: A Companion to Braunwald's Heart Disease*. Philadelphia: WB Saunders, 1996:923.
6. Nichols K, Yao SS, Kamran M, et al. Clinical impact of arrhythmias on gated SPECT cardiac myocardial perfusion and function assessment. *J Nucl Cardiol* 2001;8:19.
7. Johnson LL, Verdesca SA, Aude WY, et al. Postischemic stunning can affect left ventricular ejection fraction and regional wall motion on post-stress gated sestamibi tomograms [Comment]. *J Am Coll Cardiol* 1997;30:1641.
8. Anonymous. Updated imaging guidelines for nuclear cardiology procedures, part 1: American Society of Nuclear Cardiology. *J Nucl Cardiol* 2001;8:G39.
9. Nichols K, Dorbala S, DePuey EG, et al. Influence of arrhythmias on gated SPECT myocardial perfusion and function quantification. *J Nucl Med* 1999;40:924.
10. Cullom SJ, Case JA, Bateman TM. Electrocardiographically gated myocardial perfusion SPECT: Technical principles and quality control considerations. *J Nucl Cardiol* 1998;5:418.
11. Sandler H, Dodge HT. The use of single plane angiocardiograms for the calculation of left ventricular volume in man. *Am Heart J* 1968;75:325.
12. Nichols K, DePuey EG, Rozanski A. Automation of gated tomographic left ventricular ejection fraction. *J Nucl Cardiol* 1996;3:475.
13. DePuey EG, Nichols K, Dobrinsky C. Left ventricular ejection fraction assessed from gated technetium-99m-sestamibi SPECT. *J Nucl Med* 1993;34:1871.
14. Katz A, Force T, Folland E. Echocardiographic assessment of ventricular systolic function. In: Marcus ML, Braunwald E, eds. *Marcus Cardiac Imaging: A Companion to Braunwald's Heart Disease*. Philadelphia: WB Saunders, 1996:297.
15. Dulce MC, Mostbeck GH, Friese KK, et al. Quantification of the left ventricular volumes and function with cine MR imaging: Comparison of geometric models with three-dimensional data. *Radiology* 1993;188:371.
16. Germano G, Kiat H, Kavanagh PB, et al. Automatic quantification of ejection fraction from gated myocardial perfusion SPECT. *J Nucl Med* 1995;36:2138.
17. Smith WH, Kastner RJ, Calnon DA, et al. Quantitative gated single photon emission computed tomography imaging: A counts-based method for display and measurement of regional and global ventricular systolic function. *J Nucl Cardiol* 1997;4:451.
18. Germano G, Erel J, Lewin H, et al. Automatic quantitation of regional myocardial wall motion and thickening from gated technetium-99m sestamibi myocardial perfusion single-photon emission computed tomography. *J Am Coll Cardiol* 1997;30:1360.
19. Faber TL, Cooke CD, Folks RD, et al. Left ventricular function and perfusion from gated SPECT perfusion images: An integrated method. *J Nucl Med* 1999;40:650.
20. Vallejo E, Dione DP, Bruni WL, et al. Reproducibility and accuracy of gated SPECT for determination of left ventricular volumes and ejection fraction: Experimental validation using MRI [Comment]. *J Nucl Med* 2000;41:874.
21. Vallejo E, Dione DP, Sinusas AJ, et al. Assessment of left ventricular ejection fraction with quantitative gated SPECT: Accuracy and correlation with first-pass radionuclide angiography. *J Nucl Cardiol* 2000;7:461.
22. Nichols K, Santana CA, Folks R, et al. Comparison between ECTb and QGS for assessment of left ventricular function from gated myocardial perfusion SPECT. *J Nucl Cardiol* 2002;9:285.
23. Tadamura E, Kudoh T, Motooka M, et al. Use of technetium-99m sestamibi ECG-gated single-photon emission tomography for the evaluation of left ventricular function following coronary artery bypass graft: Comparison with three-dimensional magnetic resonance imaging. *Eur J Nucl Med* 1999;26:705.
24. DePuey EG, Rozanski A. Using gated technetium-99m-sestamibi SPECT to characterize fixed myocardial defects as infarct or artifact. *J Nucl Med* 1995;36:952.

25. Taillefer R, DePuey EG, Udelson JE, et al. Comparative diagnostic accuracy of Tl-201 and Tc-99m sestamibi SPECT imaging (perfusion and ECG-gated SPECT) in detecting coronary artery disease in women. *J Am Coll Cardiol* 1997;29:69.

26. Smanio PE, Watson DD, Segalla DL, et al. Value of gating of technetium-99m sestamibi single-photon emission computed tomographic imaging. *J Am Coll Cardiol* 1997;30:1687.

27. Chae SC, Heo J, Iskandrian AS, et al. Identification of extensive coronary artery disease in women by exercise single-photon emission computed tomographic (SPECT) thallium imaging. *J Am Coll Cardiol* 1993;21:1305.

28. Rehn T, Griffith LS, Achuff SC, et al. Exercise thallium-201 myocardial imaging in left main coronary artery disease: Sensitive but not specific. *Am J Cardiol* 1981;48:217.

29. Christian TF, Miller TD, Bailey KR, et al. Noninvasive identification of severe coronary artery disease using exercise tomographic thallium-201 imaging. *Am J Cardiol* 1992;70:14.

30. Sharir T, Bacher-Stier C, Dhar S, et al. Identification of severe and extensive coronary artery disease by postexercise regional wall motion abnormalities in Tc-99m sestamibi gated single-photon emission computed tomography. *Am J Cardiol* 2000;86:1171.

31. Yamagishi H, Shirai N, Yoshiyama M, et al. Incremental value of left ventricular ejection fraction for detection of multivessel coronary artery disease in exercise (201)Tl gated myocardial perfusion imaging. *J Nucl Med* 2002;43:131.

32. Emmett L, Iwanochko RM, Freeman MR, et al. Reversible regional wall motion abnormalities on exercise technetium-99m-gated cardiac single photon emission computed tomography predict high-grade angiographic stenoses. *J Am Coll Cardiol* 2002;39:991.

33. Sharir T, Germano G, Kavanagh PB, et al. Incremental prognostic value of post-stress left ventricular ejection fraction and volume by gated myocardial perfusion single photon emission computed tomography. *Circulation* 1999;100:1035.

34. Sharir T, Germano G, Kang X, et al. Prediction of myocardial infarction versus cardiac death by gated myocardial perfusion SPECT: Risk stratification by the amount of stress-induced ischemia and the poststress ejection fraction. *J Nucl Med* 2001;42:831.

35. Kroll D, Farah W, McKendall GR, et al. Prognostic value of stress-gated Tc-99m sestamibi SPECT after acute myocardial infarction. *Am J Cardiol* 2001;87:381.

36. Danias PG, Ahlberg AW, Clark BA III, et al. Combined assessment of myocardial perfusion and left ventricular function with exercise technetium-99m sestamibi gated single-photon emission computed tomography can differentiate between ischemic and nonischemic dilated cardiomyopathy. *Am J Cardiol* 1998;82:1253.

37. Inglese E, Brambilla M, Dondi M, et al. Assessment of myocardial viability after thallium-201 reinjection or rest-redistribution imaging: A multicenter study: The Italian Group of Nuclear Cardiology. *J Nucl Med* 1995;36:555.

38. Bonow RO, Dilsizian V, Cuocolo A, et al. Identification of viable myocardium in patients with chronic coronary artery disease and left ventricular dysfunction. Comparison of thallium scintigraphy with reinjection and PET imaging with 18F-fluorodeoxyglucose [Comment]. *Circulation* 1991;83:26.

39. Udelson JE, Coleman PS, Metherall J, et al. Predicting recovery of severe regional ventricular dysfunction: Comparison of resting scintigraphy with ^{201}Tl and ^{99m}Tc-sestamibi. *Circulation* 1994;89:2552.

40. Ragosta M, Beller GA, Watson DD, et al. Quantitative planar rest-redistribution ^{201}Tl imaging in detection of myocardial viability and prediction of improvement in left ventricular function after coronary bypass surgery in patients with severely depressed left ventricular function. *Circulation* 1993;87:1630.

41. Maes AF, Borgers M, Flameng W, et al. Assessment of myocardial viability in chronic coronary artery disease using technetium-99m sestamibi SPECT. Correlation with histologic and positron emission tomographic studies and functional follow-up. *J Am Coll Cardiol* 1997;29:62.

42. Sinusas AJ, Bergin JD, Edwards NC, et al. Redistribution of ^{99m}Tc-sestamibi and ^{201}Tl in the presence of a severe coronary artery stenosis. *Circulation* 1994;89:2332.

43. Galassi AR, Centamore G, Fiscella A, et al. Comparison of rest-redistribution thallium-201 imaging and reinjection after stress-redistribution for the assessment of myocardial viability in patients with left ventricular dysfunction secondary to coronary artery disease. *Am J Cardiol* 1995;75:436.

44. Dilsizian V, Smeltzer WR, Freedman NM, et al. Thallium reinjection after stress-redistribution imaging. Does 24-hour delayed imaging after reinjection enhance detection of viable myocardium? *Circulation* 1991;83:1247.

45. Afridi I, Kleiman NS, Raizner AE, et al. Dobutamine echocardiography in myocardial hibernation: Optimal dose and accuracy in predicting recovery of ventricular function after coronary angioplasty [Comment]. *Circulation* 1995;91:663.

46. Tamaki N, Yonekura Y, Yamashita K, et al. Positron emission tomography using fluorine-18 deoxyglucose in evaluation of coronary artery bypass grafting. *Am J Cardiol* 1989;64:860.

47. Schelbert HR. Positron emission tomography for the assessment of myocardial viability. *Circulation* 1991;84:I122.

48. Gould KL. Clinical cardiac positron emission tomography: State of the art. *Circulation* 1991;84:I22.

49. Bax JJ, Wijns W, Cornel JH, et al. Accuracy of currently available techniques for prediction of functional recovery after revascularization in patients with left ventricular dysfunction due to chronic coronary artery disease: Comparison of pooled data. *J Am Coll Cardiol* 1997;30:1451.

50. Levine MG, McGill CC, Ahlberg AW, et al. Functional assessment with electrocardiographic gated single-photon emission computed tomography improves the ability of technetium-99m sestamibi myocardial perfusion imaging to predict myocardial viability in patients undergoing revascularization. *Am J Cardiol* 1999;83:1.

51. Maruyama A, Hasegawa S, Paul AK, et al. Myocardial viability assessment with gated SPECT Tc-99m tetrofosmin % wall thickening: Comparison with F-18 FDG-PET. *Ann Nucl Med* 2002;16:25.

52. Stollfuss JC, Haas F, Matsunari I, et al. 99mTc-tetrofosmin SPECT for prediction of functional recovery defined by MRI in patients with severe left ventricular dysfunction: Additional value of gated SPECT. *J Nucl Med* 1999;40:1824.

53. Zafrir N, Vidne B, Sulkes J, et al. Usefulness of dobutamine radionuclide ventriculography for prediction of left ventricular function improvement after coronary artery bypass grafting for ischemic cardiomyopathy [Comment]. *Am J Cardiol* 1999;83:691.

54. Baer FM, Voth E, Schneider CA, et al. Comparison of low-dose dobutamine-gradient-echo magnetic resonance imaging and positron emission tomography with [18F]fluorodeoxyglucose in patients with chronic coronary artery disease: A functional and morphological approach to the detection of residual myocardial viability. *Circulation* 1995;91:1006.

55. Leoncini M, Marcucci G, Sciagra R, et al. Prediction of functional recovery in patients with chronic coronary artery disease and left ventricular dysfunction combining the evaluation of myocardial perfusion and of contractile reserve using nitrate-enhanced technetium-99m sestamibi gated single-photon emission computed tomography and dobutamine stress. *Am J Cardiol* 2001;87:1346.

56. Leoncini M, Sciagra R, Maioli M, et al. Usefulness of dobutamine Tc-99m sestamibi-gated single-photon emission computed tomography for prediction of left ventricular ejection fraction outcome after coronary revascularization for ischemic cardiomyopathy. *Am J Cardiol* 2002;89:817.

57. Yoshinaga K, Morita K, Yamada S, et al. Low-dose dobutamine electrocardiograph-gated myocardial SPECT for identifying viable myocardium: Comparison with dobutamine stress echocardiography and PET. *J Nucl Med* 2001;42:838.

58. Kumita S, Cho K, Nakajo H, et al. Assessment of left ventricular diastolic function with electrocardiography-gated myocardial perfusion SPECT: Comparison with multigated equilibrium radionuclide angiography. *J Nucl Cardiol* 2001;8:568.

59. Nakajima K, Higuchi T, Taki J, et al. Accuracy of ventricular volume and ejection fraction measured by gated myocardial SPECT: Comparison of 4 software programs. *J Nucl Med* 2001;42:1571.

60. Soudry G, Dibos PE. Gated myocardial perfusion scan leading to diagnosis of unsuspected massive pulmonary embolism. *Ann Intern Med* 2000;132:845.

61. Ioannidis JP, Trikalinos TA, Danias PG. Electrocardiogram-gated single-photon emission computed tomography versus cardiac magnetic resonance imaging for the assessment of left ventricular volumes and ejection fraction: A meta-analysis. *J Am Coll Cardiol* 2002;39:2059.

62. Baba A, Hano T, Ohmori H, et al. Assessment of left ventricular function by thallium-201 quantitative gated cardiac SPECT. *Kaku Igaku—Japanese J Nucl Med* 2002;39:21.

63. Itti E, Rosso J, Damien P, et al. Assessment of ejection fraction with Tl-201 gated SPECT in myocardial infarction: Precision in a rest-redistribution study and accuracy versus planar angiography. *J Nucl Cardiol* 2001;8:31.

64. Vourvouri EC, Poldermans D, Bax JJ, et al. Evaluation of left ventricular function and volumes in patients with ischaemic cardiomyopathy: Gated single-photon emission computed tomography versus two-dimensional echocardiography. *Eur J Nucl Med* 2001;28:1610.

65. Higuchi T, Nakajima K, Taki J, et al. Assessment of left ventricular systolic and diastolic function based on the edge detection method with myocardial ECG-gated SPET. *Eur J Nucl Med* 2001;28:1512.

66. Yoshioka J, Hasegawa S, Yamaguchi H, et al. Left ventricular volumes and ejection fraction calculated from quantitative electrocardiographic-gated 99m Tc-tetrofosmin myocardial SPECT. *J Nucl Med* 1999;42:183.

67. Nichols K, Tamis J, DePuey EG, et al. Relationship of gated SPECT ventricular function parameters to angiographic measurements. *J Nucl Cardiol* 1998;5:295.

68. Nichols K, DePuey EG, Rozanski A, et al. Image enhancement of severely hypoperfused myocardia for computation of tomographic ejection fraction. *J Nucl Med* 1997;38:1411.

69. Atsma DE, Bavelaar-Croon CD, Germano G, et al. Good correlation between gated single photon emission computed myocardial tomography and contrast ventriculography in the assessment of global and regional left ventricular function. *Int J Cardiac Imaging* 2000;16:447.

70. Wright GA, McDade M, Keeble W, et al. Quantitative

gated SPECT myocardial perfusion imaging with 201Tl: An assessment of the limitations. *Nucl Med Comm* 2000;21:1147.

71. Bax JJ, Lamb H, Dibbets P, et al. Comparison of gated single-photon emission computed tomography with magnetic resonance imaging for evaluation of left ventricular function in ischemic cardiomyopathy. *Am J Cardiol* 2000;86:1299.

72. Bavelaar-Croon CD, Kayser HW, van der Wall EE, et al. Left ventricular function: Correlation of quantitative gated SPECT and MR imaging over a wide range of values. *Radiology* 2000;217:572.

73. Cwajg E, Cwajg J, Keng F, et al. Comparison of global and regional left ventricular function assessed by gated-SPECT and 2-D echocardiography. *Revista Portuguesa de Cardiologia* 2000;19:139.

74. Nichols K, Lefkowitz D, Faber T, et al. Echocardiographic validation of gated SPECT ventricular function measurements. *J Nucl Med* 2000;41:1308.

75. He ZX, Cwajg E, Preslar JS, et al. Accuracy of left ventricular ejection fraction determined by gated myocardial perfusion SPECT with Tl-201 and Tc-99m sestamibi: Comparison with first-pass radionuclide angiography. *J Nucl Cardiol* 1999;6:412.

76. Vaduganathan P, He ZX, Vick GW III, et al. Evaluation of left ventricular wall motion, volumes, and ejection fraction by gated myocardial tomography with technetium 99m-labeled tetrofosmin: A comparison with cine magnetic resonance imaging. *J Nucl Cardiol* 1999;6:3.

77. Inubushi M, Tadamura E, Kudoh T, et al. Simultaneous assessment of myocardial free fatty acid utilization and left ventricular function using 123I-BMIPP-gated SPECT. *J Nucl Med* 1999;40:1840.

78. Everaert H, Bossuyt A, Franken PR. Left ventricular ejection fraction and volumes from gated single photon emission tomographic myocardial perfusion images: Comparison between two algorithms working in three-dimensional space. *J Nucl Cardiol* 1997;4:472.

79. Chua T, Yin LC, Thiang TH, et al. Accuracy of the automated assessment of left ventricular function with gated perfusion SPECT in the presence of perfusion defects and left ventricular dysfunction: Correlation with equilibrium radionuclide ventriculography and echocardiography. *J Nucl Cardiol* 2000;7:301.

80. Abe M, Kazatani Y, Fukuda H, et al. Left ventricular volumes, ejection fraction, and regional wall motion calculated with gated technetium-99m tetrofosmin SPECT in reperfused acute myocardial infarction at super-acute phase: Comparison with left ventriculography. *J Nucl Cardiol* 2000;7:569.

81. Manrique A, Koning R, Cribier A, et al. Effect of temporal sampling on evaluation of left ventricular ejection fraction by means of thallium-201 gated SPECT: Comparison of 16- and 8-interval gating, with reference to equilibrium radionuclide angiography. *Eur J Nucl Med* 2000;27:694.

82. Williams KA, Taillon LA. Left ventricular function in patients with coronary artery disease assessed by gated tomographic myocardial perfusion images: Comparison with assessment by contrast ventriculography and first-pass radionuclide angiography. *J Am Coll Cardiol* 1996;27:173.

83. Rozanski A, Nichols K, Yao SS, et al. Development and application of normal limits for left ventricular ejection fraction and volume measurements from 99mTc-sestamibi myocardial perfusion gates SPECT. *J Nucl Med* 2000;41:1445.

CHAPTER 23

Evaluation of Ventricular Performance with Scintigraphic Techniques

Kim A. Williams

INTRODUCTION

The noninvasive assessment of resting left ventricular (LV) performance is an integral part of the evaluation of patients with known or suspected cardiac disease, having important diagnostic, therapeutic, and prognostic significance.[1-11] Although scintigraphic measures of cardiac function historically included measurement of ejection fraction (EF), estimation of cardiac output and valvular regurgitant fraction and detection of intracardiac shunts have also been performed. Other than EF, these uses have been largely supplanted by echocardiographic and magnetic resonance imaging (MRI) techniques over the past two decades.

Gated equilibrium radionuclide angiography (ERNA, often called multiple gated acquisition [MUGA], equilibrium radionuclide ventriculography [RNV]) was introduced nearly 30 years ago. It was routinely utilized in the evaluation of patients with known or suspected LV dysfunction, post–myocardial infarction (MI), valvular

disease, and for monitoring the cardiotoxic effects of chemotherapeutic drugs. Exercise radionuclide angiography (RNA), particularly with the first-pass radionuclide angiographic (FPRNA) technique was widely used to diagnose or evaluate known coronary artery disease (CAD),[5-9] competing favorably with and often complementing planar myocardial perfusion imaging (MPI). However, since its introduction, RNA has evolved little, while competing modalities, such as gated single photon emission computed tomography (SPECT) MPI, echocardiography, and cardiac magnetic resonance have been introduced and become increasingly sophisticated and cost effective.

TECHNICAL ASPECTS

Image Acquisition

If ERNA is to be performed in addition to FPRNA, after placement of a large-bore (14- or 16-gauge) antecubital intravenous line, 1.5 mg of stannous pyrophosphate is mixed with 30 mL of the patient's blood for approximately 60 seconds, and is then reinfused. Resting FPRNA is usually performed after a 10-minute delay to allow further red blood cell uptake of stannous ion. Technetium 99m (Tc-99m) pertechnetate (25–30 millicuries) in a volume of < 1 mL is then flushed rapidly with at least 30 mL of normal saline through the indwelling catheter. This can be followed within a few minutes by planar and/or tomographic (SPECT) ERNA images. For FPRNA, Tc-99m DTPA is often used if no equilibrium images are required. Perfusion agents, such as Tc-99m sestamibi or tetrofosmin, but not teboroxime (which has high pulmonary extraction, limiting FPRNA image quality), may be utilized if perfusion images are desired.[12–14]

FPRNA images are usually obtained using a single- or multicrystal high-count rate gamma camera fitted with a high-sensitivity parallel-hole collimator (e.g., SIM 400, Scinticor, Milwaukee, WI; or ElGems CardiaL [formerly Elscint], Haifa, Israel). Images are acquired in the anterior or the right anterior oblique (RAO) projection using 25 (± 4) frames per cardiac cycle.

Analysis of First-Pass Radionuclide Angiography

FPRNA data is analyzed using the frame method for LVEF using commercially available computer software,[15–17] as shown in Figures 23-1 through 23-3. This software creates a representative LV volume curve by summing frames of several (usually 5–10) cardiac cycles, which are aligned by matching their end-diastoles (histogram peaks) and end-systoles (histogram valleys) during the operator-defined levophase of radioactive tracer transit. The pulmonary-frame background-corrected representative cycle is then examined with a fixed region of interest (ROI) in order to obtain the final first-pass LV time–activity curve. This region of interest is drawn over the LV as defined by a first harmonic Fourier transformation phase image, which distinguishes clearly the LV from the aortic counts. End-diastole is taken as the first frame of the representative cycle, and

end-systole is defined as the frame with the minimum counts in the histogram. Historically, the LVEF was taken as the end-diastolic counts minus the end-systolic counts, divided by the background subtracted end-diastolic counts.

A second ROI (end-diastolic) can be derived from a Fourier transformation amplitude image with masking of the lower 10% of image intensity, which extends the region of interest in a basal direction, usually 1 to 4 pixels, depending on the vigor of ventricular contraction, up to the amplitude signal of the aortic root. The remainder of this ROI is drawn to match the first region of interest (end-systolic). The dual ROI LVEF is determined as the end-diastolic ROI counts minus the end-systolic ROI counts, divided by the background- subtracted end-diastolic ROI counts. This results in accounting for valve plane motion during the cardiac cycle, using Fourier-guided dual ROI analysis of FPRNA, giving EFs that are highly reproducible and similar in value to ERNA.[17]

Gated Planar Equilibrium Blood Pool Image Analysis

Electrocardiogram (ECG)-gated planar equilibrium blood pool images (Figure 23-4) can be performed with any of several blood pool agents, such as Tc-99m–labeled red blood cells (described above) and Tc-99m–labeled human serum albumin. These images are best when acquired using high-resolution collimation. Images for planar LVEF calculation are obtained in the best septal (shallow) left anterior oblique (LAO) view. This angle, usually 25 to 60 degrees, must be carefully set using a persistence mode prior to acquisition. For regional wall motion assessment, the best septal view plus and minus 45 degrees should be obtained (approximately "anterior" and "lateral" views). Each of these planar-gated image should be acquired for 6 to 10 minutes' duration, dividing each cardiac cycle into a minimum of 32 frames. A smaller number of frames (e.g., 16) are adequate for assessment of EF due to the usual length of the isovolumic ejection period (at end-diastole) and relaxation period (at

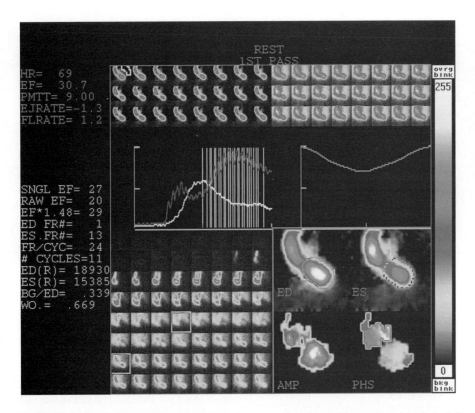

Figure 23-1. FPRNA (anterior projection) images are shown, with the serial images at the lower left, demonstrating tracer transit from the superior vena cava, to right atrium, to right ventricle to the pulmonary phase, left heart phase, and systemic circulation. Using regions of interest (ROIs) drawn over the LV and left lung (far upper left image), histograms are obtained (shown above serial images), which show overlapping RV counts with systoles (curve valleys) and diastoles (curve peaks) from which the cardiac cycles (CYC) are derived which comprise the representative cycle. Each cardiac cycle is marked. The pulmonary curve is used to compute the pulmonary mean transit time (PMTT). The length of the representative cycle in frames (FR) is used to derive the heart rate (HR). The images of the raw representative cycle are shown at upper right. This is subjected to the frame method of background subtraction (i.e., using the background to end-diastolic image ratio (BG/ED) and the washout factor (WO) needed to set the pulmonary area to zero counts), in order to derive the corrected representative cycle (upper left images) from which single ROI ejection fraction (SNGL EF), which is higher than the raw EF, but lower than the dual ROI derived EF, which is used to account for valve plane motion. The Fourier amplitude (AMP) and phase (PHS) images at the lower right demonstrate reduced apical amplitude and delayed contraction of the apex, respectively. **(See also Color Insert).**

end-systole). However, more frames are desirable if quantitative assessment of diastolic performance (e.g., the peak-diastolic filling rate obtained from the first derivative of the ventricular time–activity curve) is needed.

For LVEF, automated regions of interest are generated on the planar-gated equilibrium blood pool data throughout the cardiac cycle using the commercially available software. For most systems, this method automatically identifies the LV master region of interest by Fourier phase imaging, requiring little or no operator intervention, followed by automated edge detection. Most systems employ a first- and second-derivative tech-

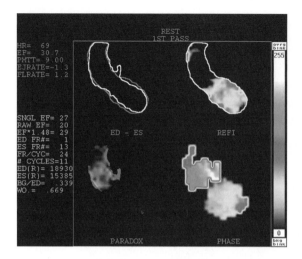

Figure 23-2. FPRNA (anterior projection) functional images are shown, with end-diastolic and end-systolic perimeter image at the upper left (ED-ES), a paradox image (lower left), regional ejection fraction index (REFI, upper right), and Fourier phase images (lower right) shown. The Fourier phase image demonstrates delayed contraction of the majority of the apex, with a small area of paradoxical movement (aneurysmal) evident at the apex on the PARADOX (ES counts – ED counts) image. These functional images allow assessment of regional function without the need for visual interpretation of cine images. (**See also Color Insert**).

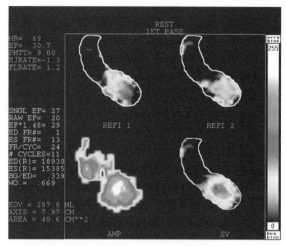

Figure 23-3. Additional FPRNA (anterior projection) functional images are shown, with regional ejection fraction index for the first and second halves of systole (REFI1 and REFI2, upper frames), an alternative method of determining the presence of delayed contraction. Note that the apical region has more ejection fraction in the latter half of systole, compared with the inferobasal wall. Fourier amplitude (AMP, lower left) and stroke volume (SV, ED – ES, lower right) images are shown. The graphic extending from the valve plane to the apex on the SV image is used to compute the LV volume using the Sandler and Dodge equation for the anterior projection. (**See also Color Insert**).

nique for edge detection. An automated periventricular background ROI must be adjusted routinely in order to avoid inclusion of high-count structures (e.g., spleen, descending aorta), which would artifactually increase the LVEF if included.

Gated Tomographic Equilibrium Blood Pool Image Acquisition, Reconstruction, and Analysis

ECG-gated projections for SPECT reconstruction are usually obtained using high-resolution collimation in a fashion similar to gated SPECT perfusion imaging (Figure 23-5), scanning from RAO 45-degree to left posterior oblique (LPO) 45-degree projections. A total of 45 to 60 projections of 20 to 30 seconds' duration, at 4-

degree or 3-degree steps (respectively) should give adequate count density. At each projection, either 8 or 16 frames per cardiac cycle should be acquired.

After collimator sensitivity and center of rotation correction, low-pass prefiltered projections are reconstructed into transaxial slices of the blood pool for each of the 8 or 16 frames of the cardiac cycle. Transaxial slices (e.g., two-pixel thickness) can be reconstructed using a Butterworth back-projection filter (e.g., a critical frequency of 0.5 and order of 14.0). The transaxial slice sets can then be reoriented in cardiac planes (i.e., short axis, horizontal long axis, and vertical long axis) for each of the 8 frames of the cardiac cycle.

Multiple methods of quantifying blood pool SPECT images have been published using either

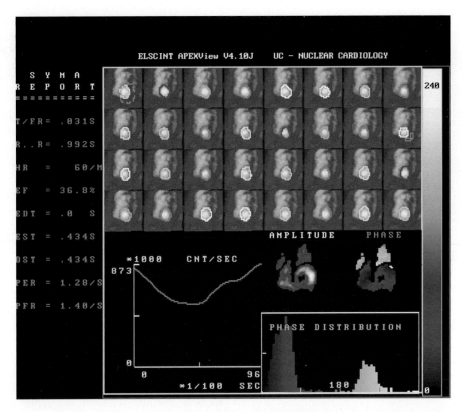

Figure 23-4.   ERNA analysis is shown for images obtained in the left anterior oblique 45-degree projection. The 32 ECG-gated frames are analyzed using a guiding region of interest (ROI, frame 1) obtained either manually or using Fourier phase and amplitude images to automatically locate and outline the LV. Automated LV edge detection is performed using a combination of first and second derivative of count profiles inside the guiding or master ROI. Background correction is performed based on the counts per pixel within a small periventricular ROI (frame 16) drawn carefully to avoid the ventricle or the spleen. The counts within the 32 ROIs are shown after background correction in the lower left histogram. The first derivative of this ventricular volume curve is used to compute the peak filling and emptying rates (PFR and PER). The Fourier phase and amplitude functional images demonstrate inferoapical and septal hypokinesis with late contraction, when compared with the RV and the basal lateral portion of the LV. (*See also Color Insert*).

three-dimensional images or midventricular horizontal and vertical long-axis slices, which can be analyzed for wall motion or EF.[18-24] If 8 frames are acquired, the 8 slices can be expanded to 16 frames by weighted frame interpolation and temporal filtering. These slices are analyzed for single and biplane LVEF using a center of mass combination first and second derivative automated edge detection algorithm commonly employed for planar-gated blood pool analysis. The LVEF and RVEF can be calculated for each long axis as the end-diastolic counts minus the end-systolic counts, divided by the end-diastolic counts, combining them for a biplane EF.

The three-dimensional techniques are useful for blood pool volume rendering, which is used for delineation of myocardial (actually endocardial) topography. This technique is limited by the accuracy of automated valve plane definition since there is often little count density change at the

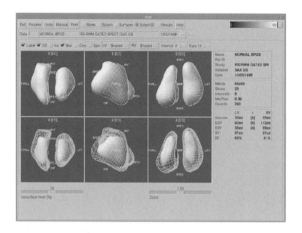

Figure 23-5. Gated tomographic ERNA analysis is shown after three-dimensional reconstruction of the left and right ventricles and surface rendering. This display (BPQS, Cedars Sinai, Los Angeles) is termed *Splash3D*. All three synchronized pairs of 3D views are displayed. The lower views can be gated, and each of these views can be rotated interactively. It is also possible to superimpose an isosurface in this mode for rapid display of regional wall motion. (*See also Color Insert*).

mitral or tricuspid valve planes. However, this method has been validated against standard approaches, such as cardiac magnetic resonance.[24] Due to the uniformly high contrast and lack of overlap between cardiac blood pool and extracardiac structures, no background subtraction algorithm should be employed for these analyses.

Gated SPECT Myocardial Perfusion Imaging

Gated SPECT MPI (Figure 23-6) has become one of the most powerful tools available in nuclear cardiology. Acquisition of SPECT data, synchronized with the electrocardiographic R wave, is generally performed using 8 or 16 gating intervals and allows evaluation of both global (EF) and regional (myocardial wall motion and wall thickening) cardiac function. These 8 sets of projection images are generally summed in order to obtain a single planar projection set ("ungated") for perfusion evaluation and comparison with nongated perfusion images obtained at rest.

Gated SPECT acquisition is now recommended for all perfusion studies whenever possible. Recent estimates indicate that over 90% of all SPECT studies in the United States are currently performed using the gated acquisition technique, up from only about 3% in 1993.[25] While it was initially held that gated perfusion SPECT acquisitions were possible only in conjunction with Tc-99m sestamibi or other Tc-99m–based agents,[25–31] recent published experience from multiple sites indicates that gated thallium 201 (Tl-201) SPECT imaging is eminently feasible, especially if a multidetector camera is used.[32–34]

Gated SPECT MPI is most often performed with poststress ECG gating. Ungated SPECT perfusion imaging is usually reserved for resting images in some institutions or for patients with cardiac arrhythmias. Although the projection images for SPECT reconstruction images are usually acquired using high-resolution collimation, some systems employ high-quality general-purpose cast (rather than foil) collimators. Similar to gated tomographic ERNA acquisition described earlier, a total of 180 degrees of projection images are usually obtained, scanning from RAO 45 degrees to LPO 45 degrees. A total of 60 projections of 15 to 30 seconds' duration at 3-degree steps will give adequate count density, for a usual total of 15 to 25 minutes acquisition time. The acquisition time is, of course, reduced when utilizing multiple-headed gamma cameras. At each projection, either 8 or 16 ECG-gated frames per cardiac cycle should be acquired.

For image processing, a wide range of SPECT reconstruction filters and settings have been utilized, depending on the tracer characteristics, the amount of myocardial tracer activity, the system and collimator characteristics, and the software used for analysis. After collimator sensitivity and center of rotation correction, low-pass prefiltered projections are reconstructed into transaxial slices for each of the 8 or 16 frames of the cardiac cycle for gated SPECT, as well as the single ungated or summed gated projection set. Transaxial slices are typically reconstructed using

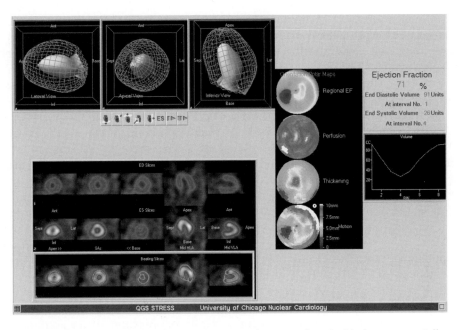

Figure 23-6. Gated SPECT myocardial perfusion images are shown analyzed with the commercially available QGS program (Cedars-Sinai) used for display and automated calculation of ejection fraction and volume. Changes in volume are tracked from ED to ES, for calculation of wall motion and regional thickening, displayed in polar map format. Three-dimensional surface rendered diagrams (above) and actual SPECT slices with fitted edges (below) are also shown. These images were obtained with Tl-201 in a normal patient. (**See also Color Insert**).

a Butterworth backprojection filter (e.g., with a cutoff frequency of 0.35 and an order of 10.0). The transaxial slice sets are then reoriented in cardiac planes (i.e., short axis, horizontal long axis, and vertical long axis) for each of the frames of the cardiac cycle. Midventricular horizontal and vertical long-axis slices can be analyzed for regional wall motion or EF. If 8 frames are acquired, these 8 slices can be expanded to 16 frames by weighted frame interpolation and temporal filtering for a smoother cinematic display. Two- and three-dimensional techniques for display of gated perfusion SPECT have also been described and validated for EF.[25–30]

Gated SPECT has been utilized extensively for determination of EF and wall motion, adding incremental diagnostic and prognostic information. The addition of wall motion has improved the specificity of myocardial perfusion SPECT by distinguishing myocardial scarring from attenua-

tion artifacts, both of which may result in "fixed" defects.[31]

The exponential increase in the use of gated SPECT perfusion has been fueled by the increased availability of automatic and semiautomatic algorithms for the quantification of cardiac function. DePuey et al.[28] described a method based on the automated detection of endocardial borders. Williams et al.[27] developed a method based on digitally subtracting and inverting the perfusion images and analyzing the change in counts occurring in the ventricular chamber, using an edge-detection method identical to that commonly used in gated ERNA. Germano et al.[26,29] developed a totally automated method of fitting geometric shapes to the endocardial borders to obtain systolic and diastolic volumes and EFs. Smith et al.[30] have used partial volumes effect to quantitate regional thickening and estimate LVEF,[30] without need for any edge detection algorithm. Each of these techniques has been well "correlated" with standard methods of performing EF, but each demonstrating varying degrees of "substitutability."[27]

For these reasons, the gated SPECT policy statement of the American Society of Nuclear Cardiology encourages the use of gated SPECT with every perfusion study in which gating is feasible (*http://www.asnc.org/policy/ecg-gating.htm*). This reflects the improved quality control and diagnostic accuracy of interpreting perfusion images in light of regional and global LV performance, as well as the incremental value of gated SPECT over perfusion imaging alone for prognosis.[31,35–37]

Recent published experience from multiple sites indicates that gated Tl-201 SPECT imaging is possible,[26,32–35] although these images are poorer in counts and higher in scatter. The best results occur with multi-headed gamma camera imaging, higher Tl-201 tracer doses, and smaller patients in order to obtain adequate count density in the study. On some systems, alteration of backprojection filters (e.g., Butterworth critical frequency of 0.25) may be useful. Due to poorer ventricular cavity resolution, Tl-201 gated SPECT EFs and volumes may not be as reproducible as Tc-99m sestamibi.[33]

Functional Images in Nuclear Cardiology

Each of the scintigraphic modalities described above, whether planar or gated SPECT ERNA, FPRNA, or gated SPECT MPI, consists of a series of digital images. These series can be evaluated by computer techniques, which allow automated analyses and aid image interpretation, particularly for the assessment of regional function. The resultant images are so-called "functional images."

Functional images may be as simple as a subtraction (e.g., end-diastole image − end-systole image = stroke volume image) or more complex computer calculations (e.g., Fourier transformation phase and amplitude images).[38–41] The Fourier transformation process fits the changes that occur in each pixel (picture element) to a cosine wave, which is characterized by the height of change throughout the cycle (amplitude) and the relative timing of the wave (phase).

The amplitude images may be used to detect regions of decreased wall motion on blood pool or FPRNA images or to quantitate myocardial wall thickening on gated SPECT perfusion images. The presence of amplitude on Fourier transformation of perfusion polar maps has been shown to correlate with perfusion residual myocardial perfusion defect reversibility.[38]

The phase images are used to detect alterations in regional timing, such as the dyskinesis (outward wall motion) of an aneurysmal myocardial segment, or the often subtle degrees of late contraction (tardokinesis), typical of myocardial ischemia or prior infarction. It has also been utilized to detect the location of ventricular tachycardia or insertion of an accessory conduction bypass tract in Wolff–Parkinson–White syndrome.[39] In fact, a delay in segmental right ventricular (RV) activation compared with the LV detected on Fourier phase images of gated blood pool RNA is consistent with arrhythmogenic RV dysplasia and has been correlated with a poor prognosis.[39–41]

CLINICAL APPLICATIONS

Thus, the assessment of LV size, systolic function, diastolic function, regional wall motion, and timing of mechanical activation remain diagnostically and prognostically important uses of RNA. The exercise FPRNA LVEF has particularly greater prognostic value in patients with ischemic heart disease than many other clinical, noninvasive, and invasively derived variables.[5–9] An exercise LVEF of 0.50 (50%) has been identified as the inflection point below which patients with CAD demonstrate a probability of cardiac death, which increases as the EF decreases.[7] However, the direct applicability of these numerical data when the EF is obtained with other protocols or techniques, such as the more widely utilized ERNA technique, is uncertain.

Features of FPRNA versus ERNA

The evaluation of LV systolic function has become one of the most common applications of nuclear imaging, using FPRNA, planar ERNA and, more recently, gated SPECT perfusion and SPECT ERNA.

The use of ERNA is far more widespread than FPRNA. Recently, however, there has been some renewed interest in FPRNA, at least in part because of the availability of Tc-99m–labeled perfusion tracers, which allow simultaneous evaluation of myocardial perfusion and ventricular function.[12–14,42–49]

FPRNA has some distinct advantages. These include (1) the acquisition of data in < 30 seconds; (2) the evaluation of RV function with less overlap of the activity from other chambers;[50] (3) the use of multiple radiopharmaceuticals, including bone, renal, and myocardial scintigraphic agents;[13] (4) a proven robust measurement of stress ventricular function at the true point of peak exercise;[5,7,9] and (5) the presence of a wealth of prognostic information available for management of patients with ischemic heart disease based on stratification by FPRNA exercise LVEFs.[5,7,9]

Despite these advantages, widespread use of FPRNA has been limited by the need for large-bore intravenous access, absence of significant tricuspid regurgitation,[50] impeccable bolus technique,[27] and a high-count rate capable, often dedicated, gamma camera.[15–17]

Good correlation coefficients between FPRNA and other EF techniques have been found.[27,51–54] However, it has been reported that FPRNA may underestimate invasively and noninvasively derived EFs by as much as 12 to 25%.[27,51–53] One potential reason for this underestimation is the use of a single fixed ROI drawn at end-diastole, which will not account for valve plane motion (base toward apex) during systole.[27,53] This shortening motion of the heart is more pronounced in vigorously contracting ventricles.[55–58] If this valve plane motion is not taken into account during the analysis of LVEF, inclusion of counts from above the aortic valve plane within the LV ROI during systole will result in a lower calculated LVEF. Thus, recent studies and software implementations utilize dual regions of interest for FPRNA, which has improved the substitutability of FPRNA EFs for those obtained with other techniques.[17]

Clinical Role of the Scintigraphic Techniques

Each noninvasive imaging technique has unique strengths and limitations. Detection of regional global ventricular dysfunction can be performed with many noninvasive methods, but the nuclear imaging techniques are inherently quantitative, rather than relying on visual estimation of ventricular size and function. Factors to consider upon test selection include local expertise, local access, cost, and the need for reproducible quantitative measurements. The ability to distinguish systolic from diastolic dysfunction should also be considered. The RNA techniques can be used to compute quantitative estimates of LV, as well as RV EFs, and absolute volumes with geometric or count-based methods.

In terms of feasibility, quantitation LV chamber volume and EFs are obtainable in essentially 100% of patients. If venous access is poor, FPRNA cannot be performed, but ERNA requires no bolus, and therefore can be performed with a minimally sized intravenous catheter or direct venous punctures. If ERNA is difficult due to poor tagging of red cells (e.g., with heparin infusion), a Tc-99m–labeled perfusion agent may be employed for planar or gated SPECT perfusion imaging. As noted earlier, the latter test has become the most commonly performed scintigraphic ejection EF, as a diagnostically and prognostically important appendage to myocardial perfusion SPECT.

Assessment of Systolic Function

The assessment of systolic function is an important component of the initial evaluation of all patients with the clinical symptoms of right- or left-sided congestive heart failure (CHF), ischemic heart disease, and in patients who are undergoing potentially cardiotoxic treatments, such as doxorubicin. Systolic dysfunction is usually defined by the presence of an LVEF < 50%, while a normal RVEF is 10 to 15 units lower than that of the LV. However, it should be recalled that the EF is an ejection phase index, which is dependent on loading conditions of the ventricle. Preload (i.e., fiber stretch) deficiency or inappropriate afterload (e.g., severe hypertension) may result in lowering of EF in the absence of any real decrease in inotropic state or contractile reserve. Compensatory dilatation of the ventricle is present in most patients with systolic dysfunction. Assessment of ventricular volume indices has both diagnostic and therapeutic implications. The presence of ventricular enlargement in the absence of systolic dysfunction in the patient with clinical symptoms of heart failure raises the possibility of heart failure secondary to high-output states, such as anemia or valvular heart disease. For example, when systolic function deteriorates in the RV or LV, this is an indicator of the need to proceed with mitral or aortic (respectively) valvular replacement surgery.[59,60] In the absence of dilatation or systolic dysfunction, heart failure symptoms suggest the presence of pulmonary disease (RV dysfunction), pericardial disease (biventricular dysfunction), or predominant diastolic dysfunction.

Assessment of Diastolic Function

The presence and severity of diastolic dysfunction should be assessed in every patient presenting with evidence for heart failure, since it is the predominant abnormality in as many as 30 to 40% of such patients.[61] Most often, this sways both the diagnostic considerations (e.g., hypertension, diabetes mellitus, hypertrophic myopathies, or myocardial infiltration) and the therapeutic options (e.g., antihypertensives, tight glucose control). This may indicate the need for further procedures, such as myocardial biopsy.

In RNA studies, the rate of change (first derivative) of counts in diastole can be analyzed to calculate indices of diastolic filling, including the peak LV filling rate, time to peak filling, and atrial contribution to filling.[62] In practice, Doppler blood flow velocity indices of transmitral flow are used much more commonly to assess LV diastolic filling parameters. For RNA, a peak diastolic filling rate of > 2.4 end-diastolic volumes per second (EDV/s) is considered normal. Age- and gender-specific criteria for diagnosing LV diastolic dysfunction using Doppler blood flow velocity from transmitral flow based on large population studies have been defined that are applicable to clinical practice.[63] However, large population-based criteria, adjusted for age and gender, for abnormal diastolic function have not yet been established for RNA.

CONCLUSION

This chapter details the technical aspects and the wide range of clinical diagnostic possibilities available by dynamic imaging of myocardial function using scintigraphic techniques. The technical aspects contained should be useful to the cardiologist intent on supervising the performance of these tests, as well as providing their interpretation. For further details and updates on study performance, image interpretation, and test reporting, the reader is referred to *http://www.asnc.org/policy/g53-84imagingguidelines.pdf*.

REFERENCES

1. Greenberg H, McMaster P, Dwyer EM, and the Multicenter Postinfarction Research Group. Left ventricular dysfunction after acute myocardial infarction: The results of a prospective multicenter study. *J Am Coll Cardiol* 1984;4:867–874.
2. Nesto RW, Cohn LH, Collins JJ Jr et al. Inotropic contractile reserve: A useful predictor of increased 5 year survival and improved post-operative left ventricular function in patients with coronary artery disease and reduced ejection fraction. *Am J Cardiol* 1982;50:39–44.
3. Ritchie JL, Hallstrom AP, Troubaugh GB, et al. Out-of-hospital sudden coronary death: Rest and exercise left ventricular function in survivors. *Am J Cardiol* 1985;55:645–651.
4. Williams KA, Sherwood DF, Fisher KM. The frequency of asymptomatic and electrically silent exercise-induced

regional myocardial ischemia during first-pass radionuclide angiography with upright bicycle ergometry. *J Nucl Med* 1992;33:359–364.

5. Lee KL, Pryor DB, Pieper KS, Prognostic value of radionuclide angiography in medically treated patients with coronary artery disease: A comparison with clinical and catheterization variables. *Circulation* 1990;82:1705–1717.

6. Muhlbaier LH, Pryor DB, Rankin JS, et al. Observational comparison of event-free survival with medical and surgical therapy in patients with coronary artery disease: 20 years of follow-up. *Circulation* 1992;86(5 Suppl):II198–204.

7. Jones RH, Johnson SH, Bigelow C, et al. Exercise radionuclide angiocardiography predicts cardiac death in patients with coronary artery disease. *Circulation* 1991;84(3 Suppl):152–58.

8. Johnson SH, Bigelow C, Lee KL, et al. Prediction of death and myocardial infarction by radionuclide angiocardiography in patients with suspected coronary artery disease. *Am J Cardiol* 1991;67(11):919–926.

9. Pryor DB, Harrell FE Jr, Lee KL, et al. Prognostic indicators from radionuclide angiography in medically treated patients with coronary artery disease. *Am J Cardiol* 1984;53(1):18–22.

10. Zhu WX, Gibbons RJ, Bailey KR, Gersh BJ. Predischarge exercise radionuclide angiography in predicting multivessel coronary artery disease and subsequent cardiac events after thrombolytic therapy for acute myocardial infarction. *Am J Cardiol* 1994;74:554–559.

11. Borer JS, Hochreiter C, Herrold EM, et al. Prediction of indications for valve replacement among asymptomatic or minimally symptomatic patients with chronic aortic regurgitation and normal left ventricular performance. *Circulation* 1998;97:525–534.

12. Berman DS, Kiat H, Maddahi J. The new ^{99m}Tc myocardial perfusion imaging agents: ^{99m}Tc-sestamibi and ^{99m}Tc-teboroxime. *Circulation* 1991;84 (3 Suppl):17–21.

13. Williams KA, Taillon LA, Draho JM, Foisy MF. First-pass radionuclide angiographic studies of left ventricular function with Tc-99m-teboroxime, Tc-99m-sestamibi and Tc-99m-DTPA. *J Nucl Med* 1993;35:394–399.

14. Jones RH, Borges-Neto S, Potts JM. Simultaneous measurement of myocardial perfusion and ventricular function during exercise from a single injection of Tc-99m sestamibi in coronary artery disease. *Am J Cardiol* 1990;66:68E–71E.

15. Gal R, Grenier RP, Carpenter J, et al. High count rate first-pass radionuclide angiography using a digital gamma camera. *J Nucl Med* 1986;27:198–206.

16. Gal R, Grenier RP, Schmidt DH, Port SC. Background correction in first-pass radionuclide angiography: Comparison of several approaches. *J Nucl Med* 1986;27:1480–1486.

17. Williams KA, Bryant TA, Taillon LA. First-pass radionuclide angiographic analysis with two regions of interest: Improved "substitutability" for gated equilibrium ejection fractions. *J Nucl Med* 1998;39(11):1857–1861.

18. Faber TL, Stokely EM, Templeton GH, et al. Quantification of three-dimensional left ventricular segmental wall motion and volumes from gated tomographic radionuclide ventriculograms. *J Nucl Med* 1989;30:638–649.

19. Bartlett ML, Srinivasan G, Barker WC, et al. Left ventricular ejection fraction: comparison of results from planar and SPECT gated blood-pool studies. *J Nucl Med* 1996;37:1795–1799.

20. Chin BB, Bloomgarden DC, Xia W, et al. Right and left ventricular volume and ejection fraction by tomographic gated blood-pool scintigraphy. *J Nucl Med* 1997;38:942–948.

21. Groch MW, Marshall RC, Erwin WD, et al. Quantitative gated blood pool SPECT for the assessment of coronary artery disease at rest. *J Nucl Cardiol* 1998;5:567–573.

22. Van Kriekinge SD, Berman DS, Germano G. Automatic quantification of left ventricular ejection fraction from gated blood pool SPECT. *J Nucl Cardiol* 1999; 6:498–506.

23. Vanhove C, Franken PR, Defrise M, et al. Automatic determination of left ventricular ejection fraction from gated blood-pool tomography. *J Nucl Med* 2001; 42:401–407.

24. Nichols K, Saouaf R, Ababneh AA, et al. Validation of SPECT equilibrium radionuclide angiographic right ventricular parameters by cardiac magnetic resonance imaging. *J Nucl Cardiol* 2002; 9:153–160.

25. Wintergreen Summary: Panel on instrumentation and quantification. *J Nucl Cardiol* 1999;6(1):94–103.

26. Germano G, Erel J, Kiat H, et al. Quantitative LVEF and qualitative regional function from gated thallium-201 perfusion SPECT. *J Nucl Med* 1997; 38(5):749–754.

27. Williams KA, Taillon LA. Left ventricular function in patients with coronary artery disease using gated tomographic myocardial perfusion images: Comparison with contrast ventriculography and first-pass radionuclide angiography. *J Am Coll Cardiol* 1996;27:173–181.

28. DePuey EG, Nichols K, Dobrinsky C. Left ventricular ejection fraction assessed from gated technetium-99m-sestamibi SPECT. *J Nucl Med* 1993;34(11):1871–1876.

29. Germano G, Kiat H, Kavanagh PB, et al. Automatic quantification of ejection fraction from gated myocardial perfusion SPECT. *J Nucl Med* 1995; 36(11): 2138–2147.

30. Smith WH, Kastner RJ, Calnon DA, et al. Quantitative gated single photon emission computed tomography imaging: A counts-based method for display and

measurement of regional and global ventricular systolic function. *J Nucl Cardiol* 1997;4(6):451–463.

31. DePuey EG, Rozanski AR. Using gated technetium-99m sestamibi SPECT to characterize fixed myocardial defects as infarct or artifact. *J Nucl Med* 1995; 36:952–955.

32. Manoury C, Chen CC, Chua KB, Thompson CJ. Quantification of left ventricular function with thallium-201 and technetium-99m-sestamibi myocardial gated SPECT. *J Nucl Med* 1997;38:958–961.

33. Lee DS, Ahn JY, Kim SK, et al. Limited performance of quantitative assessment of myocardial function by thallium-201 gated myocardial single-photon emission tomography. *Eur J Nucl Med* 2000;27:185–191.

34. Germano G, Erel J, Kiat H, et al. Quantitative LVEF and qualitative regional function from gated thallium-201 perfusion SPECT. *J Nucl Med* 1997;38:749–754.

35. Taillefer R, DePuey EG, Udelson JE, et al. Comparative diagnostic accuracy of Tl-201 and Tc-99m sestamibi SPECT imaging (perfusion and ECG-gated SPECT) in detecting coronary artery disease in women. *J Am Coll Cardiol* 1997;29:69–77.

36. Smanio PEP, Watson DD, Segalla DL, et al. Value of gating of technetium 99m sestamibi single-photon emission computed tomographic imaging. *J Am Coll Cardiol* 1997;30:1687–1692.

37. Chua T, Kiat H, Germano G, et al. Gated technetium 99m sestamibi for simultaneous assessment of stress myocardial perfusion, post-exercise regional ventricular function and myocardial viability. *J Am Coll Cardiol* 1994;23:1107–1114.

38. Le Guludec D, Bourguignon M, Sebag C, et al. Phase mapping of radionuclide gated biventriculograms in patients with sustained ventricular tachycardia or Wolff–Parkinson–White syndrome. *Int J Card Imaging* 1987;2:117–126.

39. Casset-Senon D, Babuty D, Alison D, et al. Delayed contraction area responsible for sustained ventricular tachycardia in an arrhythmogenic right ventricular cardiomyopathy: Demonstration by Fourier analysis of SPECT equilibrium radionuclide angiography. *J Nucl Cardiol* 2000;7:539–542.

40. Casset-Senon D, Philippe L, Babuty D, et al. Diagnosis of arrhythmogenic right ventricular cardiomyopathy by Fourier analysis of gated blood pool single-photon emission tomography. *J Cardiol* 1998;82:1399–1404.

41. Le Guludec D, Gauthier H, Porcher R, et al. Prognostic value of radionuclide angiography in patients with right ventricular arrhythmias. *Circulation* 2001; 103:1972–1976.

42. Williams KA, Taillon LA. Gated planar technetium-99m-sestamibi myocardial perfusion image inversion for quantitative scintigraphic assessment of left ventricular function. *J Nucl Cardiol* 1995;2:285–295.

43. Baillet GY, Mena IG, Kuperus JH, et al. Simultaneous technetium-99m MIBI angiography and myocardial perfusion imaging. *J Nucl Med* 1989;30:38–44.

44. Larock MP, Cantineau R, Legrand V, et al. 99mTc-MIBI (RP-30) to define the extent of myocardial ischemia and evaluate ventricular function. *Eur J Nucl Med* 1990;16:223–230.

45. Elliott AT, McKillop JH, Pringle SD, et al. Simultaneous measurement of left ventricular function and perfusion. *Eur J Nucl Med* 1990;17:310–314.

46. Villanueva-Meyer J, Mena I, Narahara KA. Simultaneous assessment of left ventricular wall motion and myocardial perfusion with technetium-99m-methoxy isobutyl isonitrile at stress and rest in patients with angina: Comparison with thallium-201 SPECT. *J Nucl Med* 1990;31:457–463.

47. Sporn V, Perez-Balino N, Holman BL, et al. Simultaneous measurement of ventricular function and myocardial perfusion using the technetium-99m isonitriles. *Clin Nucl Med* 1988;13:77–81.

48. Bisi G, Sciagra R, Bull U, et al. Assessment of ventricular function with first-pass radionuclide angiography using technetium 99m hexakis-2-methoxyisobutylisonitrile: A European multicentre study. *Eur J Nucl Med* 1991;18:178–183.

49. Boucher CA, Wackers FJ, Zaret BL, Mena IG. Technetium-99m sestamibi myocardial imaging at rest for assessment of myocardial infarction and first-pass ejection fraction: Multicenter Cardiolite Study Group. *Am J Cardiol* 1992;69:22–27.

50. Williams KA, Walley PE, Ryan JW. Detection and assessment of severity of tricuspid regurgitation using first-pass radionuclide angiography and comparison with pulsed Doppler echocardiography. *Am J Cardiol* 1990;66:333–339.

51. Nusynowitz ML, Benedetto AR, Walsh RA, Starling MR. First-pass anger camera radiocardiography: Biventricular ejection fraction, flow, and volume measurements. *J Nucl Med* 1987;28:950–959.

52. Folland ED, Hamilton GW, Larson SM, et al. The radionuclide ejection fraction: A comparison of three radionuclide techniques with contrast angiography. *J Nucl Med* 1977;18:1159–1166.

53. Nichols K, DePuey EG, Gooneratne N, et al. First-pass ventricular ejection fraction using a single-crystal nuclear camera. *J Nucl Med* 1994;35:1301–1302.

54. Vainio P, Jurvelin J, Kuikka J, et al. Analysis of left ventricular function from gated first-pass and multiple gated equilibrium acquisitions. *Int J Cardiac Imaging* 1992;8:243–247.

55. Simonson J, Schiller N. Decent of the base of the left ventricle: An echocardiographic index of left ventricular function. *J Am Soc Echocardiogr* 1989:2:25–35.

56. Alam M, Rosenhamer G. Atrioventricular plane displacement and left ventricular function. *J Am Soc Echocardiogr* 1992;5:427–433.

57. Arts T, Hunter WC, Douglas AS, et al. Macroscopic three-dimensional motion patterns of the left ventricle. *Adv Exper Med Biol* 1993;346:383–392.

58. Qi P, Thomsen C. Stahlberg F, Henriksen O. Normal left ventricular wall motion measured with two-dimensional myocardial tagging. *Acta Radiologica* 1993;34:450–456.

59. Wencker D, Borer JS, Hochreiter C, et al. Preoperative predictors of late postoperative outcome among patients with nonischemic mitral regurgitation with "high risk" descriptors and comparison with unoperated patients. *Cardiology* 2000;93:37–42.

60. Borer JS, Hochreiter C, Herrold EM, et al. Prediction of indications for valve replacement among asymptomatic or minimally symptomatic patients with chronic aortic regurgitation and normal left ventricular performance. *Circulation* 1998;97:525–534.

61. Ruzumna P, Gheorghiade M, Bonow RO. Mechanisms and management of heart failure due to diastolic dysfunction. *Curr Opin Cardiol* 1996;11:269–275.

62. Muntinga HJ, van den BF, Knol HR, et al. Normal values and reproducibility of left ventricular filling parameters by radionuclide angiography. *Int J Card Imaging* 1997;13:165–171.

63. Schirmer H, Lunde P, Rasmussen K. Mitral flow derived Doppler indices of left ventricular diastolic function in a general population: The Tromso study. *Eur Heart J* 2000;21:1376–1386.

CHAPTER 24

Understanding Statistical Analysis and Data Interpretation in Studies of Noninvasive Cardiovascular Testing

Rory Hachamovitch
Louise E.J. Thomson

INTRODUCTION

Statistical analysis is an intrinsic part of any research study or published manuscript; limited, if any, conclusions can be drawn from a clinical investigation without the use of statistical analysis. Yet, physicians and investigators are rarely exposed to this subject in a systematic manner. The physicians reading the literature require adequate knowledge of epidemiology, statistics, and study design in order to interpret and apply what they read to clinical practice.

GOALS OF RESEARCH STUDIES AND THEIR MEASUREMENT

In large part, the objective of medical research is to define the pattern and determinants of disease and, ideally, its optimal treatment. This process can be simply stated as the process of detecting and estimating effects. In this context, an *effect* is generally defined as the amount of change in an outcome (e.g., disease frequency) detected in the setting of a particular influencing factor. For patients with prior myocardial infarction, we may say that the *effect* of beta blocker use compared to none is a reduction in the risk of reinfarction or cardiac death.

Characteristics believed to have a causal role in the disease process are referred to as *exposures*; thus, exposures can be demographic (race, age), biochemical (cholesterol, Lp(a)), behavioral (smoking, diet), therapeutic (medications, interventions), testing results (abnormal exercise electrocardiogram [ECG], inducible ischemia by noninvasive testing), and so on.

In this context, the goals of research studies can be simplified to:

1. Quantitating the amount or frequency of disease: the frequency of disease in a population, the amount of inducible ischemia, or frequency of events in patients with abnormal noninvasive testing.

2. Quantitating the relationship between an exposure of interest and a disease by comparing the frequency of the disease as a function of the exposure. For example, presence of coronary artery disease (CAD) as a function of cardiac risk factors or cardiac death as a function of inducible ischemia.

Based on these two goals, two types of measures can be described: (1) measures of disease frequency: describing disease in a population with respect to how much or how often; and (2) measures of effect of the exposure: comparing the frequency of disease in subgroups with versus without the exposure of interest. The specific measures chosen to address study questions are a function of the study design, the endpoints and characteristics examined, and several other potential factors.

TYPES OF VARIABLES

Before discussing the analysis or presentation of data, the types of variables that can be encountered must be introduced (Table 24-1). Data can be separated into two major categories: *continuous* and *discrete*.

Continuous variables, as the name implies, exist along a continuum as a series of values within a range (potentially including zero) along this continuum. Also, the difference between continuous variable values has meaning (i.e., the difference between a systolic blood pressure of 100 and 150 mm Hg is a valid measure, has meaning and is a continuous variable in itself). Other examples of continuous variables include age, minutes of exercise performed, and income.

Discrete variables exist within defined categories (known as categorical variables) and thus are usually represented as ordered numerical data and restricted to integer values. Discrete variables can be dichotomous, having one of two values, such as a yes–no (history of prior CAD) or a binary coding of a characteristic (male vs. female, normal vs. abnormal). Discrete variables can also

Table 24-1

Types of Variables

1. Continuous:

- Variable can assume all possible values along a continuum within a specified range.
- Values represent distance between categories or points (e.g., the difference between two values has meaning).
- Zero value exists.
- Examples: age, income, minutes exercise.

2. Discrete (categorical)

Values of variable fall into a limited number of categories with no intermediate levels.

Subtypes:

1. Dichotomous: Binary; male vs. female, alive vs. dead, normal test vs. abnormal test.

2. Multichotomous: Multiple categories for variable (e.g., normal, mildly abnormal, moderately abnormal, and severely abnormal test results). Multichotomous variables can be further subtyped:

a. Nominal: No inherent order to the categories, thus assigned ranks have no meaning (e.g., race, discharge diagnosis, blood type).

b. Ordinal: Categories have a natural order or progression thus values can be assigned. However, the values of the assigned ranks do not reflect the difference between levels (e.g., disease staging, New York Hospital Association [NYHA] congestive heart failure [CHF] class).

c. Numerical: Categories have a natural order or progression, but the rank is quantitative, not qualitative as (b). For example, number of anginal episodes; this is numerical, thus differences between categories have meaning, but is not continuous, since half an anginal episode cannot exist.

be multichotomous, that is, have more than two categories. Several subtypes of multichotomous variables exist. A discrete, multichotomous variable with no natural order to its categories is referred to as *nominal*. For example, blood type and ethnicity are discrete, multichotomous, and nominal data variables—different categories exist, but there is no logical or natural order to these categories. *Ordinal* data is that which can be ordered in a logical fashion, albeit without meaning to the distance or difference between these categories. For example, if we order the categories of scan results (normal; mildly, moderately, and severely abnormal), the difference between normal and mildly abnormal cannot be compared to the difference between moderately and severely abnormal scan categories. Finally, multichotomous variables can be *numerical*, having order (meaning to the difference between the levels), but not being continuous. For example, the number of anginal episodes experienced by a patient is categorical and can be ordered, and the difference between categories has meaning (i.e., four episodes is twice as many as two episodes). However, it is not possible to have half an episode, nor does half an episode have meaning. Thus, although similar to a continuous variable, it is not truly a continuous variable.

SELECTION OF ENDPOINTS— WHAT DO WE WANT THE TEST TO DO?

Endpoints and Outcomes

The endpoints or outcomes that are studied and analyzed can be generally divided into three types or categories (Table 24-2). Endpoints or outcomes studied and assessed in cardiovascular studies have traditionally been anatomical or events based. Paradigm shifts in understanding mechanisms of acute coronary syndromes and recent developments in noninvasive imaging technology are contributing forces toward the use of less conventional measures of outcome.

Anatomic Endpoints

The way in which anatomic endpoints are used varies widely in the literature. Presence or absence of CAD may be the defined endpoint, which can then be further classified according to the *location* (left main disease vs. other) or *severity* (lesions > 50% vs. > 70%) of stenoses. Endpoint measures such as the presence of left main CAD or three-vessel CAD are especially suited to

Table 24-2

Categories of Potential Study Endpoints

Anatomy Based

- Summary, aggregate, or composite variable (score for summarizing overall disease incorporating both location, number and severity of stenoses)
- Location (left main CAD)
- Presence of CAD ($\geq$ 50% vs. $\geq$ 70% threshold)
- Presence of multivessel CAD ($\geq$ 50% or $\geq$ 70% lesions in > 1 coronary artery or a $\geq$ 50% lesion in the left main coronary artery)
- Presence of severe CAD (e.g., two-vessel CAD with proximal left anterior artery lesion, three-vessel or left main CAD)
- Presence of three-vessel or left main CAD
- Presence of plaque and the characteristics thereof

Prognosis or Events Based

- Death
- Cardiac death
- Myocardial infarction
- Stroke
- Referral to catheterization
- Referral to coronary artery bypass surgery or percutaneous transluminal coronary angioplasty
- Hospitalization for
  - Unstable angina
  - Congestive heart failure
  - Other cardiac event
- Recurrent angina
- Emergency room visit for chest pain
- Repeat noninvasive testing

Function and Symptom Based

- Exercise tolerance
- Exercise time until occurrence of symptoms
- Anginal status or class
- Quality of life
- Activities of daily living

identifying subsets of patients with severe and extensive disease within populations with known CAD. The use of a composite score can further augment the definition of patients with severe and extensive CAD, while also creating a continuum of scores resulting in a finer grading scheme for CAD.

Improvements in imaging technology may permit evaluation of plaque characteristics over time. This outcome can be used to enhance the above scoring schemes or can be an appropriate outcome measure when evaluating therapies such as lipid lowering or intracoronary irradiation.

Events as Outcome Measures

Studies assessing prognosis use a wide range of events as endpoints (Table 24-2). The selection of endpoints for a study is dependent on the size and characteristics of the population to be enrolled. In studies evaluating low-risk or small populations, insufficient numbers of events may occur to allow detection of a difference between groups when cardiac death or myocardial infarction (MI) is the sole endpoint. However, the inclusion of endpoints such as rehospitalization or revascularization may allow detection of differences between therapies or management strategies.

The type of question being asked also determines which event measures are appropriate. For example, the extent and severity of measured ischemia may be the most clinically relevant outcome measure in a study focusing on early disease detection or management of very mild CAD in a low-risk population.

A Paradigm Shift

The risk of development of unstable coronary syndromes has been found to be independent of conventional measures of stenosis severity and instead dependent on the presence of unstable plaque. Given this paradigm shift, the challenge now becomes to identify patients with unstable plaque using rapidly developing computed tomography (CT), magnetic resonance imaging (MRI), or positron-emission tomography (PET)

technology. These new tests are likely to be applied to asymptomatic, relatively low-risk populations. The use of traditional outcome measures then becomes inappropriate as outlined above.

Newer technologies are also allowing very early plaque detection through improvements in image resolution with MRI/CT and measurement of plaque's "fellow traveler," coronary calcium, by electron beam computed tomography (EBCT). If the goal of imaging is to identify patients at risk of developing symptomatic CAD, the use of "softer" outcome measures as surrogate markers of CAD development (such as the development of anginal chest discomfort, worsening functional status, emergency department visits for chest pain) is likely to provide clinically useful information.

In the past, the use of these soft endpoints has been criticized. However, therapeutic options for prevention of disease progression and thrombosis-related outcomes (stroke and MI) are now available, and the use of traditional endpoints may not adequately assess these therapies or noninvasive testing in these populations. Thus, we may see a proliferation of studies aimed at identification of softer endpoints and their incorporation into hierarchical models as a part of technology assessment.

UNCONVENTIONAL OUTCOMES—THE IMPORTANCE OF FUNCTIONAL VARIABLES

As we have more success in prevention of early death from ischemic heart disease, there is a growing population with CAD in whom the focus of care is the management of chronic illness rather than a cure. The use of functional endpoints is appropriate for the detection of subtle changes in disease status and to allow evaluation of the quality of the patient's life. Thus, functional endpoints are being used in a number of current studies and have become increasingly relevant in cardiovascular clinical trials.

Quality of life has become an essential outcome variable that is considered a significant endpoint of medical care. Quality-of-life measures in cardiovascular studies have historically focused on reduction of anginal symptoms and return to work. The Seattle Angina Questionnaire (SAQ) has gained popularity, particularly for serial evaluation of anginal symptoms. A number of other evaluation instruments have been developed for CAD patients and widely applied such as the Duke Activity Status Index for assessment of functional status and the Minnesota Living with Heart Failure questionnaire.

Health-related quality of life is characterized by its application to well-being. Satisfaction with life is determined by how the individual's life is affected by disease, accidents, and treatments. Regarding the psychometric approach and evaluation of global aspects of quality of life, there are four areas highly relevant for patients with CAD: physical, functional, emotional, and social well-being. Use of quality-of-life measures is appropriate for the quantitation of patient symptoms or functional status, whereas prognostic endpoints measure numbers of events. These two broad categories of endpoints provide different but complementary descriptions of treatment outcomes. Consequently, it would be very useful to be able to distill the multifactorial quality-of-life measures into a single value that could be combined with the hard endpoint of mortality to describe the overall outcome of a treatment.

Measures of Effect

To illustrate the meaning and use of various measures of disease effect, we will utilize an example study. Many individuals have cardiac risk factors predisposing them to the development of CAD, including hypercholesterolemia, family history of premature CAD, hypertension, diabetes, and so on. To identify which patients are at risk of developing symptomatic disease within a specified time interval, a study is performed in which an asymptomatic "high-risk" (multiple risk factors) cohort is subjected to noninvasive testing using test "X." Individuals are then followed for 10 years to determine the development of symptomatic CAD (defined as cardiac death, MI,

angina, evidence of anatomic CAD by catheterization). The results of this study are shown in Table 24-3.

Of the 1,000 "high-risk" individuals enrolled, 250 developed CAD by the above criteria; 150 of these individuals had a positive test and 100 had a negative test. While 700 of 800 subjects with initial negative tests did not develop disease, only 50 of 200 individuals with a positive test did not develop disease. At first glance, it would appear that a positive test X in a "high-risk" population is associated with a dramatic difference in the risk of developing CAD. Using the definitions in Table 24-4, we will quantify this effect.

As defined in Table 24-4, the estimated risk of disease development in the setting of a positive test X is 75% as compared to 12.5% with a negative test X. Thus, the *risk ratio* or *relative risk* of developing CAD given a positive test is 6.0 (75/12.5). This measure is a relative one and does not capture the absolute change in risk associated with a positive test X.

The *risk difference* determines the absolute change in risk (see Table 24-4). This is calculated as 0.625 (0.75 – 0.125), indicating a large change in the risk of developing CAD. Note that if the risks of developing CAD associated with a positive versus a negative test X result were 7.5% and 1.25%, the relative risk would still be 6, but the risk difference would then be a relatively low, at 0.0625.

The *attributable risk percent* is that portion of the risk among the exposed individuals (e.g.,

Table 24-3

Results of Study Evaluating Development of CAD

	CAD Development		
	Present	Absent	Total
Test positive	150	50	200
Test negative	100	700	800
Total	250	750	1,000

Table 24-4

Standard 2×2 Table Defining the Relationship Between Binary Exposure and Outcome and Measures of Effect of a Binary Outcome (Cohort Study)

	Disease		
	Present	*Absent*	*Total*
Exposure present	a	b	N_1
Exposure absent	c	d	N_0
Total	M_1	M_0	T

	Estimated Risk of Disease
Exposure present	$R_1 = a/N_1$
Exposure absent	$R_2 = c/N_0$

Measure of Effect	*Definition*
Risk ratio or relative risk	$RR = R_1/R_0$
Risk difference or attributable risk	$RD = R_1 - R_0$
Disease odds ratio	$OR = (ad)/(bc)$ or $[R_1/(1 - R_1)]/[R_0/(1 - R_0)]$
Attributable risk percent (among exposed)	$AR_E\% = (RR - 1)/RR$
Attributable risk percent (population)	$AR_P\% = [N_1/T_1 \times (RR - 1)]/[N_1/T_1 \times (RR - 1) + 1]$

positive test X) that is due to the presence of the positive test (as opposed to other sources of risk for CAD). In this case, 83% $[(0.75 - 0.125)/(.75)]$ of the increased risk is attributable to the positive test. In Table 24-5 we summarize the common measures of effect for various types of variables.

The example above is a cohort study (a cohort of individuals were identified and followed), and relative risk is the appropriate means to assess effect measures. If a case control design had been used (for each "high-risk" patient with an abnormal test X, a matched "high-risk" control with a

Table 24-5

Examples of Common Measures of Effect

Outcome	*Example*	*Measure of Frequency*	*Example of Measure of Effect*
Binary	Death, MI, presence of CAD	Proportion, rate, risk	Relative risk, odds ratio, risk difference
Ordinal	Socioeconomic status (poverty, low, middle, and upper)	Proportion, rate, risk	Relative risk, odds ratio, risk difference
Nominal	Gender, racial ethnicity, religion	Proportion, rate, risk	Relative risk, odds ratio, risk difference
Continuous	Blood pressure, age, weight, amount of perfusion abnormality, ejection fraction	Mean (arithmetic, geometric), median, range	Mean difference/ratio, median difference

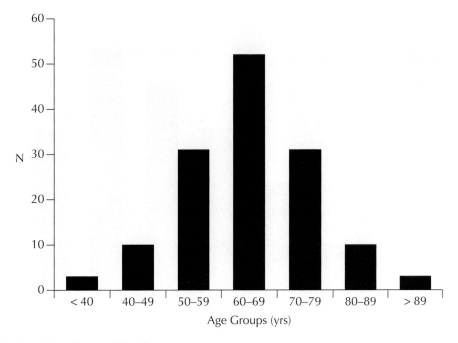

Figure 24-1.   Example of normal distribution.

negative test X would be identified), the odds ratio would have been the correct measure to use.

Statistical Comparison of Variables

The results of statistical testing are often represented by a p value. Before statistical testing, an alpha value (α) is selected, below which the p value must fall in order to be considered statistically significant. The standard approach is an α = 0.05. Generally speaking, this can be interpreted to mean that if the p value is < 0.05, there is < 5% chance of the result's being due to random chance rather than a true difference between groups being compared (incorrectly rejecting the null hypothesis when the null hypothesis is true).

Understanding Continuous Variables

Continuous variable are summarized and compared differently than are categorical variables. The average value is referred to as the *mean*, μ. The *median*, M, is the middle value when data is

ordered from smallest to largest, and the *mode* is the most common value found within your variable. The amount of difference between individual values within a population or study group (variation around a mean value) is measured by the *standard deviation*, σ. It assumes that the population studied has a normal distribution and refers to the area around the mean in both directions (examples of normal and non-normal distributions are shown in Figures 24-1 and 24-2).*

---

*Statistical tests tend to be divisible into two distinct families of tests—those that are based on underlying assumptions of normality in the distribution of the data (parametric) and those that make no assumptions regarding this distribution (nonparametric). Examples of normal and non-normal distribution of data are shown in Figures 24-1 and 24-2, respectively. Evaluation of the data to be analyzed is often required to determine which statistical tests can be used. Since the noninvasive testing literature uses almost exclusively parametric testing, the reader is now informed that alternative tests exist, but will not be covered.

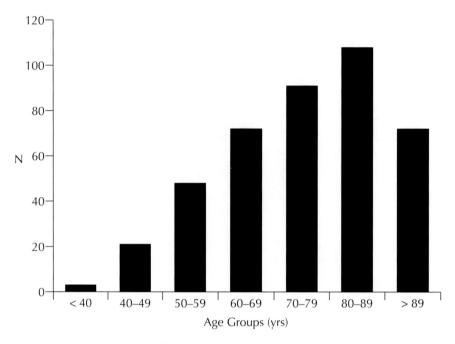

Figure 24-2. Example of non-normal distribution.

UNIVARIABLE DATA ANALYSIS

One standard deviation contains 68% of the population, 1.96 standard deviations contains 95% of the population. For example, assume age is normally distributed with mean, $\mu = 35$, and standard deviation, $\sigma = 5$. Sixty-eight percent of the study population is aged between 30 and 40 (35 $\pm$ 5), and 95% of the study population is aged between 25.2 and 44.8.

UNIVARIABLE DATA ANALYSIS

The following is a very generalized outline of the tests one can expect to encounter while reading the medical literature. The correct test to use for a particular situation depends on the number of samples and the nature of the variables being compared (see Figure 24-3). Most commonly, results from two groups are compared. Some form of t test (Student t test) is used for continuous variables. The paired t test is used when the data is normally distributed, the variable of interest is continuous, and the two groups compared consist of the same individual samples examined under different conditions or at different times (e.g., a pre- and post-measurement on the same person at two different points in time). The paired t test is used to test whether the calculated difference for each person is statistically different from zero. Individuals serve as their own controls, thus increasing the power of the test (a smaller number of samples are needed). For categorical variables, a McNemar's test is used for nonindependent groups (the equivalent of a paired t test). With independent groups, Fisher's exact test (for small samples) or a chi-square test with a 2 $\times$ 2 table (for larger samples) is appropriate. The latter, as will be discussed later, can be combined with a Mantel–Haenszel test in cases of confounding.

If more than two samples of continuous variables are being compared, the t test is replaced by an analysis of variance (effectively identical to a t test). For categorical data, the chi-square test is again used, but rather than a 2 $\times$ 2 table, the shape and size of the table varies with the data

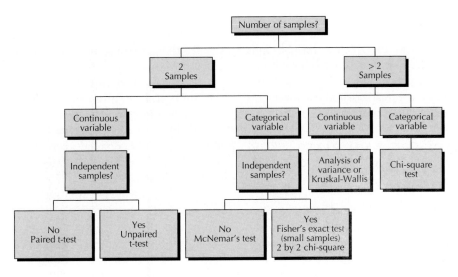

Figure 24-3. Selection of appropriate statistical test.

used (e.g., if four groups are compared with respect to a variable that could take on one of three values, a 4×3 table would be expected).

Why Look at Univariable Analyses?

The purpose of univariable analyses is twofold. First, the reader gains a sense of who was included in the study. The results of a study performed in patients with no prior CAD and few cardiac risk factors will have very different results compared to the same study performed in patients who have multiple cardiac risk factors. Thus, the univariable descriptors of the study population should be reviewed to discern whether the patients included are representative of patients seen in the reader's practice. In addition, by reviewing a univariable analysis comparing patients with versus without the endpoint of interest, the reader can begin to shape in his or her mind the phenomena driving the occurrence of the outcomes.

It is important to attempt to identify patterns in data. Cardiac risk factors may *not* be statistically significant predictors of adverse outcomes if an entire cohort has a history of prior CAD, the homogeneity of this factor thus eliminating its prognostic value. Conversely, in a cohort with no prior CAD, the risk of adverse events is less and cardiac risk factors take on a predictive role because their frequency is less and thus their value enhanced. Similarly, other patterns may emerge in the frequency and predictors of endpoints, depending on the population. Myocardial infarctions often outnumber cardiac deaths in low-risk cohorts, since patients with less extensive disease are more likely to have the former than the latter. Conversely, higher-risk cohorts (e.g., elderly patients with prior CAD referred to pharmacologic stress) will often be at greater risk of cardiac death than MI. When cardiac death is a more common event than MI, presence of scar (fixed defects on single photon emission computed tomography [SPECT]) and ejection fraction will be the most predictive variables. Conversely, if MI is the most common endpoint, markers of inducible ischemia become more predictive.

In study design, the cohort selection often dictates the likely results and pattern of predictive variables. For example, in an elderly cohort, the proportion of women will probably be high, since women develop CAD at a later age. If women predominate, variables such as diabetes mellitus become more powerful predictors, given that they are more significant predictors of adverse events in women compared to men. Thus, careful examination of the cohort and their characteristics will allow the reader insight into whether the results found are consistent with or contrary to that which would be expected. If the latter is the case, the reader should expect and search for confounding variables.

CONFOUNDING AND BIAS— WHAT DOES THE DATA ACTUALLY SHOW?

The validity of a study can be threatened by a number of factors. *Bias* is any systematic error or misinformation that results in erroneous assessment of the relationship between the outcome of interest and the exposure being evaluated. Bias may be defined further as *selection bias*—due to flawed selection of subjects—or *misclassification bias*—resulting from errors of measurement (e.g., incorrect classification of the patients disease state, exposure status or instrumentation error—the manner of test performance). Multiple other types of bias may occur, including *observer bias* (error on the part of the individual measuring results) and *recall bias* (stemming from incorrect recollection by a patient).

Examples of invalid study design due to selection bias include selection of an inappropriate population. If a consecutive series of patients undergoing stress SPECT are selected in order to determine a relationship between the results of SPECT and patient income, but all patients enrolled with higher income are male and most of the low-income patients are female, a bias is present and the relationship between the results, income, and gender will not represent that found elsewhere.

Referral Bias

Referral bias is probably the most important singular concept with respect to understanding and applying noninvasive testing literature. Particularly important is the role this bias plays in determining the sensitivity and specificity of a noninvasive test.

Sensitivity and specificity are the most widely accepted measure of test accuracy. Sensitivity addresses the question "of all individuals with disease, how many will have positive tests?" and equals the number of true positives divided by the sum of true positives and false negatives. Specificity addresses the question "of all individuals without disease, how many will have negative tests?" and is defined as the number of true negatives divided by the number of true negatives and false positives.

In using sensitivity and specificity to assess the value of a noninvasive test, it must be assumed that the study population is representative of clinical populations in whom the test may be applied and that all study participants go on to a gold standard test. Unfortunately, these assumptions are usually not valid.

Post-test referral bias, first described by Rozanski and colleagues from Los Angeles, is the clinically most important type of referral bias. Briefly, these investigators found that exercise radionuclide wall motion studies, a test found to have an excellent sensitivity and specificity when first popularized, had a dramatically lowered specificity and slightly increased sensitivity when reexamined a number of years later. Underlying this finding was the fact that physicians, increasingly confident with this noninvasive test, referred only patients with abnormal test results on to the "gold standard" of cardiac catheterization. Thus, low-risk patients were not referred to the gold standard test.

The impact of post-test referral bias on a study designed to measure the sensitivity and specificity of a test is shown in Figure 24-4. Since few patients with negative tests go on to the gold standard, the number of true negatives and false negatives will be underrepresented in the population examined. On the other hand, the numbers of true positives and false positives will be overrepresented due to the relative increase in high-risk patients sent for the gold standard test. The impact of this will be a slight increase in sensitivity and a significant reduction of specificity.

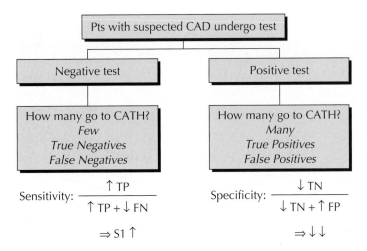

Figure 24-4. Mechanism of post-test referral bias.

For example, assume that the positive and negative predictive values of the test (positive predictive value = true positives/all positive tests and negative predictive value = true negatives/all negative studies) are 90% and 90% (an excellent test) and that half the patients presenting to the test have positive tests (50% prevalence of abnormal studies), the theoretical sensitivity and specificity of the test are 90% and 90%, respectively. However, in practice < 5% of negative studies will go to catheterization, while > 70% of positive studies are usually referred to catheterization. Thus, the observed sensitivity will be > 90%, while the observed specificity will be < 50%. Indeed, in practice the number of false positives outnumbers the true negatives! This phenomenon is observed in practice any time a gold standard utilized is performed on the basis of the result of the test under scrutiny. Sensitivity and specificity in this context become measures of physician confidence in the test under study and post-test resource utilization, rather than measures of the test performance itself. A closer examination of the post-test referral bias and its influences are shown in Figure 24-5.

The phenomenon of post-test referral bias is further propagated when noninvasive tests are compared. If a new technology is compared to an established technology with respect to an anatomic endpoint, and the basis of the referral to catheterization (the anatomic gold standard) is the established technology, this bias will not only underestimate the value of the established technology, but also act to overestimate the value of the new technology (since no post-test referral bias is present with respect to the new technology).

Normalcy Rate

A review of the literature of stress radionuclide imaging demonstrates sensitivity of the test reported consistently as > 90%, while specificity is often reported as 60%, 50%, or less. Due to the inability to accurately measure the specificity of such noninvasive testing, investigators have derived other measures to replace specificity such as the *normalcy rate*. This commonly used measure is defined as the frequency of normal studies in a population with very low (< 5%) likelihood of CAD. The measure of how frequently a test yields a normal result in low-risk patients is used as a substitute or surrogate for specificity.

Confounding

Unlike post-test referral bias, *confounding* is often difficult to identify, but can be corrected in

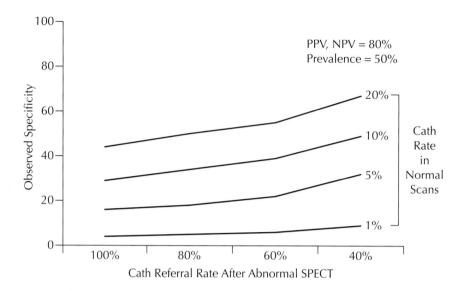

Figure 24-5.   A closer examination of post-test referral bias and its drivers. If positive and negative predictive values of 80% are assumed for a specific noninvasive test, and the prevalence of abnormal studies is 50%, the curves shown describe the relationship between the referral rate to catheterization after an abnormal test result (x axis) and the observed specificity (y axis). The different curves represent a range of values for the referral rates to catheterization after a normal test result. For any value of referral rate after a normal study, there is not a wide variation in observed specificity as a function of the referral rate after an abnormal study. On the other hand, for any value of referral rate to catheterization after an abnormal test result, changes in the referral rate to catheterization after a normal study lead to enormous changes in the observed specificity. Hence, it appears that the effect of post-test referral bias is predominantly due to the lack of referral to catheterization after a normal noninvasive test result. Further, the lower the referral rate to catheterization after a normal result (e.g., the greater the belief of the referring physician in the accuracy of the noninvasive test), the greater the distortion of the measurement of the test (amount of lowering of the observed specificity of the noninvasive test).

the analytic process. Confounding is present when an observed causal relationship between an exposure and an outcome of interest has actually been influenced or due to a separate exposure that has not been considered or detected. For example, it is observed that being male is associated with increased frequency of cardiovascular screening test use. However, the confounding factor is that CAD prevalence is greater in males than in females, and this increased prevalence is responsible for the observed increased rates of screening.

The most striking example of confounding is demonstrated by Simpson's paradox, an example of which follows. In Figure 24-6, the frequency

of referral to testing is compared between two hospitals, A and B. At the bottom of the figure, we see that the overall use of testing is greater in Hospital A than Hospital B (21.3% vs. 10.8%). Without examining the data any further, it could be concluded that Hospital A tests twice as often as Hospital B. However, when referral rates to testing in high- and low-risk patients are then examined, Hospital B tests low-risk patients three times more frequently than Hospital A (overall rates are low, consistent with a lower need for testing in low-risk patients), and high-risk patients are tested almost 50% more often! Thus, despite the high overall rate of test use in Hospital A, Hospital B has a greater rate of testing in

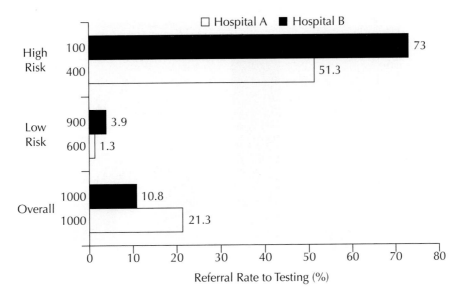

Figure 24-6.   Relationship between referral rates to testing and patient risk in Hospitals A and B.

high- and low-risk groups. This disparity can be understood by examining the patients presenting to the two hospitals. Patients presenting to Hospital B are overwhelmingly low risk; thus, the referral rates to testing are predominantly influenced by the lower rates in low-risk patients. Contrary to this, 40% of patients at Hospital A are high risk, and thus there is greater overall referral rate to testing. We can say the following with regard to confounding as it relates to this example: Confounding occurs when an extraneous factor (patient risk) is associated with both the exposure of interest (Hospital A vs. B) and the outcome of interest (referral rate). To give another example that will be used later in this chapter, physicians often refer patients on to more aggressive testing if their initial clinical impression suggests that the patient is at risk of adverse outcomes.

A number of studies suggest that men are referred to aggressive testing more frequently than women; hence, the exposure (patient sex) leads to an outcome (use of cardiovascular testing). If an increased prevalence of CAD is also associated with increased testing, and men tend to have a

greater prevalence of CAD, prevalence of CAD is a potential confounder since it promotes use of cardiovascular testing (outcome) and is also associated with the exposure (patient sex) (Figure 24-7).

Two variables are described as "confounded" if they vary together in such a way that it is impossible to determine which variable is responsible for an observed effect, unless its effect can be isolated. For example, if we had only the data shown in Figure 24-8, we would conclude that Hospital A had greater referral rates than Hospital B and that high-risk patients had greater re-

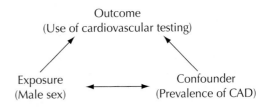

Figure 24-7.   Relationship between confounder, exposure, and outcome.

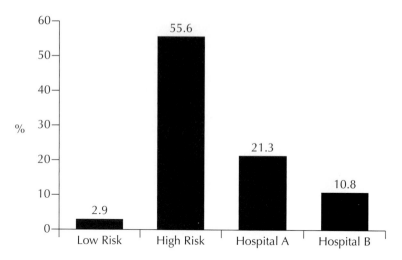

Figure 24-8. Frequency distribution in low- and high-risk patients and by hospital.

ferral rates than low-risk patients—a misinterpretation due to presence of confounding. However, with data collected about referral rates in risk groups at the two hospitals, and the nature of the presenting population (Figure 24-6), a completely different conclusion may be drawn regarding practice patterns and patient mix.

The only way to control for potential confounding is by good experimental design and rigorous checking for confounding factors at all stages of the study. However, some confounding is much more subtle, and the investigators may introduce or alter an exposure that is both predictive of the outcome of interest and associated with a variable of interest.

Several approaches exist for handling or "controlling for" potential confounding variables. One means, as shown in the preceding example, is stratification. We find, as shown in Figure 24-8, that patient risk influences the referral rate to testing. We then examine the referral rate to testing in Hospital A versus Hospital B as a function of this potentially confounding variable. The results of this were shown in Figure 24-6. The statistical test that is applied in analyzing a relationship after controlling for confounding is called the Mantel–Haenszel test. The results of

this test demonstrate whether a statistically significant difference was present between the hospitals with respect to referral rate to testing after taking into account patient risk.

A recent study that addressed the question of whether a sex-related bias still existed with respect to post-SPECT treatment is also a good example of how confounding can be overcome. Investigators from Cedars-Sinai Medical Center in Los Angeles examined 3,211 consecutive patients (1,074 women and 2,137 men) who underwent exercise SPECT for the evaluation of known or suspected CAD. The endpoint examined was referral to cardiac catheterization within 60 days after nuclear testing, a time interval shown to be associated with referral to catheterization due to the test results rather than clinical worsening by the patient. When the referral rates to catheterization were examined, men were referred to catheterization more frequently than women (10.6% vs. 7.1%; $p < 0.001$) early after nuclear testing. Previous studies, however, had shown that significant differences existed between men and women with respect to the prevalence of CAD at the time of presentation to stress testing, as well as with respect to the number of cardiac risk factors present.

Thus, the authors first stratified the referral rates to catheterization by the clinical risk of the patients, as shown in Figure 24-9. Even after stratification by clinical risk group, the difference in referral rates to catheterization between men and women remained statistically significant. However, when the authors adjusted for the amount of ischemia present on the stress nuclear images, the pattern of referral to catheterization changed dramatically. There was no difference between men and women with respect to referral rates to catheterization in the setting of normal scans, abnormal scans without ischemia, or abnormal scans with mild ischemia (Figure 24-10); however, in the setting of abnormal scans with severe ischemia, women were found to have a statistically significantly greater rate of referral to catheterization compared to men. In this example, the nuclear scan result was the major confounding factor. Indeed, of the 1,074 women in this study, 777 had normal scans (72%) while of the 2,137 men in the study, 48% had normal scans, a statistically significant difference between men and women with respect to the prevalence of normal scans.

This type of analysis, and adjusting for confounding, can also be performed by means of multivariable modeling.

MULTIVARIABLE MODELING

Multivariable modeling is a mathematical analytic tool that can be applied for better understanding of the predictive value of a set of variables with respect to an outcome (e.g., prediction of risk) and to examine the interrelationship between variables with respect to the outcome (i.e., identification of confounding or bias). Thus, investigators can assess or measure the predictive value of one or more variables of interest with respect to an outcome of interest. Multivariable modeling yields information regarding which variables are predictive of the outcome, whether the predictive value of a model (an aggregate of these variables) has enhanced predictive value over individual variables, and, within a model, quantitates the value of variable(s) with respect to endpoint prediction (i.e., the weight of the variable). Applying this approach to nonrandomized data, models can adjust for differences in underlying patient characteristics in order to answer defined clinical questions.

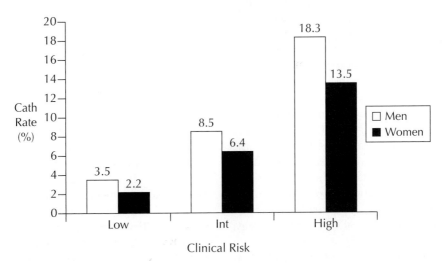

Figure 24-9.   Referral rates to catheterization as a function of patient risk in men and women.

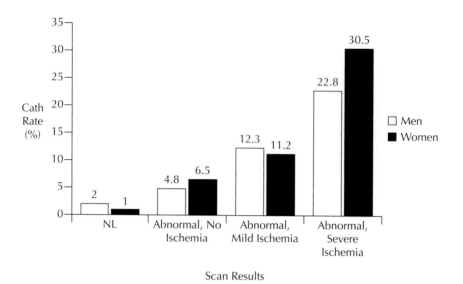

Figure 24-10. Referral rates to catheterization as a function of scan findings (normal vs. abnormal, no ischemia vs. abnormal, mild ischemia vs. abnormal, severe ischemia) in men and women.

An advantage of this type of analysis is the preservation of all available statistical power from an entire data set, as opposed to stratification when data are subdivided. However, this type of analysis is less clinically intuitive. Many physicians are also of the opinion that regression methods do not mirror clinical reasoning, a process based on "heuristics"—so called rules of thumb. Also, the reader must make assumptions regarding the statistical expertise of the investigators and whether the correct model was performed. Multivariable models themselves are based on complex mathematical formulae that make a number of assumptions. These assumptions require close examination and testing to ensure the validity of the model. Ideally, manuscripts utilizing multivariable models detail the manner in which these assumptions were tested.

Despite the disadvantages, these models can be applied to many situations, including the prediction of events (death, MI), anatomy (significant epicardial CAD), cost of care, length of stay, and quality of life. It is not an exaggeration to say that virtually any clinical phenomenon that can be measured, can also be modeled.

There are two principal reasons to perform multivariable modeling:

1. To assess a phenomenon of interest and quantitate the predictive capacity of one or more variables toward an endpoint of interest
2. To assess validity (i.e., to determine whether a bias is present) with respect to an outcome of interest, and to quantitate any bias and adjust for it

Which Model Should Be Used?

Depending on the type of outcome being used and the analysis required, a number of multivariable approaches currently exist. Selection of the appropriate model for an analysis is dependent on the endpoint being examined. If a study uses a binary endpoint (e.g., determining the presence of CAD coded as yes–no, predicting the occurrence of referral to catheterization), the correct model is a *logistic regression model*. A modified version of logistic regression, *ordinal logistic*, is used when the endpoint has a series of categories, for example, no CAD, one-vessel disease, two-vessel disease, three-vessel disease.

Endpoints represented by continuous variables (predicting the percentage of stenosis present on catheterization in an artery) are best handled by *linear regression*. Finally, a special type of multivariable modeling is *survival analysis*. Unlike the preceding models, this unique form of analysis requires two pieces of information—the duration of time a patient was followed and whether an event occurred during this period (one continuous variable, one binary variable).

Model Interpretation

When reading a study that utilized a multivariable model, the presented results may vary depending on the reasons for the model use and the questions it sought to answer. A plethora of data are produced by multivariable modeling, only a fraction of which is usually presented. Those elements commonly reported include:

- χ^2: The chi-square statistic is generated by many statistical tests, and its size reflects the statistical significance of a result. It is a surrogate measure of the quantity of information present in a model. That is, the larger the χ^2, the greater the amount of information contained in the model. A number of different χ^2s are generated, and it is the χ^2 representing the statistical test of the overall value of the model that is shown, with an accompanying p value representing whether the model as a whole is statistically significant with respect to endpoint prediction.
- β *estimate:* All models can report a coefficient for each variable in the model (usually referred to as a β coefficient). The coefficients derived from a model are of primary importance, as they define the relationship between the outcome of interest and the exposure studied (e.g., amount of scan abnormality and the risk of adverse events). It must be kept in mind that this

coefficient represents the relationship between the variable and the outcome of interest *after adjusting for all other variables in the model*, and hence is referred to as an adjusted (versus unadjusted) estimate.

The precise mathematical relationship between the coefficient and the outcome studied varies with the model used. For example, a *logistic regression analysis* using referral to catheterization as the endpoint of interest and evaluating the predictive value of patient sex finds the β coefficient associated with this variable (for male sex) to be 0.4492. A positive value for the coefficient reflects increased risk, while a negative value is associated with a lowered risk. Since this coefficient is positive, male sex is associated with a greater likelihood of referral to catheterization. The odds ratio associated with this covariate (odds ratio = e^{β}) is 1.57. Thus, the presence of male sex has this odds ratio, indicating that a man has a 57% greater likelihood of referral to catheterization based on this population (1-odds ratio).

Similarly, for a continuous variable such as patient age, an odds ratio of 1.019 would indicate that for each *unit of age* (in this case, years) the risk of the outcome increases by 1.9% per year (as compared to the preceding example in which the odds ratio gives the change for presence versus absence of the variable). The likelihood of referral to catheterization increases by 19% for every 10 years of age, based on these results.

If a *linear regression model* were used, the interpretation of the coefficient would change as well. For example, in a study wherein patients undergo stress perfusion testing and cardiac catheterization, a linear regression model is utilized to determine whether patient sex alters the amount of stress-induced ischemia (measured as a percentage of the total myocardium). Variables in the model include patient sex, cardiac risk factors, exercise tolerance test (ETT) results, and the results of catheterization. After adjusting for the amount of anatomic CAD present, as well as for the presence of cardiac risk factors, the authors find that the coefficient for patient sex (male = 1, female = 0) is 3.1225 and the variable patient sex is statistically significant in the model (the p for the individual variable, as opposed to the p for the model, is < 0.05). This value for the coefficient indicates that after taking into account (adjusting for) the amount of anatomic CAD and the presence of cardiac risk factors, men have 3.1% more ischemia than women.

Given the coefficients for the variables in the model, the amount of ischemic myocardium as a function of various combinations of values for the variables can be predicted. For example, if variables in the model other than patient sex include presence of hypertension (coefficient = 1.25), the number of vessels with CAD (coefficient = 5.5) and patient age (coefficient = 0.02), and the intercept for the overall model is 8, an 80-year-old man with hypertension and one-vessel CAD would be predicted to have 11.45% of the total myocardium ischemic [(1 × 3.1 for male) + (1 × 1.25 for hypertension) + (1 × 5.5 for one-vessel CAD) + (80 × 0.02 for age)]. With presence of two-vessel CAD, the predicted ischemic myocardium increases to 16.95% (addition of another 5.5 for the extra vessel with CAD). Similar estimates can be made for other types of models as well, with varying degrees of complexity.

Stepwise Variable Selection

Stepwise regression refers to the entry of variables into a multivariable model in predefined steps. Using this approach, one can determine the predictive value of a first set of variables, fix them in a model, and then determine whether a second set of variable(s) will add further to the model. This approach has been applied in the nuclear cardiology predominantly in the assessment of incremental prognostic value.

Incremental Prognostic Value and Its Measurement

This topic is most easily understood if the concept of "quantification of the available informa-

tion" is accepted, as described earlier. If we are measuring whether nuclear imaging adds information over and above everything else we know from data acquired prior to the SPECT study (clinical, physical exam, history, and ETT data), a rectangular puzzle can be used to represent the individual contributing portions of clinical of information—patient sex, age, symptoms, hypertension, and so on. However, when these variables are combined in a model, the total amount of information is far greater (i.e., the total area of the rectangle represents the equivalent of a measurement of a global χ^2 of the model or, more appropriately, the model's C index). The *incremental or added value* of nuclear testing is determined by examining whether the overall amount of information known about the risk of adverse outcomes is increased by the test information. There are two possible outcomes (Figures 24-11, 24-12): (1) The amount of information added by the nuclear scan (gray piece) is greater than that added by any one variable but the total information does not change. The nuclear scan puzzle piece in gray is larger than other pieces but the total puzzle size remains the same; thus, the nuclear information is redundant. Alterna-

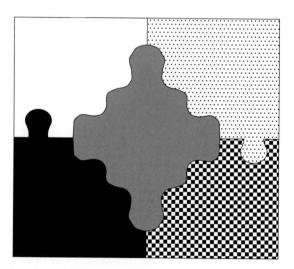

Figure 24-11. Jigsaw puzzle representing contributions of various variables to an overall estimate of information regarding a phenomenon.

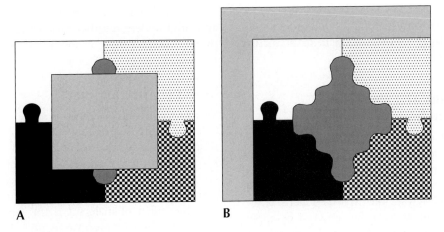

Figure 24-12. Jigsaw puzzle representing absence (**A**) versus presence (**B**) of incremental value.

tively, (2) the nuclear scan may contribute a considerable amount of new, unique information—enlarging the overall puzzle size with some overlap with the other pieces.

How Do We Do This Statistically?

First, a model is created of all prescan information, considering clinical variables, such as pa-

tient sex, age, and anginal status for the prediction of early catheterization. The model's weight or value is determined by its global χ^2. Subsequently, a stepwise approach fixes this initial set of variables in the model, and then has the model consider addition of variables from the nuclear test. If these additional variables result in an increase in the global χ^2, *incremental value* is said to be present (Figure 24-13). Conversely, failure

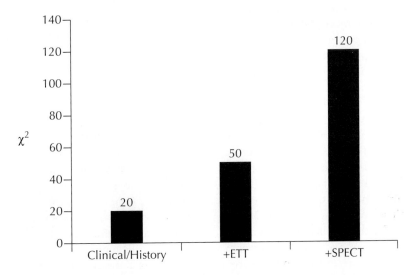

Figure 24-13. Relationship between clinical history, ETT and SPECT data, and χ^2 from a multivariable model.

of the nuclear variables to add statistically significant additional information to the model indicates redundancy of the scan data in predicting early catheterization.

Determining the Presence of Confounding

As discussed earlier, minimizing or controlling for the presence of confounding is an important part of any analysis and enhances the perceived validity of a study. Rather than using comparison of 2 × 2 tables with the Mantel–Haenszel approach, the same end can be achieved by applying multivariable modeling.

Returning to the previously used example of how confounding can be overcome, the Cedars-Sinai Medical Center in Los Angeles addressed the question of whether a sex-related bias still existed with respect to early post-SPECT treatment. Using the endpoint of referral to cardiac catheterization within 60 days after nuclear testing, men were referred more frequently than women (10.6% vs. 7.1%; $p < 0.001$). However, after adjustment for the amount of ischemia present on the stress nuclear images, there was no difference in the referral rates to catheterization between men and women, excepting the setting of severe ischemia when women were referred to catheterization more frequently. This analysis could have been performed using logistic regression modeling (appropriate for the binary endpoint of catheterization). For example, if a β coefficient for patient sex as a single variable model (0 = female, 1 = male) is 0.4492 with an odds ratio of 1.57, it indicates a greater rate of catheterization in men compared to women. If both patient sex and the amount of ischemia present are included in the model, the new β coefficient for patient sex reflects the role of ischemia. If very different results for patient sex are obtained, such as β coefficient (-0.2620) and odds ratio (0.77), the implication is that after adjusting for the amount of ischemia present, men are actually *less likely* than women to be referred to catheterization. A significant change in

the β coefficient (and thus odds ratio) of a variable after adding another variable to a model indicates the presence of confounding of the former by the latter.

Variable Interactions

One of the many assumptions made in multivariable modeling is that, the predictive value of a single variable for the endpoint (its β coefficient) is constant over the range of values of other, potentially confounding, variables. For example, for patient sex and hypertension as predictors CAD risk, the effect of male sex is the same over the range of values of blood pressure. If this is not the case, blood pressure is said to be an *effect modifier* of patient sex. Multivariable modeling can simply examine such interactions between variables. The investigator enters into the model the product of the two variables to be examined for an interaction. For example, to determine whether a particular SPECT result has equal prognostic implications for both men and women, a model can be created using the endpoint of interest. Entered into the model are the SPECT result, patient sex, as well as an interaction between variables (e.g., sex × scan result). An *interaction term* represents a new variable that in this example is the product of two variables for each patient studied. If the interaction term is found to be statistically significant in a model that also includes the two variables used in the interaction, there is presence of *effect modification* between the two variables.

Overfitting: How Many Variables Can Be Examined?

The application of multivariable modeling to clinical research requires the occurrence of a reasonable number of endpoints (outcomes). Unfortunately, for multivariable modeling, the endpoints of interest (especially with survival analysis) occur relatively rarely ($< 5\%$, usually about 1.5–2.5%). The generally accepted threshold is that for every variable entered into the model, 10 outcomes of interest occur (although some argue for a higher ratio, e.g., 20 to one). If 13 cardiac deaths and 16 nonfatal MIs occur during follow-up in a study of 1,000 patients, these 29 events would mandate that only 3 variables be entered into the model. Nonobservance of this rule is overfitting, a common occurrence in the literature that significantly compromises model validity and increases estimation error in determination of the β estimate.

There are several ways to handle this issue. First, the use of aggregate variables or scores can decrease the number of variables. For example, instead of using four to eight cardiac risk factors in a model, calculating the likelihood of CAD using various standard formulae results in a single variable in place of multiple. There are statistical methods referred to as data reduction techniques, such as principle components analysis or factorial analysis (both beyond the scope of the current review). These methods begin with multiple variables and proceed to create a new smaller set, to reduce the number of variables to be entered into a model.

Survival Analysis: Special Considerations

The first application of multivariable modeling in cardiovascular disease was in therapeutic interventions, namely, the measurement of the impact of interventions on survival. When noninvasive testing is considered, however, there is no direct link between test results and subsequent outcome. Importantly, treatment received after the test significantly alters outcome independently of the noninvasive test results. The approach to handling this issue has generally been to remove or censor from survival analyses those patients who undergo revascularization shortly after the noninvasive test being studied (within 60 or 90 days after the noninvasive test), the rationale being that natural history is altered by the revascularization procedure and that inclusion of these patients would adversely alter the analysis of the noninvasive test. Multivariable models used for survival analysis are designed to handle such censored data or unequal follow-up intervals among

patients. However, how should patients be handled when the natural history has been influenced by intervention? Potential modifications of the currently used approaches include accounting for treatments or interventions in the model (i.e., risk adjustment for revascularization).

There are two other areas of potential difficulty in survival analysis deserving consideration. First, newer aggressive medical management strategies using agents such as hydroxymethyl-glutaryl coenzyme A (HMG CoA) reductase inhibitors have been shown to rival the strength of revascularization to lower the risk of cardiac death or MI. To date, no studies have tracked the use of these agents; however, the measured value of noninvasive testing in the newer literature may well be altered by their use, and adjustment for them may be needed in future studies. Second, post-test referral bias will probably impact on the prognostic analysis of noninvasive testing. As described in detail earlier, preferential referral of patients with positive test results to the gold standard of catheterization results in reduction in test specificity (see section on post-test referral bias). Preferential referral of highest-risk patients to catheterization and thus revascularization on the basis of the noninvasive test leads to these patients being censored from the analysis. The overall event rate, and particularly that in the population with strongly positive test results, is artificially lowered by this phenomenon. This leads to a reduction in the *measured* value of noninvasive testing in this setting. As is the case for measuring sensitivity and specificity in the setting of post-test referral bias, there is no adequate means to measure the loss of prognostic information. These issues need to be better examined in the future.

As stated, two pieces of information are considered in a survival model—the time to an event and whether or not the event occurred. In a study examining survival free of cardiac death or MI after stress SPECT, a patient followed for 750 days with no event has a time variable value of 750 (if measured in days) and 0 for event (a binary variable). On the other hand, a patient followed for

355 days, with an MI on day 188, has a time variable value of 188 and an event value of 1.

Many of the basic concepts we have discussed regarding multivariable modeling hold true for all types of models. However, survival analysis differs significantly from other types of multivariable modeling in that particular allowances need to be made:

- If follow-up is obtained only to a certain date, what is said about the patient's condition after this date?
- How are unequal follow-up intervals among patients handled?
- How does one adjust for the patients who, on the basis of the test being studied, have had interventions that would alter their survival?
- What about different outcomes that may or may not be related?

One of the basic assumptions made by survival analysis is that if patients are followed for long enough, all will experience the event of interest. Thus, a patient followed with no event occurring is included with all follow-up information available, but the patient is not considered in the analysis of survival at a time point beyond that maximum follow-up time. So, for example, on a survival curve, the number of patients usually decreases as time passes.

Censoring

Patients who, although alive, are removed from a survival analysis at a particular time point are said to be *censored* from the analysis. There are a number of situations in which this may happen. Figure 24-14 shows eight patients (A through H) who had stress SPECT and follow-up, with their follow-up represented by a solid horizontal line and the reason for termination shown at the right end of the line. The initial and end dates for inclusion to the study are represented by vertical dotted lines. Patient A has follow-up data beginning before the initial study date (the analysis may be limited to include only the follow-up data between the two inclusion dates), but follow-up ended be-

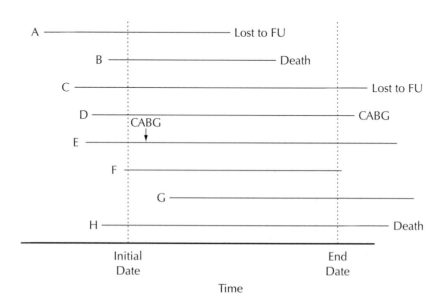

Figure 24-14.   Examples of follow-up intervals and events in patients for a prognosis study.

tween the two dates. We may or may not know whether the patient is still alive after the end of this line, but, for purposes of the analysis (since we do not have this data with certainty), the patient will be censored (removed) from the analysis after the time point when follow-up ended. We see with patient E that although we have extensive follow-up information, a coronary artery bypass graft (CABG) was performed shortly after follow-up began. If this CABG was performed because a workup was prompted by the results of the SPECT study (usually, procedures occurring within 60–90 days after the SPECT study are attributed to this), the prognosis of the patient will be better than in those individuals with similar SPECT results but no revascularization. There are two ways of handling this situation. The approach that has predominated to date is to censor these patients at the time of their revascularization. This approach tends to underestimate the power of the test due to the loss of higher-risk patients to revascularization. The underestimation of test value, however, would be greater if we would include these patients.

Competing Risk

It is assumed that the events used as endpoints in a Cox Proportional Hazards model are independent from each other. If the risk factors that promote cardiac death, MI and noncardiac death are all different, then these events can be used as separate endpoints. However, cardiac death and MI are clearly not independent from each other since similar factors promote the occurrence of each. Since cardiac death is a terminating event, it can be used as a separate endpoint. However, MI cannot be used as a separate endpoint for multivariable modeling, but must be combined with cardiac death (e.g., cardiac death or MI).

Proportional Hazards

The basic assumption underlying the Cox Proportional Hazards model, for which it is named, is that of proportional hazard or risk. It is assumed that for any variable considered in the model, the relative risk of one subgroup versus the other is constant over time. For example, in a Cox Proportional Hazards model using cardiac death as an endpoint, the relative risk associated with an abnormal scan is the same at one week after study as one year after study—there is no additional progression of CAD in patients with abnormal compared to normal scans. Thus, the hazard ratio (the equivalent of an odds ratio or relative risk produced by a Cox Proportional Hazards model) for an abnormal scan must be constant over time. Medically, this is a troublesome assumption since many of these variables would be associated with increased risk over time (e.g., wouldn't patients with angina tend to have an increasing risk compared to patients without angina as time passed?). This assumption must be examined for every variable to be considered in a model.

If this assumption is tested and found to be lacking, two possible solutions remain. First, a different model can be used, for example, a parametric survival model that does not make these assumptions regarding proportional hazards. The more commonly used solution is to use what is referred to as time-dependent covariates. Rather than enter the variable to be considered (e.g., SSS), one enters the product of the variable and the time to event (SSS × time). The interpretation of models using time-dependent covariates is more complex and less intuitive, but it is the only way to handle failure of the proportional hazards assumption.

REFERENCES

The information contained in this chapter is based on numerous sources. The purpose of this reference section is to allow the reader to find sources for further reading and study. In addition, concepts covered within this chapter are elucidated more thoroughly.

RECOMMENDED READINGS

Biostatistics

Glantz SA. *Primer of Biostatistics.* New York: McGraw-Hill, 1987.

An excellent basic self-teaching text for those interested in learning the basics of biostatistics.

Rosner B. *Fundamentals of Biostatistics.* Boston: PWS-Kent Publishing, 1990.

One of a number of standard texts used in first level statistics courses.

Epidemiology

Hennekens, CH, Buring JE. *Epidemiology in Medicine.* New York: Lippincott Williams and Wilkins, 1987.

Rothman KJ. *Epidemiology: An Introduction.* London: Oxford University Press, 2002.

These short, yet comprehensive, overviews of epidemiology cover both theory and practice of medical epidemiology. The most basic and important statistical approaches in analyzing data, while remaining understandable throughout.

Kleinbaum DG, Kupper LL, Morgenstern H. *Epidemiologic Research Principles and Quantitative Methods.* New York: John Wiley & Sons, 1982.

A classic text covering the principles and methods of planning, analysis, and interpretation of epidemiologic research studies. It remains an excellent source of information on quantitative (including statistical) issues arising from epidemiologic investigations, as well as on the questions of study design, measurement and validity.

Rothman KJ, Greenland S, eds. *Modern Epidemiology*, 2nd ed. New York: Lippincott Williams and Wilkins, 1998.

This text, considered a landmark work by some, comprehensively covers the entirety of epidemiology in a cohesive fashion. The authors, both leading epidemiologists, and 15 additional contributors cover a broad range of concepts and methods ranging from the basic to the advanced, and covers the breadth of the field as well (infectious disease epidemiology, ecologic studies, disease surveillance, analysis of vital statistics, screening, clinical epidemiology, environmental and occupational epidemiology, reproductive and perinatal epidemiology, genetic epidemiology, and nutritional epidemiology).

Multivariable Modeling

Kleinbaum, DG. *Logistic Regression: A Self-Learning Text* (Statistics in the Health Sciences). New York: Springer Verlag, 1994.

Kleinbaum, DG. *Survival Analysis: A Self-Learning Text* (Statistics in the Health Sciences). New York: Springer Verlag, 1996.

These two books by Kleinbaum are both an easy-to-follow self-teaching introduction to the main concepts and techniques of logistic regression and survival analysis, respectively. The emphasis is practical, yet gives a reasonable amount of background theory. Since it is annotated throughout with

examples of analyses, it makes an excellent first book on this subject.

The following reviews are excellent and widely cited. We recommend these as well as sources of information. Included are papers criticizing the medical literature from a statistical perspective that we recommend as well.

Concato J, Feinstein AR, Holford TR. The risk of determining risk with multivariable models. *Ann Intern Med* 1993;118:201–210.

Glantz SA. Biostatistics: How to detect, correct and prevent errors in the medical literature. *Circulation* 1980;61:1–7.

Greenland S. Modeling and variable selection in epidemiologic analysis. *Am J Public Health* 1989; 79:340–349.

Harrell FE Jr, Lee KL, Califf RM, et al. Regression modelling strategies for improved prognostic prediction. *Stat Med* 1984;3:143–152.

Harrell FE Jr, Lee KL, Matchar DB, Reichert TA. Regression models for prognostic prediction: Advantages, problems, and suggested solutions. *Cancer Treat Rep* 1985;69:1071–1077.

Harrell FE Jr, Lee KL, Pollock BG. Regression models in clinical studies: Determining relationships between predicors and response. *J Nat Cancer Inst* 1988;80:1198–1202.

Harrell FE Jr, Lee KL, Mark DB. Multivariable prognostic models: Issues in developing models, evaluating assumptions and adequacy, and measuring and reducing errors. *Stat Med* 1996;15:361–387.

Reviews of Statistical, Epidemiological, and Cost-Effectiveness Research

Hachamovitch R, Shufelt C. Statistical analysis of medical data. Part I: Univariable analysis. *J Nucl Cardiol* 2000;7(2):146–152.

Shufelt C, Hachamovitch R. Statistical analysis of medical data. Part II. *J Nucl Cardiol* 2000;7(3):263–266.

Hachamovitch R, Shufelt C. Statistical analysis of medical data. Part III: Multivariable analysis. *J Nucl Cardiol* 2000;7(5):484–495.

Shaw LJ, Hachamovitch R, Eisenstein EL, et al. A primer of biostatistic and economic methods for diagnostic and prognostic modeling in nuclear cardiology: Part I. *J Nucl Cardiol* 1996;3:538–545.

Shaw LJ, Eisenstein EL, Hachamovitch R, et al. A primer of biostatistic and economic methods for diagnostic and prognostic modeling in nuclear cardiology: Part II. *J Nucl Cardiol* 1997;4:52–60.

The following are specific papers defining original methods that are recommended.

Bland JM, Altman DG. Statistical methods for assessing agreement between two methods of clinical measurement. *Lancet* 1986;1:307–310.

Index

Page numbers appearing in **boldface** indicate tables and illustrations